Master Techniques in Orthopaedic Surgery

Relevant Surgical Exposures

Master Techniques in Orthopaedic Surgery

Editor-in-Chief
Bernard F. Morrey, MD

Founding Editor
Roby C. Thompson, Jr., MD

Volume Editors

Surgical Exposures
Bernard F. Morrey, MD
Matthew C. Morrey, MD

The Hand
James Strickland, MD
Thomas Graham, MD

The Wrist
Richard H. Gelberman, MD

The Elbow
Bernard F. Morrey, MD

The Shoulder
Edward V. Craig, MD

The Spine
David S. Bradford, MD
Thomas L. Zdeblick, MD

The Hip
Robert L. Barrack, MD

Reconstructive Knee Surgery
Douglas W. Jackson, MD

Knee Arthroplasty
Paul A. Lotke, MD
Jess H. Lonner, MD

The Foot & Anke
Harold B. Kitaoka, MD

Fractures
Donald A. Wiss, MD

Pediatrics
Vernon T. Tolo, MD
David L. Skaggs, MD

Soft Tissue Surgery
Steven L. Moran, MD
William P. Cooney, MD

Master Techniques in Orthopaedic Surgery

Relevant Surgical Exposures

Editors

Bernard F. Morrey
Professor of Orthopaedic Surgery
Mayo Clinic School of Medicine
Emeritus Chairman of Orthopaedics
Mayo Clinic
Rochester, Minnesota

Matthew C. Morrey
Senior Resident of Orthopaedic Surgery
Mayo Clinic
Rochester, Minnesota

 Wolters Kluwer | Lippincott Williams & Wilkins
Health

Philadelphia • Baltimore • New York • London
Buenos Aires • Hong Kong • Sydney • Tokyo

Acquisitions Editor: Robert Hurley
Managing Editor: David Murphy, Jr.
Developmental Editor: Keith Donnellan, Dovetail Content Solutions
Project Manager: Bridgett Dougherty
Senior Manufacturing Manager: Benjamin Rivera
Director of Marketing: Sharon Zinner
Creative Director: Doug Smock
Production Service: Maryland Composition

Printed in the USA

Library of Congress Cataloging-in-Publication Data

Relevant surgical exposures / editors, Bernard F. Morrey and Matthew C. Morrey.
   p. ; cm. — (Master techniques in orthopaedic surgery)
 Includes bibliographical references.
 ISBN-13: 978-0-7817-9891-4
 ISBN-10: 0-7817-9891-4
 1. Orthopedic surgery. I. Morrey, Bernard F., 1943- II. Morrey, Matthew C. III. Series: Master techniques in orthopaedic surgery (3rd ed.)
 [DNLM: 1. Orthopedic Procedures—methods. WE 190 R382 2008]
 RD731.R42 2008
 617.4'7—dc22

                           2007037789

Care has been taken to confirm the accuracy of the information presented and to describe generally accepted practices. However, the authors, editors, and publisher are not responsible for errors or omissions or for any consequences from application of the information in this book and make no warranty, expressed or implied, with respect to the currency, completeness, or accuracy of the contents of the publication. Application of the information in a particular situation remains the professional responsibility of the practitioner.

    The authors, editors, and publisher have exerted every effort to ensure that drug selection and dosage set forth in this text are in accordance with current recommendations and practice at the time of publication. However, in view of ongoing research, changes in government regulations, and the constant flow of information relating to drug therapy and drug reactions, the reader is urged to check the package insert for each drug for any change in indications and dosage and for added warnings and precautions. This is particularly important when the recommended agent is a new or infrequently employed drug.

    Some drugs and medical devices presented in the publication have Food and Drug Administration (FDA) clearance for limited use in restricted research settings. It is the responsibility of the health care provider to ascertain the FDA status of each drug or device planned for use in their clinical practice.

To purchase additional copies of this book, call our customer service department at (800) 638-3030 or fax orders to (301) 223-2320. International customers should call (301) 223-2300.

Visit Lippincott Williams & Wilkins on the Internet: at LWW.com. Lippincott Williams & Wilkins customer service representatives are available from 8:30 am to 6 pm, EST.

                                 10 9 8 7 6 5 4 3 2 1

This volume is dedicated to my partners in the Department of Orthopaedic Surgery at the Mayo Clinic. I have been a member of this institution for 30 years and without question the compassion, intelligence, camaraderie, and commitment to patient care has characterized our team throughout this period. This volume is comprised of contributions almost exclusively from my colleagues in the department. I wish to publicly express my heartfelt appreciation to them; truly, without their support and inspiration this book would not have been possible.

Contents

Contents

Series Preface

Since its inception in 1994, the *Master Techniques in Orthopaedic Surgery* series has become the gold standard for both physicians in training and experienced surgeons. Its exceptional success may be traced to the leadership of the original series editor, Roby Thompson, whose clarity of thought and focused vision sought "to provide direct, detailed access to techniques preferred by orthopaedic surgeons who are recognized by their colleagues as 'masters' in their specialty," as he stated in his series preface. It is personally very rewarding to hear testimonials from both residents and practicing orthopaedic surgeons on the value of these volumes to their training and practice.

A key element of the success of the series is its format. The effectiveness of the format is reflected by the fact that it is now being replicated by others. An essential feature is the standardized presentation of information replete with tips and pearls shared by experts with years of experience. Abundant color photographs and drawings guide the reader through the procedures step-by-step.

The second key to the success of the *Master Techniques* series rests in the reputation and experience of our volume editors. The editors are truly dedicated "masters" with a commitment to share their rich experience through these texts. We feel a great debt of gratitude to them and a real responsibility to maintain and enhance the reputation of the *Master Techniques* series that has developed over the years. We are proud of the progress made in formulating the third edition volumes and are particularly pleased with the expanded content of this series. Six new volumes will soon be available covering topics that are exciting and relevant to a broad cross-section of our profession. While we are in the process of carefully expanding *Master Techniques* topics and editors, we are committed to the now-classic format.

The first of the new volumes is the present text—*Relevant Surgical Exposures*—which I have had the honor of editing. The second new volume is *Essential Procedures in Pediatrics*. Subsequent new topics to be introduced are *Soft Tissue Reconstruction, Management of Peripheral Nerve Dysfunction, Advanced Reconstructive Techniques in the Joint*, and finally *Essential Procedures in Sports Medicine*. The full library thus will consist of 16 useful and relevant titles.

I am pleased to have accepted the position of series editor, feeling so strongly about the value of this series to educate the orthopaedic surgeon in the full array of expert surgical procedures. The true worth of this endeavor will continue to be measured by the ever-increasing success and critical acceptance of the series. I remain indebted to Dr. Thompson for his inaugural vision and leadership, as well as to the *Master Techniques* volume editors and numerous contributors who have been true to the series style and vision. As I indicated in the preface to the second edition of *The Hip* volume, the words of William Mayo are especially relevant to characterize the ultimate goal of this endeavor: "The best interest of the patient is the only interest to be considered." We are confident that the information in the expanded *Master Techniques* offers the surgeon an opportunity to realize the patient-centric view of our surgical practice.

Bernard F. Morrey, MD

Preface

The first volumes of *Master Techniques in Orthopaedic Surgery* appeared in the mid-1990s. The original concept featured 10 titles with the now-classic structure of focused techniques, well documented and well illustrated. All 10 are in their second editions. When I assumed the position of series editor, we added those titles we felt would fill the void in the orthopaedic surgeons' armamentarium as they were heading to the operating room.

I was personally very excited to organize and contribute to this particular volume for several reasons. First, it provided an opportunity to focus on those surgical exposures believed to be most important or useful, that is, relevant. It is not a broad-based approach, which would not help the surgeon determine what really works for more complicated cases. Second, it allowed the application of the *Master Technique* format consisting of clear illustrations rendered in an elegant, uniform, standardized style. The contents thus are a blend of well-received traditional exposures and promising new minimally-invasive techniques. The most rewarding aspect, however, is that my coeditor is my son, Matthew, who began his career as a medical illustrator and now is a resident in the Department of Orthopaedic Surgery at the Mayo Clinic. His expertise as a professional medical illustrator and orthopaedic surgeon gives him the unique ability to present essential features of exposures through dissection, photography, and his highly-detailed anatomic drawings. It is my sincere hope that those aspects of this effort that I find so gratifying will also be useful to orthopaedic surgeons in training and practice. We have very carefully tried to keep our eye on the common goal of the series: to provide material that is useful and practical to our colleagues on the front line caring for patients with musculoskeletal problems. I am honored and feel privileged to have had the opportunity to prepare this text, and hope that my orthopaedic colleagues find this useful in their practice.

Bernard F. Morrey, MD

Acknowledgments

I acknowledge with great appreciation the sustained support of Dean Fisher, who heads our anatomy lab, for making fresh cadaver material readily available for our dissections, often with very limited notice. The organizational and typing skills of Donna Riemersma are demonstrated in this text and in virtually all of the manuscripts and textbooks that emerge from our department. I, as always, extend a most sincere appreciation to Sherry Koperski, my secretary of 20 plus years, for all the contacts and communications that a text such as this necessitates. Of course, I must express my sincere and special appreciation to Bob Adams, my physician assistant colleague of 30 years. Bob has in this volume, as in others, arranged for cadavers, assisted in the dissections, and offered any service necessary to complete the task. His dedication is reflected not just in this text but also in research, education, and particularly in my clinical practice.

This text, however, has special significance since the coeditor is a medical illustrator and orthopaedic surgical resident, and is also my son, Matthew. Finally, I must acknowledge with words that could never adequately express it, my undying appreciation of the support and patience of my wife, Carla. So, to Carla and Matthew, and to our other children, Mike, Mark, and Maggie and their spouses, I publicly thank them and am forever grateful for their love and generous support.

Contributors

Julie E. Adams, MD
Hand Surgery Fellow
The Philadelphia Hand Center
Thomas Jefferson University
Philadelphia, Pennsylvania

Joseph R. Cass, MD
Associate Professor of Orthopaedic Surgery
Mayo Clinic School of Medicine
Rochester, Minnesota

Stephen D. Cassivi, MD
Associate Professor of Surgery
Division of General Thoracic Surgery
Mayo Clinic School of Medicine
Surgical Director of Lung Transplantation
William J. von Liebig Transplant Center
Mayo Clinic
Rochester, Minnesota

William P. Cooney III, MD
Professor Emeritus
Department of Orthopaedic Surgery
Mayo Clinic School of Medicine
Mayo Clinic
Rochester, Minnesota

Bradford L. Currier, MD
Professor of Orthopaedic Surgery
Mayo Clinic School of Medicine
Orthopaedic Surgeon
St. Mary's Hospital
Rochester, Minnesota

Mark B. Dekutoski, MD
Associate Professor of Orthopaedics
Mayo Clinic School of Medicine
Mayo Foundation
Rochester, Minnesota

David G. Dennison, MD
Instructor of Orthopaedics
Department of Orthopaedic Surgery
Mayo Clinic School of Medicine
Consultant in Orthopaedic Surgery
Mayo Clinic
Rochester, Minnesota

Robert K. Eastlack, MD
Clinical Instructor of Orthopaedic Surgery
University of California–San Diego
Active Staff in Orthopaedic Sugery
Sharp Memorial, Scripps Mercy, UCSD/VA Hospitals
San Diego, California

Jason C. Eck, DO, MS
Assistant Professor of Orthopaedic Surgery
Mayo Clinic School of Medicine
Rochester, Minnesota

Ziya L. Gokaslan, MD, FACS
Donlin M. Long Professor of Neurosurgery and Oncology
Vice Chairman of Neurosurgery
Director of Neurosurgical Spine Program
John Hopkins Medical Institutions
Baltimore, Maryland

Paul M. Huddleston, MD
Instructor of Orthopaedics
Department of Orthopaedic Surgery
Mayo Clinic School of Medicine
Orthopaedic Surgeon
St. Mary's Hospital
Rochester, Minnesota

Harold B. Kitaoka, MD
Professor of Orthopaedic Surgery
Mayo Clinic School of Medicine
Rochester, Minnesota

Steven L. Moran, MD
Associate Professor of Orthopaedics and Plastic Surgery
Mayo Clinic School of Medicine
Division of Hand and Microvascular Surgery
Mayo Clinic
Rochester, Minnesota

Bernard F. Morrey, MD
Professor of Orthopaedic Surgery
Mayo Clinic School of Medicine
Emeritus Chairman of Orthopaedics
Mayo Clinic
Rochester, Minnesota

Matthew Morrey, MD
Senior Resident of Orthopaedic Surgery
Mayo Clinic
Rochester, Minnesota

Mark W. Pagnano, MD
Associate Professor of Orthopaedics
Mayo Clinic School of Medicine
Consultant in Orthopaedics
Mayo Clinic
Rochester, Minnesota

David S. Ruch, MD
Professor of Orthopaedic Surgery
Director of Hand, Upper Extremity, and Microvascular
   Surgery Fellowship Program
Duke University Medical Center
Durham, North Carolina

S. Andrew Sems, MD
Clinical Instructor of Orthopaedic Surgery
Mayo Clinical School of Medicine
Senior Associate Consultant of Orthopaedic Surgery
Mayo Clinic
Rochester, Minnesota

John W. Sperling, MD, MBA
Associate Professor of Orthopaedic Surgery
Mayo Clinic School of Medicine
Rochester, Minnesota

Scott P. Steinmann, MD
Associate Professor of Orthopaedic Surgery
Mayo Clinic School of Medicine
St. Mary's Hospital
Rochester, Minnesota

Michael E. Torchia, MD
Associate Professor of Orthopaedics
Department of Orthopaedic Surgery
Mayo Clinic School of Medicine
Consultant for Orthopaedic Surgery
St. Mary's Hospital
Rochester, Minnesota

Luther H. Wolff III, MD
Director of Adult Reconstruction and Traumatology
St. Francis Orthopaedic Institute
Columbus, Georgia

Nikolaos P. Zagoreos, MD
Orthopaedic Hand Fellow
Department of Surgery
Duke University
Durham, North Carolina

Scott Zietlow, MD
Associate Professor of Surgery
Mayo Clinic School of Medicine
Chair, Division of Trauma, Critical Care, and General
Surgery
Mayo Clinic
Rochester, Minnesota

Figure Credits

Figure 1.43. Reproduced by permission of Mayo Foundation for Medical Education and Research from Bishop AT, Berger RA. Treatment with Reverse Flow Vascularized Pedicle Bone Grafts. In: Gelberman RH, ed. *Master Techniques in Orthopaedic Surgery: The Wrist*, 2nd ed. Philadelphia: Lippincott Williams & Wilkins, 2002; 149–159.

Figure 1.44. Reproduced with permission from Umlas ME, Gelberman RH. Surgical Management of de Quervain's Disease. In: Gelberman RH, ed. *Master Techniques in Orthopaedic Surgery: The Wrist*, 2nd ed. Philadelphia: Lippincott Williams & Wilkins, 2002; 445–453.

Figure 1.45A. Reproduced with permission from Herbert TJ, Krimmer H. Scaphoid Fractures: Internal Fixation. In: Gelberman RH, ed. *Master Techniques in Orthopaedic Surgery: The Wrist*, 2nd ed. Philadelphia: Lippincott Williams & Wilkins, 2002; 111–453.

Figure 1.49B. Reproduced by permission of Mayo Foundation for Medical Education and Research from Bishop AT, Berger RA. Treatment with Reverse Flow Vascularized Pedicle Bone Grafts. In: Gelberman RH, ed. *Master Techniques in Orthopaedic Surgery: The Wrist*, 2nd ed. Philadelphia: Lippincott Williams & Wilkins, 2002; 149–159.

Figure 3.1. Reproduced by permission of Mayo Foundation for Medical Education and Research from Morrey BF. Limited and Extensile Triceps Reflecting and Exposures of the Elbow. In: Morrey BF, ed. *Master Techniques in Orthopaedic Surgery: The Elbow*, 2nd ed. Philadelphia: Lippincott Williams & Wilkins, 2002; 3–25.

Figure 3.3A. Reproduced by permission of Mayo Foundation for Medical Education and Research from Morrey BF. Ulnohumeral Arthoplasty. In: Morrey BF, ed. *Master Techniques in Orthopaedic Surgery: The Elbow*, 2nd ed. Philadelphia: Lippincott Williams & Wilkins, 2002; 369–380.

Figure 3.3B. Reproduced by permission of Mayo Foundation for Medical Education and Research from Morrey BF. Limited and Extensile Triceps Reflecting and Exposures of the Elbow. In: Morrey BF, ed. *Master Techniques in Orthopaedic Surgery: The Elbow*, 2nd ed. Philadelphia: Lippincott Williams & Wilkins, 2002; 3–25.

Figure 3.3D. Reproduced by permission of Mayo Foundation for Medical Education and Research from Jupiter J. The Surgical Management of Intraarticular Fractures of the Distal Humerus. In: Morrey BF, ed. *Master Techniques in Orthopaedic Surgery: The Elbow*, 2nd ed. Philadelphia: Lippincott Williams & Wilkins, 2002; 65–81.

Figure 3.3F. Reproduced by permission of Mayo Foundation for Medical Education and Research from Coonrad RW, Morrey BF. Management of Olecranon Fractures and Nonunion. In: Morrey BF, ed. *Master Techniques in Orthopaedic Surgery: The Elbow*, 2nd ed. Philadelphia: Lippincott Williams & Wilkins, 2002; 103–126.

Figure 3.5. Reproduced by permission of Mayo Foundation for Medical Education and Research from Morrey BF. Limited and Extensile Triceps Reflecting and Exposures of the Elbow. In: Morrey BF, ed. *Master Techniques in Orthopaedic Surgery: The Elbow*, 2nd ed. Philadelphia: Lippincott Williams & Wilkins, 2002; 3–25.

Figure 3.6A-E. Reproduced with permission from Morrey BF, Mansat P. Capsular Release for Flexion Contracture: The Column Procedure. In: Morrey BF, ed. *Master Techniques in Orthopaedic Surgery: The Elbow*, 2nd ed. Philadelphia: Lippincott Williams & Wilkins, 2002; 381–389.

Figures 3.7A (right) and 3.7C (left). Reproduced by permission of Mayo Foundation for Medical Education and Research from Morrey BF. Radial Head Fractures. In: Morrey BF, ed. *Master Techniques in Orthopaedic Surgery: The Elbow*, 2nd ed. Philadelphia: Lippincott Williams & Wilkins, 2002; 83–102.

Figures 3.7A (left), 3.7C (center), and 3.7C (right). Reproduced with permission from Morrey BF. Radial Head Fractures. In: Morrey BF, ed. *Master Techniques in Orthopaedic Surgery: The Elbow*, 2nd ed. Philadelphia: Lippincott Williams & Wilkins, 2002; 83–102.

Figure 3.7D. Reproduced by permission of Mayo Foundation for Medical Education and Research from Morrey BF. Limited and Extensile Triceps Reflecting and Exposures of the Elbow. In: Morrey BF, ed. *Master Techniques in Orthopaedic Surgery: The Elbow*, 2nd ed. Philadelphia: Lippincott Williams & Wilkins, 2002; 3–25.

Figure 3.9B. Reproduced with permission from Morrey BF. Limited and Extensile Triceps Reflecting and Exposures of the Elbow. In: Morrey BF, ed. *Master Techniques in Orthopaedic Surgery: The Elbow*, 2nd ed. Philadelphia: Lippincott Williams & Wilkins, 2002; 3–25.

Figures 3.9D (right) and 3.9E. Reproduced by permission of Mayo Foundation for Medical Education and Research from Morrey BF. Limited and Extensile Triceps Reflecting and Exposures of the Elbow. In: Morrey BF, ed. *Master Techniques in Orthopaedic Surgery: The Elbow*, 2nd ed. Philadelphia: Lippincott Williams & Wilkins, 2002; 3–25.

Figures 3.10A, 3.10B, 3.10C (right), and 3.10D (right). Reproduced by permission of Mayo Foundation for Medical Education and Research from Morrey BF. Limited and Extensile Triceps Reflecting and Exposures of the Elbow. In: Morrey BF, ed. *Master Techniques in Orthopaedic Surgery: The Elbow*, 2nd ed. Philadelphia: Lippincott Williams & Wilkins, 2002; 3–25.

Figure 3.11A and 3.11B. Reproduced with permission from Morrey BF. Semiconstrained Total Elbow Replacement. In: Morrey BF, ed. *Master Techniques in Orthopaedic Surgery: The Elbow*, 2nd ed. Philadelphia: Lippincott Williams & Wilkins, 2002; 313–342.

Figure 3.11C. Reproduced by permission of Mayo Foundation for Medical Education and Research from Morrey BF. Limited and Extensile Triceps Reflecting and Exposures of the Elbow. In: Morrey BF, ed. *Master Techniques in Orthopaedic Surgery: The Elbow*, 2nd ed. Philadelphia: Lippincott Williams & Wilkins, 2002; 3–25.

Figure 3.13A. Reproduced with permission from ElAttrache NS, Jobe FW. Treatment of Ulnar Collateral Ligament Injuries in Athletes. In: Morrey BF, ed. *Master Techniques in Orthopaedic Surgery: The Elbow*, 2nd ed. Philadelphia: Lippincott Williams & Wilkins, 2002; 229–247.

Figures 3.13C, 13.13D, 3.13F (right), and 3.13G. Reproduced by permission of Mayo Foundation for Medical Education and Research from Morrey BF. Limited and Extensile Triceps Reflecting and Exposures of the Elbow. In: Morrey BF, ed. *Master Techniques in Orthopaedic Surgery: The Elbow*, 2nd ed. Philadelphia: Lippincott Williams & Wilkins, 2002; 3–25.

Figures 5.23, 5.24AB, 5.25AB, and 5.26AB. Reproduced with permission from Tibone JE. Capsular Repair for Recurrent Posterior Instability. In: Craig EV, ed. *Master Techniques in Orthopaedic Surgery: The Shoulder*, 2nd ed. Philadelphia: Lippincott Williams & Wilkins, 2004; 273–287.

Figures 5.27, 5.28, and 5.29. Reproduced with permission from Kalandiak SP, Tapscott RS, Wirth MA, Rockwood Jr CA. Anteroinferior Capsular Shift for Involuntary Multidirectional Instability. In: Craig EV, ed. *Master Techniques in Orthopaedic Surgery: The Shoulder*, 2nd ed. Philadelphia: Lippincott Williams & Wilkins, 2004; 241–272.

Figures 5.30A–C and 5.31. Reproduced with permission from Zarins B. Bankart Repair of Anterior Shoulder Dislocation and Subluxation. In: Craig EV, ed. *Master Techniques in Orthopaedic Surgery: The Shoulder*, 2nd ed. Philadelphia: Lippincott Williams & Wilkins, 2004; 209–224.

Figures 6.25, 6.27, 6.28, 6.29, and 6.31. Reproduced with permission from Bartlett CS, Malkani AL, Sen MK, Helfet DL. Acetabular Fractures: Extended Iliofemoral Approach. In: Wiss DA, ed. *Master Techniques in Orthopaedic Surgery: Fractures*, 2nd ed. Philadelphia: Lippincott Williams & Wilkins, 2006; 729–752.

Figures 6.26 and 6.30. Modified with permission from Bartlett CS, Malkani AL, Sen MK, Helfet DL. Acetabular Fractures: Extended Iliofemoral Approach. In: Wiss DA, ed. *Master Techniques in Orthopaedic Surgery: Fractures*, 2nd ed. Philadelphia: Lippincott Williams & Wilkins, 2006; 729–752.

Figure 7-2. Reproduced with permission from Bezwada HP, Ragland PS, Thomas CM, Mont MA. Core Decompression and Nonvascularized Bone Grafting. In: Barrack RL, Rosenberg AG, eds. *Master Techniques in Orthopaedic Surgery: The Hip*, 2nd ed. Philadelphia: Lippincott Williams & Wilkins, 2006; 159–174.

Figure 7.11. Reproduced with permission from Schmalzreid T, Antoniades J. Hemiarthroplasty. In: Barrack RL, Rosenberg AG, eds. *Master Techniques in Orthopaedic Surgery: The Hip*, 2nd ed. Philadelphia: Lippincott Williams & Wilkins, 2006; 153–158.

Figures 7.59, 7.60, 7.61A and B, 7.62, 7.63, 7.64, 7.66, 7.67, 7.68A, and 7.69. Reproduced with permission from Silverton CD. Trochanteric Osteotomy. In: Barrack RL, Rosenberg AG, eds. *Master Techniques in Orthopaedic Surgery: The Hip*, 2nd ed. Philadelphia: Lippincott Williams & Wilkins, 2006; 49–70.

Figure 9.4. Reproduced with permission from Lotke PA. Anterior Medial Exposure. In: Lotke PA, Lonner JH, eds. *Master Techniques in Orthopaedic Surgery: Knee Arthroplasty*, 2nd ed. Philadelphia: Lippincott Williams & Wilkins, 2006; 3–14.

Figure 11.10B. Reproduced with permission from Dahm DL, Kitaoka HB. Peroneal Tendon Repair and Reconstruction. In: Kitaoka HB, ed. *Master Techniques in Orthopaedic Surgery: The Foot and Ankle*, 2nd ed. Philadelphia: Lippincott Williams & Wilkins, 2002; 293–310.

Figures 11.16A, 11.16B (left), 11.16D, and 11.16E. Reproduced with permission from Kitaoka HB. Chevron Osteotomy. In: Kitaoka HB, ed. *Master Techniques in Orthopaedic Surgery: The Foot and Ankle*, 2nd ed. Philadelphia: Lippincott Williams & Wilkins, 2002; 29–44.

Figures 11.17A (left), 11.17B, and 11.17C. Reproduced with permission from Pfeffer GB. Cheilectomy. In: Kitaoka HB, ed. *Master Techniques in Orthopaedic Surgery: The Foot and Ankle*, 2nd ed. Philadelphia: Lippincott Williams & Wilkins, 2002; 119–134.

Figures 12.1, 12.2, 12.6, 12.8B, and 12.10B. Reproduced with permission from Bono CM, Garfin SR. Anterior Cervical Approach. In: Bradford DS, Zdeblick, eds. *Master Techniques in Orthopaedic Surgery: The Spine*, 2nd ed. Philadelphia: Lippincott Williams & Wilkins, 2004; 3–28.

Figure 12.14. Reproduced with permission from Patel CK, Fischgrund JS Herkowitz HN. Anterior Cervical Discectomy and Spine Fusion. In: Bradford DS, Zdeblick, eds. *Master Techniques in Orthopaedic Surgery: The Spine*, 2nd ed. Philadelphia: Lippincott Williams & Wilkins, 2004; 29–45.

Figure 12.25. Reproduced with permission from Gill SS, Heller JG. Cervical Laminoplasty. In: Bradford DS, Zdeblick, eds. *Master Techniques in Orthopaedic Surgery: The Spine*, 2nd ed. Philadelphia: Lippincott Williams & Wilkins, 2004; 111–128.

Figures 13.1, 13.2, 13.3, 13.4, 13.10, and 13.11. Reproduced with permission from Alpert TJ. Anterior exposures of cervicothoracic junction and thoracic spine. In: Albert TJ, Balderston RA, Northrup BE, eds. *Surgical Approaches to the Spine*. Philadelphia: WB Saunders, 1997.

Figures 13.5, 13.6, 13.7, and 13.8. Reproduced with permission from Bono CM, Garfin SR. Anterior Cervical Approach. In: Bradford DS, Zdeblick, eds. *Master Techniques in Orthopaedic Surgery: The Spine*, 2nd ed. Philadelphia: Lippincott Williams & Wilkins, 2004; 3–28.

Figures 13.12 and 13.13. Reproduced with permission from Cohen ZR, Fourney DR, Gokaslan ZL, Walsh GL, Rhines LD. Anterior stabilization of the upper thoracic spine via an "interaortocaval subinnominate window": case report and description of operative technique. *J Spinal Disord Tech* 2004;17(6):543–548. Illustrations by Ian Suk.

Figures 13.15, 13.16, 13.17, and 13.18. Reproduced with permission from McGuire Jr RA. Anterior Thoracolumbar Extensile Approach. In: Bradford DS, Zdeblick, eds. *Master Techniques in Orthopaedic Surgery: The Spine*, 2nd ed. Philadelphia: Lippincott Williams & Wilkins, 2004; 159–181.

Figures 14.20, 14.25, and 14.26B. Reproduced with permission from McLain RF. Transpedicular Fixation. In: Bradford DS, Zdeblick, eds. *Master Techniques in Orthopaedic Surgery: The Spine*, 2nd ed. Philadelphia: Lippincott Williams & Wilkins, 2004; 293–311.

1 Hand and Wrist

PART 1. Dorsal Approach to the Wrist Joint

Julie E. Adams and Scott P. Steinmann

Dorsal approaches to the wrist joint are useful to address fractures, dislocations, ligamentous injuries, arthritis, and other pathology such as congenital anomalies or neoplasms (1–3). Moreover, one can perform compartment releases, tenosynovectomy, and posterior interosseous nerve (PIN) neurectomy through a dorsal approach (1,4).

ANATOMIC CONSIDERATIONS

The superficial nature of the wrist relative to the dorsum of the hand facilitates easy exposure (2). The dorsal aspect of the wrist is characterized by a loose skin and subcutaneous tissue. A thin superficial fascia covers the dorsal aspect of the wrist and hand including fatty and fibrous layers, cutaneous nerves, and venous and lymphatic vessels. When approaching the wrist joint, the vessels should be preserved whenever possible to facilitate venous return from the hand which is largely dependent upon these cutaneous vessels (3). The dorsal nerves and subcutaneous veins should be raised in continuity with the skin and subcutaneous tissues. The dorsal aspect of the hand is supplied by branches of the superficial branch of the radial nerve and the dorsal sensory branch of the ulnar nerve in a variable pattern with an inconsistent contribution of the lateral and posterior antebrachial cutaneous nerves (5–7). These cutaneous nerves should be identified and preserved. Use of vessel loops to isolate and protect the nerves may be helpful.

The extensor retinaculum is the next deepest structure encountered. The wrist and finger extensors travel beneath the extensor retinaculum in six dorsal compartments, delineated by fibrous septae attaching from the extensor retinaculum to the periosteum of the radius. Palmer et al investigated the anatomy and biomechanical role of the extensor retinaculum of the wrist (8). This fibrous thickening of the antebrachial fascia lies in a band over the dorsal aspect of the wrist joint and is continuous with the volar carpal ligament palmarly and the dorsal fascia over the distal hand and metacarpal region (8). Fibrous septae traversing from the retinaculum palmarly to insert upon the radial periosteum or wrist capsule create five fibro-osseous tunnels and one fibrous canal, the 5th compartment. From radial to ulnar, the compartments are as follows: first dorsal compartment: abductor pollicis longus and extensor pollicis brevis; second dorsal compartment: extensor carpi radialis longus and brevis; third dorsal compartment: extensor pollicis longus; fourth dorsal compartment: extensor digitorum communis and extensor indicis proprius; fifth dorsal compartment: extensor digiti minimi; and sixth dorsal compartment: extensor carpi ulnaris.

Deep to the extensor tendons lies the capsule of the wrist joint. The capsule is comprised of ligamentous tissue and nonligamentous tissues. The major dorsal wrist ligaments are the dorsal radioulnar ligament, the dorsal radiocarpal ligament, and the dorsal intercarpal ligament. The dorsal radioulnar ligament spans from the radius at the dorsal margin of the sigmoid notch over the distal radioulnar joint (DRUJ) to attach to the head of the ulna and along the styloid process. It contributes to the extensor carpi ulnaris subsheath and the triangular fibrocartilaginous complex (TFCC). Similarly, the dorsoradioulnar ligament attaches to the radius at a site ulnar to the Lister's tubercle then spans the radiocarpal joint obliquely to attach to the dorsal horn of the lunate and to form the lunotriquetral interosseous ligament superficially. The dorsal intercarpal ligament is confluent with the dorsal radiocarpal ligament at their insertions upon the triquetrum. It courses distally and obliquely from the triquetrum to the dorsal ridge of the distal half of the scaphoid and to the dorsal cortex of the trapezoid (2). To expose the dorsal aspect of the wrist, a dorsal capsular flap (the Mayo flap) can be raised by elevating a split dorsal radiotriquetral and dorsal intercarpal ligament with a radial based flap.

DORSAL SURGICAL APPROACH

Position

The patient is positioned in the supine position with the forearm pronated. The arm is exsanguinated and a tourniquet inflated.

Landmarks

Superficial landmarks are palpable. The radial styloid lies in a lateral position when the hand and forearm are in the anatomic position. The ulnar styloid process is medially and posteriorly located when the hand and forearm are in the anatomic position. The extensor carpi ulnaris (ECU) lies in a dorsal groove radial to this landmark. Distally, the eight carpal bones are aligned in two rows. The anatomic snuff box is outlined when the thumb is abducted. The scaphoid bone lies in the floor and ulnar deviation of the wrist causes it to slide outward from beneath the radial styloid to become palpable. Lister's tubercle or the dorsal tubercle of the radius lies about one third the distance across the dorsum of the wrist from the radial styloid. The scaphoid-lunate junction (and scapholunate ligament) is located just distal to Lister's tubercle. The capitate lies at the base of the 3rd metacarpal bone. When the wrist is in a neutral position, the depression in the capitate becomes palpable (9).

Technique

The skin incision may be longitudinal or transverse. We prefer a longitudinal incision that may be extended distally and proximally (3,10) (**Fig. 1-1**). The incision may be centered in the radial and ulnar dimension and extends longitudinally from 2 to 3 cm proximal to the radiocarpal joint to 2 cm distal to Lister's tubercle, depending on the pathology to be addressed. Although not in Langer's lines and indeed, the longitudinal incision is perpendicular to Langer's lines, incisional contracture is not problematic as the skin overlying the dorsum of the wrist is quite pliable and longitudinal scarring is uncommon. Alternatively, a transverse slightly curved incision, directed in line with Langer's lines, with the concavity oriented distally may be used (2) (**Fig. 1-2**). This incision can extend from the radial styloid to the ulnar styloid, in which case mobilization of the incision allows for exposure of the carpometacarpal joints and the distal radial metaphysis (2).

Full-thickness flaps are developed down to the extensor retinaculum (**Fig. 1-3**), taking care to identify and preserve the superficial radial nerve, the dorsal sensory branch of the ulnar nerve, and any dorsal veins, and elevating them with the flaps (2,3). This is in contradistinction to the practice on the palmar aspect of the hand, where skin flaps are raised and elevated away from the neurovascular structures.

If the pathology to be addressed is in the extensor tendons, the retinaculum over the desired compartment is incised. If a posterior interosseous nerve (PIN) neurectomy is to be performed, a deeper dissection is made 2 cm proximal to the extensor retinaculum (11) (**Fig. 1-4**). The dissection proceeds through the deep fascia of the forearm. The PIN is identified as it enters the 4th extensor compartment and a 2 cm segment of the nerve, which is purely sensory at this level, is excised (11) (**Figs. 1-4 and 1-5**). The PIN and posterior interosseous artery course longitudinally from proximal to distal. Proximally, the PIN innervates the extensor pollicis longus (EPL) and extensor indicis proprius (EIP). At this level, it departs from the posterior interosseous artery and travels distally bound under

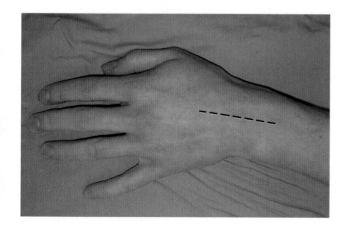

FIGURE 1-1

A longitudinal incision centered over the wrist is preferred. Incisional contractures are rarely problematic.

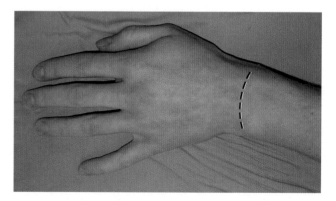

FIGURE 1-2

An alternative transverse incision in Langer's lines. This incision can extend from the radial styloid to the ulnar styloid, in which case mobilization allows for exposure of the carpometacarpal joints and the distal radial metaphysis.

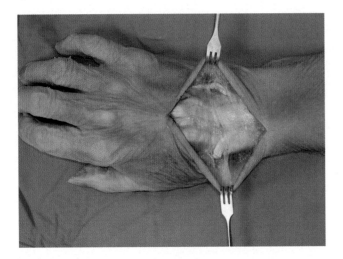

FIGURE 1-3

Full-thickness flaps are developed down to the extensor retinaculum, taking care to identify and preserve the superficial radial nerve, the dorsal sensory branch of the ulnar nerve, and any dorsal veins, and elevating them with the flaps. EDC (extensor digitorum comminus), EDM (extensor digiti minimi), EPL (extensor pollicis longus).

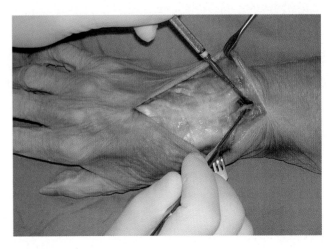

FIGURE 1-4

The posterior interosseous nerve (PIN) may be exposed for neurectomy by dissection 2 cm proximal to the extensor retinaculum.

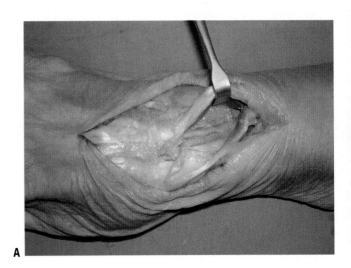

FIGURE 1-5

A,B: The PIN is identified as it enters the 4th extensor compartment and a 2 cm segment of the nerve, which is purely sensory at this level, is excised to achieve PIN neurectomy.

A

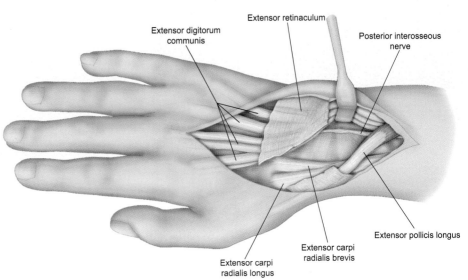

Extensor digitorum communis

Extensor retinaculum

Posterior interosseous nerve

Extensor pollicis longus

Extensor carpi radialis brevis

Extensor carpi radialis longus

B

a fascial layer to the interosseus membrane along the ulnar border of the radius (4). At the level of the Lister's tubercle, the PIN lies adjacent to the ulnar origin of the 3rd dorsal compartment. It then travels distally with the anterior interosseus artery across the radiocarpal joint. At the level of the scapholunate ligament, the PIN branches into its terminal extensions to bring sensory and proprioceptive nerve fibers to the capsule and ligaments of the dorsal aspect of the wrist (4). By denervating the PIN (and anterior interosseus nerve [AIN]), pain related to the scapholunate ligament and adjacent capsule may be attenuated.

To gain access to the wrist joint, the retinaculum overlying the 3rd dorsal compartment is incised longitudinally from the deep antebrachial fascia proximally and then distally to the distal margin of the retinaculum (**Fig. 1-6**). The EPL in the 3rd dorsal compartment is retracted radially, and the 4th extensor compartment is elevated subperiosteally or by dividing the septum between the 3rd and 4th compartments and reflecting the retinaculum as an ulnarly based flap (**Fig. 1-7**). The approach is limited by the septum between the 5th and 6th dorsal compartments. Radially, the extensor retinaculum may be elevated off of Lister's tubercle and the 2nd dorsal compartment released. Subsequently, the extensor carpi radialis brevis (ECRB) and extensor carpi radialis longus (ECRL) can be retracted radially deep to the extensor retinaculum, with the EPL retracted radially and superficial to the extensor retinaculum. This allows for exposure of approximately 90% of the dorsal wrist (2) (**Fig. 1-8**).

The wrist capsule is divided and reflected to gain access to the pathology to be addressed. Care should be taken when planning the capsulotomy to access the wrist joint. A poorly designed capsulotomy may destabilize the joint by disrupting the dorsal capsular ligaments, result in limited range of motion due to scar formation, or leave inadequate remaining tissue to facilitate closure (2). While some surgeons advocate a simple transverse or longitudinal capsulotomy in line with the skin incision (and these may be adequate in revision surgery, subtotal or complete wrist fusion, or in other cases) (1,3,10), we prefer a ligament-sparing capsulotomy with capsulotomy incisions parallel to the dorsal wrist ligaments.

Radial Capsulotomy

The radial capsulotomy provides exposure of the radial two-thirds of the radiocarpal joint and most of the midcarpal joint. The fibers of the dorsal radiocarpal and dorsal intercarpal ligaments are incised in line with their fibers in the midline of each ligament (**Fig. 1-9**) with continuation along the dorsal rim of the radius toward the radial styloid process to generate a three-sided trapezoidal flap remaining attached on the radial side. The flap of capsule is then elevated sharply off the dorsal surface of the triquetrum then off the lunate and scaphoid, with care taken to avoid injury to the lunotriquetral and scapholunate interosseous ligaments (**Fig. 1-10**). Elevation is halted upon encountering the dorsal ridge of the scaphoid to avoid damage to the vascular supply of the scaphoid.

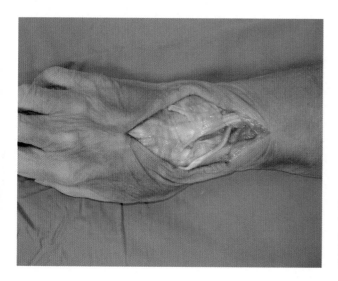

FIGURE 1-6

To gain access to the wrist joint, the retinaculum overlying the 3rd dorsal compartment is incised longitudinally from the deep antebrachial fascia proximally and then distally to the distal margin of the retinaculum.

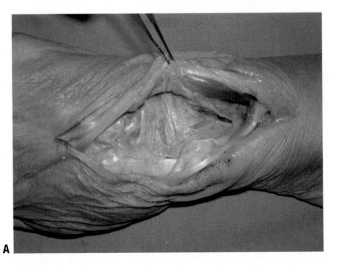

A

FIGURE 1-7

A,B: The EPL in the 3rd dorsal compartment is retracted radially, and the 4th extensor compartment is elevated subperiosteally or by dividing the septum between the 3rd and 4th compartments and reflecting the retinaculum as an ulnarly based flap.

B

Dorsal intercarpal ligament

Dorsal radiotriquetral ligament

Extensor digitorum communis

Posterior interosseous nerve

Extensor carpi radialis brevis

Extensor pollicis longus

Lister's tubercle

FIGURE 1-8

The ECRL can be retracted radially deep to the extensor retinaculum, with the EPL retracted radially and superficial to the extensor retinaculum. This allows for exposure of approximately 90% of the dorsal wrist.

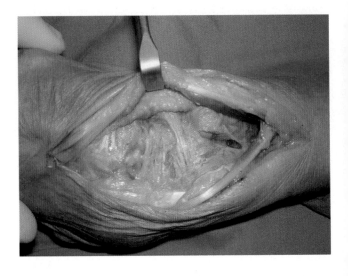

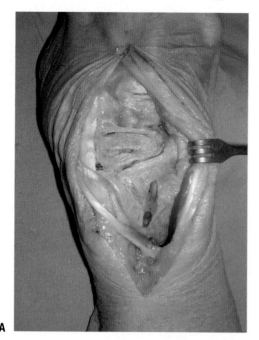

A

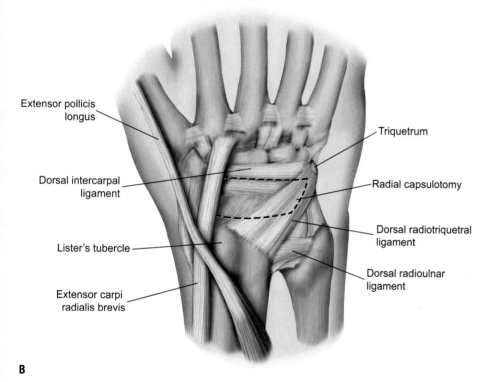

Extensor pollicis
longus

Dorsal intercarpal
ligament

Lister's tubercle

Extensor carpi
radialis brevis

Triquetrum

Radial capsulotomy

Dorsal radiotriquetral
ligament

Dorsal radioulnar
ligament

B

FIGURE 1-9

A,B: The fibers of the dorsal radiocarpal and dorsal intercarpal ligaments are incised in line
with their fibers in the midline of each ligament, with continuation along the dorsal rim of
the radius toward the radial styloid process to generate a three-sided trapezoidal flap remaining attached on the radial side. The flap of capsule is then elevated sharply off the dorsal surface of the triquetrum then off the lunate and scaphoid, with care taken to avoid injury to the lunotriquetral and scapholunate interosseous ligaments.

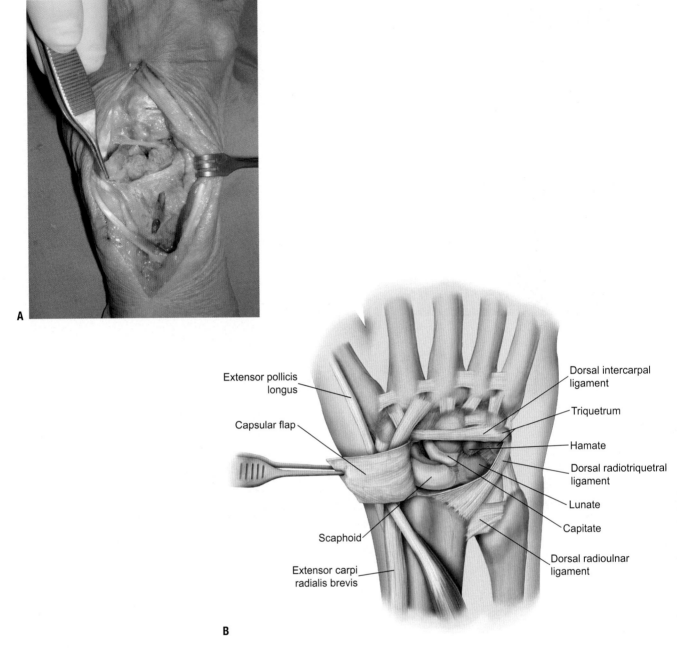

FIGURE 1-10

A,B: Elevation of capsular flaps in this manner preserves the blood supply and allows for closure of tissues following the procedure.

Any loose synovial tissue is removed to allow for visualization of the lunate, the scaphoid, the scapholunate ligament, the dorsal aspect of the radiocarpal joint, the lunotriquetral joint, the proximal capitate and triquetrum, and the hamate. Mobilization radially allows for access to the proximal trapezoid, trapezium and STT joint. Distraction of the wrist allows for access to the palmar joint capsule of the radiocarpal joint and the midcarpal ligaments (2). Closure of the capsule is facilitated using 3-0 braided absorbable sutures in a figure of eight or horizontal mattress pattern (2).

Ulnar Capsulotomy

This approach allows access to the proximal lunate and triquetrum and the ulnar aspect of the radiocarpal joint. The skin and subcutaneous dissection may proceed as outlined above for the capsulotomy to the radial aspect of the joint (2). Alternatively, only the ulnar half of the transverse inci-

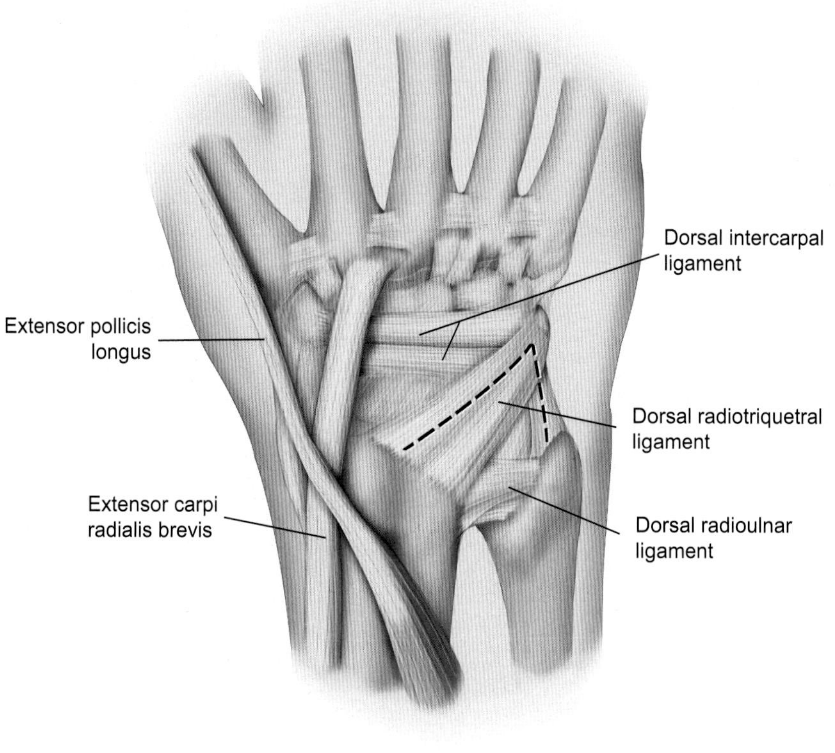

Extensor pollicis
longus

Dorsal intercarpal
ligament

Dorsal radiotriquetral
ligament

Extensor carpi
radialis brevis

Dorsal radioulnar
ligament

FIGURE 1-11

For the ulnar capsultomy, the dorsal radiocarpal ligament is incised longitudinally through its midline. The dorsal radioulnar ligament is preserved as are the 6th extensor compartment and the ECU subsheath.

sion may be made with dissection proceeding to the extensor retinaculum where the 5th extensor compartment is incised and the EDM retracted ulnarly. To expand the exposure, the septum between the 4th and 5th dorsal compartments may be incised, the 4th compartment entered and the extensor digitorum communis (EDC) and EIP tendons retracted radially.

For exposure, the septum between the 5th and 6th compartments is identified at the level of the triquetrum and reflected ulnarly or the ulnar part of the extensor retinaculum is released radial to ulnar from Lister's tubercle to the 6th extensor compartment.

The dorsal radiocarpal ligament is incised longitudinally through its midline (**Fig. 1-11**). The dorsal radioulnar ligament is preserved as are the 6th extensor compartment and the ECU subsheath. A proximally based triangular flap is elevated sharply from the triquetrum and the lunate, until the distal extent of the dorsal radioulnar ligament is encountered (**Fig. 1-12**). Synovial tissue is removed to expose the lunate, the lunotriquetral interosseous ligament, the triquetrum, and the triangular fibrocartilage complex (**Fig. 1-13**). Wrist distraction provides access to the ulnolunate and ulnotriquetral ligaments. Following completion of work, capsular closure is performed in the usual fashion with interrupted figure of eight or horizontal mattress sutures with 3-0 braided absorbable sutures (2).

SUMMARY

Dorsal exposure of the wrist joint is useful for procedures to address pathology of the carpus, the extensor tendons, the PIN, or fractures. The subcutaneous location makes this approach readily available and relatively simple. Attention to ligament sparing capsulotomy can preserve stability and motion in certain cases.

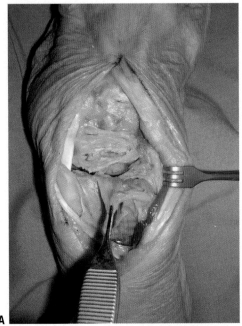

A

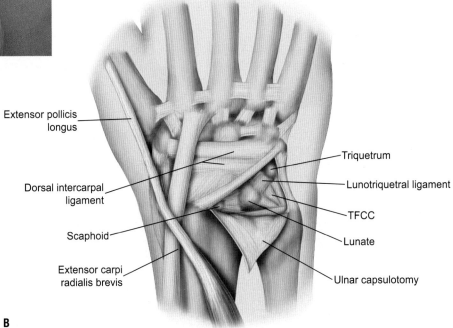

Extensor pollicis longus

Dorsal intercarpal ligament

Scaphoid

Extensor carpi radialis brevis

Triquetrum

Lunotriquetral ligament

TFCC

Lunate

Ulnar capsulotomy

B

FIGURE 1-12

A,B: A proximally based triangular flap is elevated sharply from the triquetrum and the lunate, until the distal extent of the dorsal radioulnar ligament is encountered.

FIGURE 1-13

Synovial tissue is removed to expose the lunate, the lunotriquetral interosseous ligament, the triquetrum, and the triangular fibrocartilage complex.

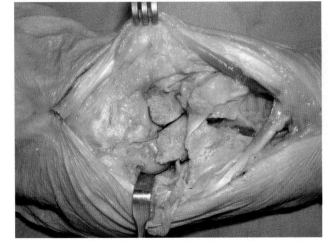

PART 2. Surgical Approach of the Ulnar Nerve at the Level of the Wrist

David Ruch and Nikolaos P. Zagoreos

The ulnar nerve runs down the volar surface of the forearm under the muscle and the tendon of the flexor carpi ulnaris (FCU) with the ulnar artery being on its radial side. Just before the wrist crease, the ulnar artery and nerve emerge from under the muscle and enter the distal ulnar tunnel canal in the wrist. At this level, the ulnar artery and nerve are located on the radial surface of the FCU.

The distal ulnar tunnel was initially described by Guyon, a French urologist, in 1861 and is also referred as Guyon's canal (1). It is essentially a triangular fibro-osseous tunnel about 3 cm long located at the carpus. The volar carpal ligament forms the roof of the canal, which is a condensation of the forearm fascia and expansion of the FCU. The transverse carpal ligament, extending between the pisiform and the hook of the hamate, forms the floor of the canal. The hook of the hamate and the medial side defines the lateral side of the canal by the pisiform. The contents of the distal ulnar tunnel are the ulnar nerve, the ulnar artery, and the ulnar veins.

The roof of the canal is a very thin layer of tissue located quite superficially, exactly below the skin and the subcutaneous tissue. The respective roof of the neighboring carpal tunnel, the transverse carpal ligament, is the floor of the Guyon's canal and is a relatively thick fibrous layer.

The longitudinal axis of the distal ulnar tunnel is angulated medially about 30 degrees to the long axis of the forearm and the wrist, since the hook of the hamate lies a little more distal to the pisiform.

Indications for volar approach of the ulnar nerve in the wrist are traumatic injuries of the ulnar nerve, compression neuropathies within the Guyon's canal, and intrinsic muscle spasticity requiring ulnar motor neurectomy.

EXPLORATION OF THE ULNAR NERVE WITHIN THE GUYON'S CANAL

Regional or general anesthesia is routinely used and the exploration is performed in a bloodless field provided by a tourniquet. The ulnar nerve can be explored through a volar approach, which is located 1 to 2 cm more medially than the typical approaches for open release of the carpal tunnel. A consideration in planning the skin incision is the location of the palmar cutaneous branch of the ulnar nerve. Although this nerve was found to be present in only 25% in previous cadaveric studies (2), injury to it can lead to painful neuromas. The ideal incision should be located in the internervous plane between the palmar cutaneous branch of the ulnar and median nerve. Unfortunately, cadaveric studies have identified that there is not such a plane. This plane is innervated by the nerve of Henle (the nerve of the ulnar artery) and multiple ulnar cutaneous branches (3). Therefore, the dissection of the skin and subcutaneous tissue should be performed carefully, possibly under loop magnification, preserving any emerging cutaneous branches.

Anatomic landmarks are the pisiform, the hook of the hamate, and the hypothenar eminence. The typical incision is curvilinear in shape with the distal limb following the radial limb of the hypothenar eminence and the proximal limb extending on the volar ulnar part of the forearm. The wrist crease should not be crossed longitudinally but rather in an angle of 60 degrees to avoid skin contractures. The total length of the incision is about 6 to 8 cm centered over the wrist crease **(Fig. 1-14)**.

The ulnar nerve and artery can be easily identified in the proximal part of the incision where they lie on the lateral surface of the tendon of the FCU **(Fig. 1-15)**. They can be traced easily distally incising all tissues more superficial to these structures. The dissection of the subcutaneous fat should be performed bluntly in order to avoid injury to any cutaneous branches. The palmaris brevis muscle is elevated slightly ulnarly and the volar carpal ligament and pisohamate ligament are incised resulting in a complete decompression of the Guyon's canal. The two branches of the ulnar nerve at the level of the pisiform are identified.

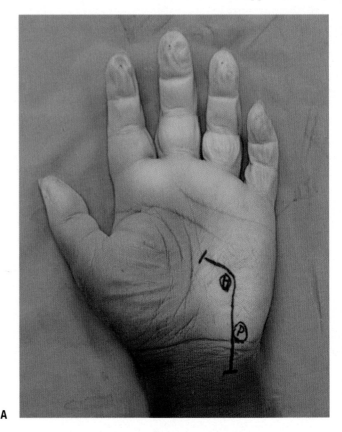

FIGURE 1-14

A,B: Incisions for the exploration of the ulnar nerve. At the level of the wrist, the incisions pass radial to the pisiform and ulnar to the hook of the hamate.

A

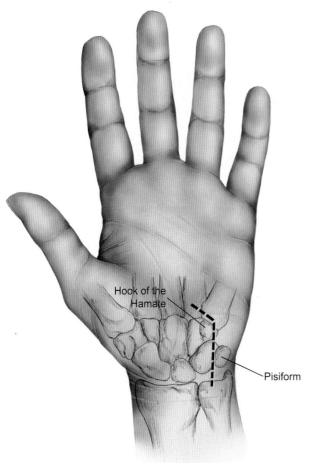

Hook of the Hamate

Pisiform

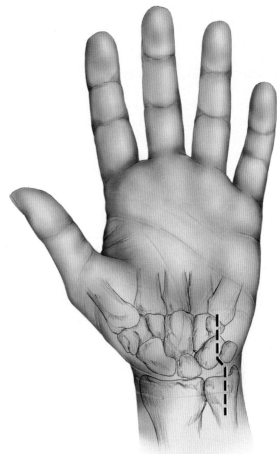

B

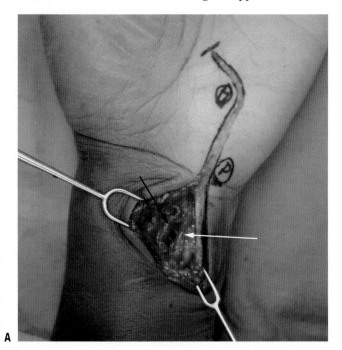

A

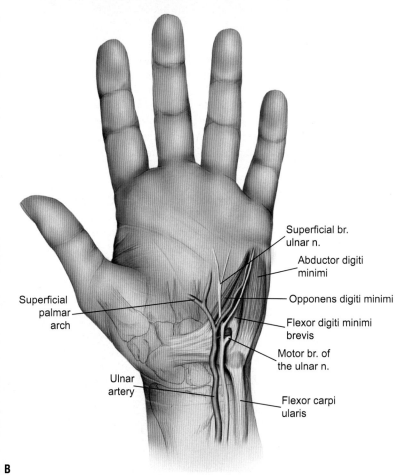

Superficial br.
ulnar n.

Abductor digiti
minimi

Opponens digiti minimi

Superficial
palmar
arch

Flexor digiti minimi
brevis

Motor br. of
the ulnar n.

Ulnar
artery

Flexor carpi
ularis

B

FIGURE 1-15

A,B: The ulnar artery (*white arrow*) and the ulnar nerve (*black arrow*) are identified at the radial margin of the flexor carpi ulnaris tendon.

The motor branch is more dorsal and more medial at the level of the bifurcation. It can be traced beneath the fibrous arch of the hypothenar muscles formed between the abductor digiti minimi and the flexor digiti minimi, through the muscle mass of the opponens digiti minimi and around the hook of the hamate. A careful exploration of the floor of the distal ulnar tunnel is performed looking for any pathology like ganglions, fibrous bands, anomalous muscle masses, fractures of the hook of the hamate, and vascular aneurysms.

The tourniquet should be deflated before closure of the wound and the ulnar artery and its branches should be examined for any injury. Thorough hemostasis should be achieved since a postoperative hematoma can result in compression neuropathy of the ulnar nerve.

An alternative surgical approach is through an open carpal tunnel syndrome incision extending slightly more proximally and distally. The ulnar nerve and artery are located on the volar medial surface of the transverse carpal ligament and can be identified tracing the superficial palmar arch proximally. Several hand surgeons prefer to decompress the Guyon's canal and the carpal tunnel simultaneously.

ANATOMY OF THE ULNAR NERVE IN GUYON'S CANAL

Around the pisiform the ulnar nerve divides into two branches, the superficial and the deep branch. The superficial branch gives immediately after the bifurcation motor branches to the palmaris brevis muscle and becomes purely sensory. It continues its course distally deep and medial to the ulnar artery providing sensory supply to the small finger and the ulnar side of the ring finger. The deep branch of the ulnar nerve bifurcation is purely motor and supplies the hypothenar muscles, all the interossei, the medial two lumbricals, and the adductor pollicis. The motor part of the ulnar nerve is located dorsally in the ulnar nerve at the level of the distal forearm and emerges from the nerve on the dorsal medial surface. The motor branch leaves the tunnel and passes beneath the fibrous arch of the hypothenar muscles and enters the interval between the abductor digiti minimi and flexor digiti muscles. It pierces the opponens digiti minimi and curves radially and dorsally around the distal part of the hook of the hamate, lying on the floor of the carpal tunnel (**Fig. 1-16**).

Compared to the carpal tunnel syndrome, ulnar tunnel syndrome is less common because the space within the Guyon's canal is much more yielding. Compression within the canal can produce motor or sensory or combined motor and sensory symptoms. The Guyon's canal can be divided in three zones to allow more accurate localization of the pathology of the compression in respect to the neurological symptoms (4).

Zone I is the most proximal and is bounded palmarly and radially by the volar carpal ligament, medially by the FCU and the pisiform, and dorsally by the transverse carpal ligament. This region includes both the sensory and the motor branches of the ulnar nerve; therefore, compression in the region results in combined motor and sensory deficits. Compressions within this region are usually produced by fractures of the hook of the hamate and ganglions (**Fig. 1-17**).

FIGURE 1-16

The deep motor branch of the ulnar nerve passes under the fibrous arch of the hypothenar muscles ulnar to the hook of the hamate. (P, pisiform; M, motor branch; SPA, ulnar branch to superficial palmar arch; FA, fibrous arch of the hypothenar muscles; S, one of the sensory branches of the ulnar nerve.)

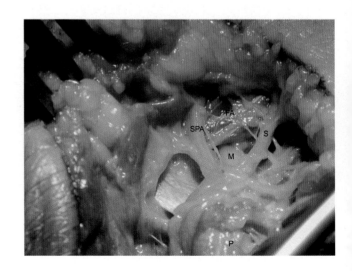

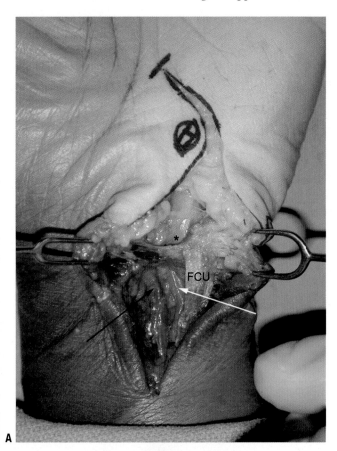

FIGURE 1-17

A,B: Zone I of the ulnar tunnel as described by Gross and Gelberman (*asterisk*). Note the neurovascular bundle passing under the proximal edge of the palmar carpal ligament. (FCU, flexor carpi ulnaris; *white arrow*, ulnar artery; *black arrow*, ulnar nerve.)

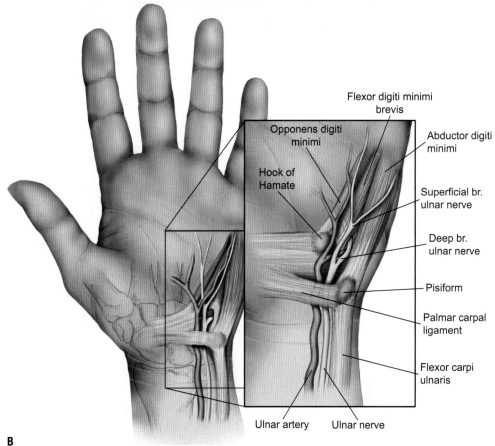

Zone II is bounded palmarly by the palmaris brevis muscle and the fibrous arch of the hypothenar muscles; dorsally by the pisiform and hamate ligaments and the oppenens digiti minimi; medially by the superficial branch of the ulnar nerve and the abductor digiti minimi; and laterally by the transverse carpal ligament, flexor digiti minimi, and the hook of the hamate. This region surrounds the motor branch of the ulnar nerve and compression within this region results in motor symptoms. Ganglions and fractures of the hook of the hamate can produce compression within this region, as well as anomalous intrinsic muscles within the canal (**Figs. 1-18 and 1-19**).

Zone III is bounded palmarly by the ulnar artery and the palmaris brevis muscle, dorsally by the hypothenar fascia, laterally by the motor branch of the ulnar nerve, and medially by the abductor digiti minimi muscle. This region surrounds the superficial branches of the ulnar nerve, and compression within this region produces exclusively sensory symptoms (**Fig. 1-19**). The most frequent causes of compression within this region are synovial inflammation, vascular lesions of the ulnar artery (thrombosis, aneurysm, or pseudoaneurysm), and anomalous size and location of abductor digiti minimi.

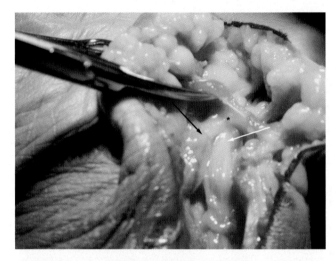

FIGURE 1-18

Demonstrates the entrance to zone II of the ulnar tunnel in which the nerve passes under the palmar brevis muscle providing innervation to the muscle (asterisk). (White arrow, ulnar artery; black arrow, ulnar nerve.)

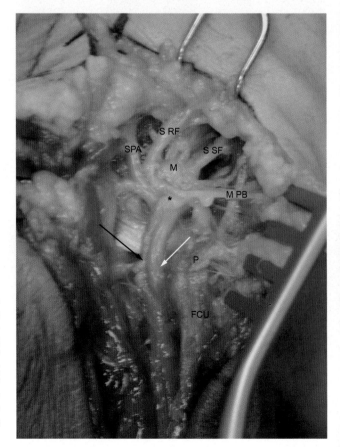

FIGURE 1-19

The ulnar nerve passes over the pisohamate and pisometacarpal ligaments which form the floor of the tunnel. Note the branches which supply the hypothenar muscles. The asterisk marks the nerve bifurcation into the deep motor branch (M) and the superficial sensory branches. (P, pisiform; FCU: flexor carpi ulnaris; white arrow, ulnar artery; black arrow, ulnar nerve; SPA, ulnar branch to superficial palmar arch; S RF, sensory branch to ulnar side of ring finger and radial side of the small finger; S SF, sensory branch to the ulnar surface of the small finger; M PB, motor branches to the palmaris brevis muscle.)

PART 3. Surgical Approaches of Flexor Tendons in Wrist and Hand

David Ruch and Nikolaos P. Zagoreos

The versatility of the human hand depends, to a great extent, on the normal function of the flexor tendons. These collagenous structures are able to transmit enormous forces from the muscles in the forearm to the fingers allowing not only powerful motions but also fine motor activities.

Unfortunately, tendon lacerations are quite common and require prompt tendon surgery and accurate surgical approach. The same approaches can be used to address clinical conditions affecting neighboring structures like the nerves, the vessels, or the bones in the hand.

The various surgical approaches needed for flexor tendon surgery will be presented, as well as brief description of the anatomy of the flexor tendons and of the special properties and considerations of the volar skin of the palm and the fingers.

GROSS ANATOMY OF FLEXOR TENDONS OF THE WRIST AND THE HAND

The flexor muscles originate in the proximal two-thirds and provide the respective flexor tendons in the distal third of the volar compartment of the forearm. Three flexor tendons insert around the area of the wrist; the flexor carpi radialis located on the radial side of the forearm inserts at the base of the second metacarpal; the FCU located in the ulnar aspect of the forearm inserts at the pisiform bone; the palmaris longus located in the most superficial layers along the midline of the forearm inserts at the palmar fascia of the hand. The palmaris longus is absent unilaterally or bilaterally in 12% and is useful in grafting because it is readily accessible and expandable.

The remaining nine flexor tendons are the flexor tendons of the fingers and the thumb; two for each of the fingers and one long flexor for the thumb. They all enter the hand through the carpal tunnel and diverge towards the respective digit where they insert.

There are two flexor tendons for each finger, the flexor digitorum superficialis (FDS) and the flexor digitorum profundus (FDP). The FDS tendons lie more anterior to the FDP within the forearm and the palm and are grouped in two layers within the carpal tunnel. The tendons of the middle and ring fingers lie volarly to those of the index and small fingers. At the palm all the tendons of the FDS lie in the same plane, volar to the tendons of the FDP.

The tendons of the FPD are all in the same plane and are usually not so distinct at the level of the palm with the exception of the tendon to the index. They become more distinct distal to the carpal tunnel. An important anatomical relationship helpful in distinguishing the tendons of the FDP from the FDS in multiple tendon lacerations within the palm is that the four lumbrical muscles take their origin from the tendons of the FDP.

At the level of the metacarpophalangeal joint, the FDS splits into bands. The FDP passes between these two bands becoming more superficial to the FDS forming the Camper's chiasm. The two bands of the FDS rotate away from the midline so that the most medial fibers become the most volar ones and the most lateral ones become the most dorsal, and insert at the two lateral edges of the base of the middle phalanx. The FDP continues more distally and inserts at the base of the distal phalanx.

The thumb has only one flexor tendon, the flexor pollicis longus (FPL), which enters the carpal tunnel in its most radial aspect. Following the carpal tunnel, the tendon courses around the scaphoid, beneath the thenar musculature, and inserts at the base of the distal phalanx of the thumb.

The tendons of the FDS and FDP for each finger enter a well-defined fibro-osseous tunnel just proximal to the respective metacarpophalangeal joint of the finger. This digital fibrous sheath consists of thick fibrous bands in oblique or transverse orientation, known as pulleys, which keep the tendons close to the phalanges and prevent bowstringing during flexion of the finger. The current nomenclature for the pulley system was established by Doyle and Blythe (1,2), who described five annular "A" (A1–A5) and three cruciate "C" (C1–C3) pulleys. A1, A3 and A5 are located over the metcarpophalangeal, proximal interphalangeal, and distal interphalangeal respectively. A2 and A4 are located over the middle part of the proximal and distal phalanx respectively. The C1 pulley is over the distal end of the proximal phalanx, the C2 pulley over the proximal end of the middle phalanx, and the C3 pulley over the distal end of the middle phalanx (**Fig. 1-20**).

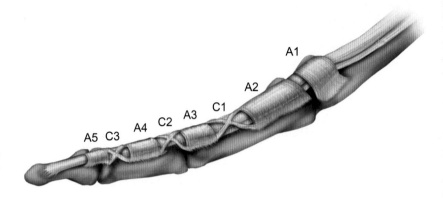

FIGURE 1-20

The fibro-osseous tunnel of each finger with the annular A1–A5 and cruciate C1–C3 pulleys.

The thumb has a similar fibro-osseous tunnel with an annular A1 pulley over the metacarpophalangeal joint, an oblique annular ligament extending from proximal ulnar to distal radial direction over the proximal phalanx of the thumb, and an annular A2 pulley over the interphalangeal joint.

The nutrition of the flexor tendons within the digital sheath comes from two sources: diffusion and vascular perfusion from the vincular system. Each tendon has a long and short vinculum, which are folds of the mesotenon running from the dorsal portion of the dorsal wall of the tendon sheath, emerging from the digital vessels. The short vinculae of the FDS and FDP, which are located respectively over the ends of the proximal and middle phalanges, are considered the important ones.

The course of the flexor tendons from their origin to the tip of the digits has been classified by Kleinert and Verdan (3) into five zones, I–V, based on their peculiar anatomy and their prognosis after primary repair. Zone I represents the region distal to the insertion of the FDS. Zone II describes the region where the FDS and the FDP share the fibro-osseous sheath of the digit, from the level of the metacarpal neck to the middle of the second phalanx. This zone is also known as the "no man's land," a term introduced by Bunnell (4) to describe the poor earlier results of flexor tendon repairs within this area. Zone III represents the region between the distal part of the transverse carpal ligament and Zone II. The tendons under the transverse carpal ligament are located within Zone IV. Finally, Zone V represents the most proximal part of the tendons within the region proximal to the carpal canal in the forearm. A similar zone system has been described for the thumb flexor tendon (**Fig. 1-21**).

VOLAR HAND SKIN AND SKIN CREASES

There are significant differences between the volar and the dorsal skin of the palm and the fingers. The volar skin is thicker and tougher to stand wear, and more firmly attached to the underlying structures. The palmar aponeurosis is a specialized thickening in the deep fascia located under the palmar skin extending from the level of the wrist joint to the level of the metacarpal heads. At that level, it divides into longitudinal fibers which continue into the fingers. Both the palmar aponeurosis and the longitudinal fibers give off superficial attachments to the skin resulting in a rather nonmobile skin allowing little plastic maneuvering. A system of creases, where the skin is adherent to the deeper layers, allows for closing of the hand without bunching up in folds.

On each finger there are two flexion creases overlying the proximal interphalangeal joint called *proximal digital creases*, but only one overlying the distal interphalangeal joint called *distal digital crease*. A single crease at the base of each finger, the *palmar digital crease*, identifies the distal end of the palm and is located over the proximal third of the proximal phalanx. On the thumb, there is double flexion crease over the interphalangeal joint called *thumb interphalangeal crease* and a wider double crease over the metacarpophalangeal joint called proximal thumb crease (**Fig. 1-22**).

Three distinct skin creases are normally seen in the palm. The *proximal palmar* or *thenar crease* designates the limit of thenar eminence and the level of motion of the thumb. The *transverse* or *midpalmar crease* begins at the midpoint of the hypothenar eminence and extends almost to the radial end of the thenar crease. It signifies the level of the metacarpal heads of the fingers. The *distal palmar crease* is situated distal to the midpalmar crease and runs from the index middle finger cleft to the ulnar border. It represents the level of motion of the metacarpophalangeal joints of the ulnar three fingers. A number of oblique and vertical skin creases of minor clinical significance exist proximal

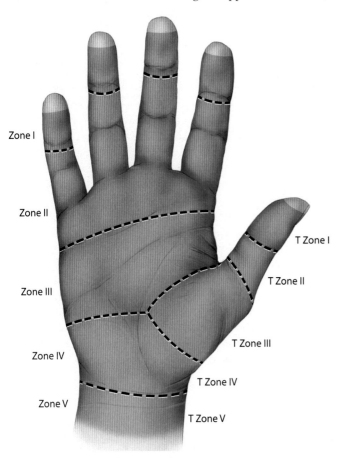

Zone I
Zone II
Zone III
Zone IV
Zone V

T Zone I
T Zone II
T Zone III
T Zone IV
T Zone V

FIGURE 1-21

The five zones of the flexor tendons.

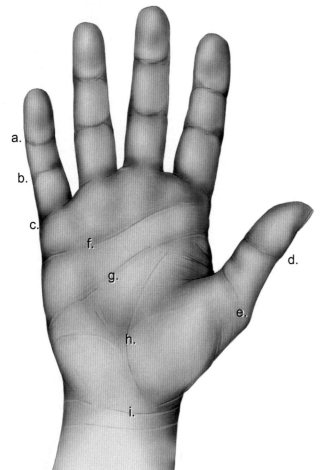

a.
b.
c.
f.
g.
d.
e.
h.
i.

FIGURE 1-22

The skin creases of the human hand. *a*, distal digital crease; *b*, proximal digital crease; *c*, palmar digital crease; *d*, thumb interphalangeal crease; *e*, proximal thumb crease; *f*, distal palmar crease; *g*, transverse or midpalmar crease; *h*, proximal palmar or thenar crease; *i*, wrist crease.

to the midpalmar crease. Finally, the distal forearm is separated from the palm with a transverse skin crease called the *wrist crease* (**Fig. 1-22**).

BASIC SURGICAL PREPARATION

A standard operating table is usually used with the ability to firmly anchor a hand board or table on its side. Most hand surgeries can be performed with the patient supine on the operating table.

Regional anesthesia in the form of supraclavicular, axillary, brachial, and peripheral nerve blocks can be used in the majority of the surgical procedures of the hand. In case of apprehensive adults or children, general anesthesia is usually preferred. The final choice of the type of anesthesia for each procedure is made by the anesthesiologist after being presented with the patient's and surgeon's concerns and wishes.

Sterling Bunnell, the father of modern hand surgery, emphasized the importance of atraumatic surgical technique in reconstructive hand surgery. He mentioned: "A jeweler can't repair a watch in a bottle of ink and neither can we repair a hand in a pool of blood" (4). A bloodless field achieved with a tourniquet allows surgical dissection with accuracy and minimal trauma. The tourniquet pressure should be at least 100 to 150 mm Hg higher than the systolic blood pressure, reaching about 250 mm Hg in adults and 200 mm Hg in children. Wilgis (5) established that the safe period of tourniquet inflation is about 2 hours since longer use may lead to tourniquet palsy. In case there is a need for a longer period than 2 hours, then the tourniquet should be deflated for 10 to 15 minutes and then reinflated.

Sharp dissection with the aid of magnifying loops or glasses using small blades and instruments is essential in the atraumatic technique advocated by Bunnell and other hand surgeons.

SKIN INCISION PRINCIPLES

There are a great number of skin incisions in the hand and the fingers. Certain basic principles should be followed at all instances. The skin incisions should never be placed within deep skin creases. The subcutaneous fat is very thin under these creases and moisture tends to accumulate leading to maceration of the skin edges. The incisions should be long enough to expose the underlying deep structures without stretching the skin edges, since the mobility of the volar skin in the hand is limited. The reflected skin edges should be thick involving the underlying fat in order to avoid devascularization of the skin edges. The direction of the dissection in the deeper tissues can follow a different orientation than the direction of the skin incision.

Straight-line incisions should be avoided; gently curved or angled incisions provide better exposure and are less noticeable cosmetically. Furthermore, they can be extended with freer choice of direction.

The plane of motion of the different parts of the hand is perpendicular to the long axis of the skin creases. Therefore, an incision should not cross a crease at or near a right angle since the resulting scar being in the line of tension during early motion will hypertrophy resulting in function impairment.

Parallel or nearly parallel incisions should be avoided because necrosis or delayed healing can occur due to limited blood supply of the bridged skin flap, especially if the incisions are too close to each other or too long.

SURGICAL EXPOSURE TO THE FLEXOR TENDONS IN THE FINGERS

Based on the principles mentioned above there are many different finger incisions. The most popular are the zigzag incision and the midlateral incision.

The Zigzag Incision

The concept of zigzag incisions was introduced by Brunner (6) and consists of several oblique incisions between the different skin creases meeting each other exactly over the creases. The angle between the different creases should be about 90 degrees (**Figs. 1-23 and 1-24A**). Angles of less than 90 degrees can lead to skin necrosis of the corners. The apex of the angles is located at the edges of the creases and should not extend more posteriorly since the neurovascular bundles could be injured during mobilization of the skin flaps.

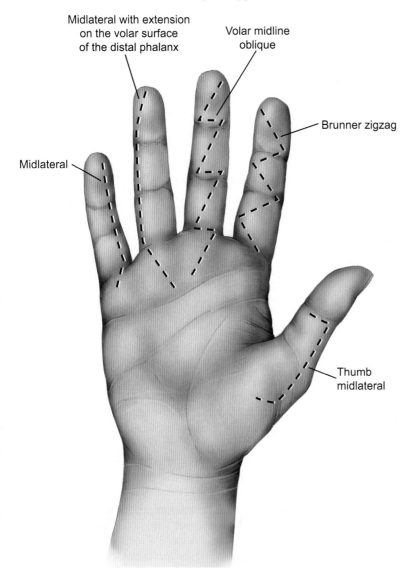

Midlateral with extension on the volar surface of the distal phalanx

Volar midline oblique

Brunner zigzag

Midlateral

Thumb midlateral

FIGURE 1-23

The different finger skin incisions from right to left: Thumb midlateral incision, the Brunner zigzag incision, volar midline oblique incision, the midlateral incisionextending on the volar surface of the distal phalanx, and the midlateral incision. All the incisions have beenextended proximally within the palm.

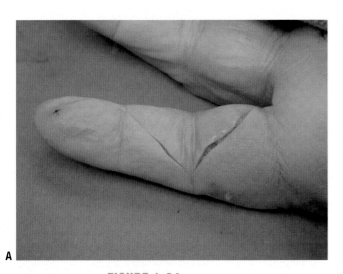
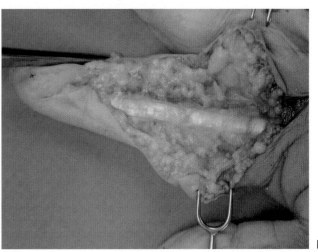

A   B

FIGURE 1-24

The volar zigzag finger incision described by Brunner. **A:** Superficial skin incision. **B:** Deeper dissection.

The skin flaps should be elevated as thick flaps with some underlying fat to avoid devascularizing the skin. Deeper surgical dissection in a longitudinal fashion can be performed along the midline where the fibrous-pulley system and the flexor tendons lie under the subcutaneous fat. The dissection should be performed very carefully along the lateral borders of the digit to avoid any injury to the neurovascular bundles. The digital vessels and the nerve are located beneath a thin fibrous layer called the Grayson's ligament. Blunt dissection in a longitudinal fashion can reveal the neurovascular bundle, the most lateral borders of the fibrous-pulley system and the bone **(Fig. 1-24B)**.

A variation of this incision is the volar midline oblique incision in which the whole skin incision is performed volarly, along the midline of the finger **(Fig. 1-23)**. It is relatively safe and easily closed. The incision crosses the skin creases transversely and slightly obliquely allowing exposure of the flexor tendon sheath in the midline of the finger between the two neurovascular bundles. Both zigzag incisions can be extended to the palmar region using the same principles and following a zigzag pattern to the distal palmar crease.

The Midlateral Incision

Important landmarks in this approach are the proximal and the distal interphalangeal creases, which tend to extend slightly more to the dorsal surface of the finger. These creases may disappear in a swollen finger. Another important landmark is the junction between the smooth volar skin and the dorsal wrinkled skin on the side of the finger.

The incision is not a true lateral incision but rather dorsolateral. A straight incision is performed connecting the more dorsal points of the finger creases. The incision can reach up to the lateral end of the fingernail distally and up to the web space proximally. An alternative way to find the connecting points for the skin incision is to flex the fingers and connect the most dorsal points of the interphalangeal creases **(Figs. 1-23 and 1-25)**. This approach can be performed on radial or ulnar side of a finger but never on both sides. The ulnar side of the index, middle, and ring fingers and the radial side of the small finger are usually preferred, since the incisions will not interfere with normal hand function postoperatively.

A dorsal skin flap should be developed to aid in closure of the incision. On the radial side of the index and middle fingers, there is dorsal branch of the digital nerve that should be preserved whenever it is encountered. The superficial skin dissection involves dissection of the subcutaneous tissue and developing a volar skin flap. Deeper dissection should proceed carefully around the proximal interphalangeal joint since the subcutaneous fat over the joint is quite thin. Following the dissection of the fat, aim the dissection volarward and expose the tendon sheath. A volar skin flap will develop which contains the neurovascular bundle. The tendon sheath and the flexor tendons can be exposed through this approach. Furthermore, the opposite neurovascular bundle can also be exposed since its position is anterolateral to the tendon sheath.

A simple variation of the midlateral approach involves a skin flap superficial and volar to the neurovascular bundle **(Fig. 1-26)**. The same incision is performed from proximally up to the distal flexor crease, but at that point the incision is curved obliquely into the pulp of the finger. The neurovascu-

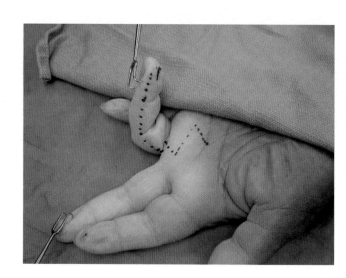

FIGURE 1-25

The midlateral finger skin incision with extension in the palm.

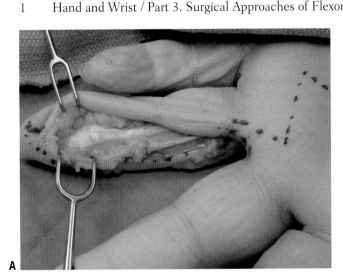

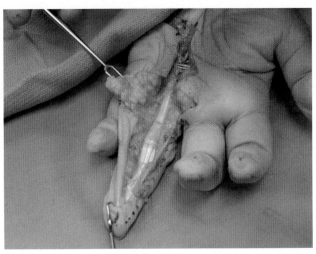

A   B

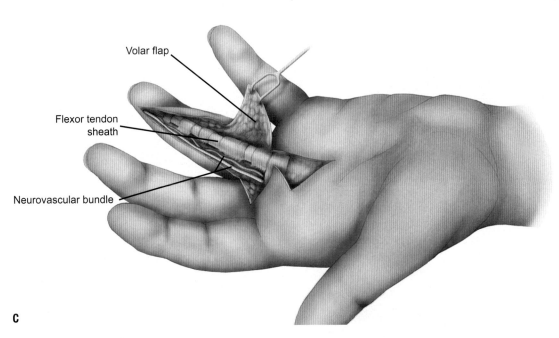

Volar flap

Flexor tendon
sheath

Neurovascular bundle

C

FIGURE 1-26

A–C: Deeper dissection of the midlateral approach of the finger. The flexor tendon sheath has
been approached raising a skin flap volar to the neurovascular bundle of the finger.

lar bundle should be exposed and protected through this incision. It can be best found over the proximal interphalangeal joint. The dissection continues volar to the neurovascular bundle and the flexor
tendon sheath is exposed. The advantage of this variation over the classical midlateral approach is
that it is easier to reach over the opposite neurovascular bundle with less skin tension.

Both midlateral approaches can be extended in the palm proximally. Although both the digital
nerve and artery are in danger, an advantage of these approaches is that the incision is offset to the
flexor tendon sheath system providing an intact skin and subcutaneous flap over it. On the contrary,
the volar zigzag and volar midline oblique incisions are relatively easier, since they do not require
mobilization of the neurovascular bundle, but the skin incision is exactly over the tendon sheath
system.

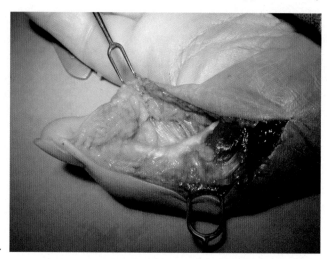

FIGURE 1-27
The midlateral thumb skin incision.

Thumb Incisions

The incisions that can be performed in the thumb are similar to the finger incisions described previously. The midlateral incision in the radial side is easier and can be extended by curving its proximal end at the midmetacarpal area and creating a flap on the palmar surface of the thumb (**Figs. 1-23 and 1-27**). Care should be taken to avoid injury of the dorsal radial branch of the superficial radial nerve which is located exactly under the skin. The lateral surface of the thumb does not contain a lot of fat, especially at the interphalangeal joint, so care should be taken to avoid incising the joint or the volar plate.

Another alternative incision is the volar zigzag incision. The two digital nerves at the level of the metacarpophalangeal joint are very superficial on either side of the flexor tendons and care should be taken to avoid injury of them.

In FPL lacerations within the thumb, the proximal stump of the tendon retracts, usually under the thenar eminence. It is advisable not to extend the thumb incisions in the thenar eminence and retrieve the tendon with an open approach through the thenar musculature, but rather to retrieve the tendon through a separate approach in the distal forearm and pass it under the thenar musculature to the thumb.

Transverse incisions along the proximal thumb crease can be performed to access the flexor tendon at the level of the metacarpophalangeal joint as well as the A1 pulley. The digital nerves are located on either side of the tendon and should always be identified and protected throughout the operative procedure.

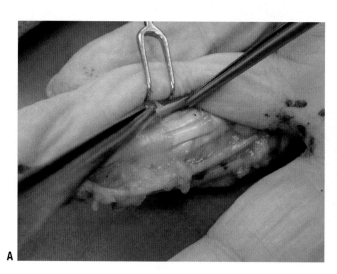

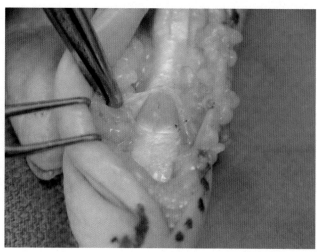

A   B

FIGURE 1-28
Incisions of the flexor tendon sheath. **A:** Ulnarly based flap of the sheath between the annular pulleys A2 and A4. **B:** Incision of the sheath distal to the annular A5 pulley.

Fibro-Osseous Sheath Incision

Injuries of the flexor tendons within the fibro-osseous sheath usually result in retraction of the proximal part of the tendon within the sheath. In order to retrieve this part of the tendon and perform the repair, the sheath should be incised at certain locations. Various studies have revealed that the most important pulleys are the annular A2 and A4. Therefore, the sheath must be opened away from these pulleys, in the C1 pulley, in the C2 pulley, or in the C3-A5 pulley complex (**Fig. 1-28**). If a wider exposure is needed, a radial- or ulnar-based flap of the sheath is created between the A2 and the A4 pulley (**Fig. 1-28A**). In case that there is need to open the annular A2 or A4 pulleys, a Z type of lengthening incision is preferred to enable repair of the pulleys. Partial resection of the A2 or A4 should be avoided.

SURGICAL EXPOSURE TO THE FLEXOR TENDONS IN THE PALM

All the principles that apply to the fingers concerning the skin and the skin creases apply to palmar incisions too. As a general principle, the incisions in the palm tend to be more transverse in the distal part and more longitudinal curving radially and parallel to the closest skin crease in the proximal part. There is a great variability of skin incisions in the palm, especially in the distal part.

The most common incisions in the distal part of the palm are the transverse incisions used in trigger fingers. The location of these incisions is exactly over the midpalmar crease in most of the patients, although they may be located slightly more distally in case of the middle, ring, and small fingers. All these transverse incisions can be extended more proximally towards the thenar crease keeping in mind that the flexor tendon course is towards the midline from distal to proximal as they exit from the carpal tunnel (**Fig. 1-29**).

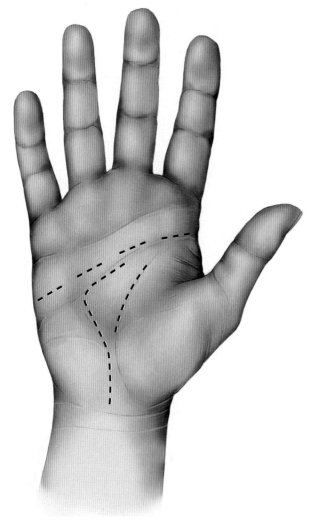

FIGURE 1-29

The different palmar skin incisions.

After the dissection of skin and subcutaneous fat, the latter is dissected from the palmar fascia trying to preserve any perforating small vessels that may supply the more superficial layers. The palmar fascia is incised in any desired orientation keeping in mind that the vital structures are under it. If wider exposure is desired, part of the palmar fascia can be excised. The tendons and the longitudinally oriented neurovascular bundles can be seen. It is advisable to always locate the neurovascular bundles at this level and protect them at all times during the flexor tendon surgical procedure.

Most of the vital structures like arteries or nerves lie under the palmar fascia in the proximal part of the palm. In the distal palm, these structures are lying between the metacarpals heads and are not protected by the palmar fascia. In the very distal part of the palm the arteries and nerves are oriented longitudinally. In the proximal part of the palm there are some structures with a transverse orientation, like the superficial palmar arch and the thenar motor branch of the median nerve.

The more proximal incision of the palm involves release of the transverse carpal ligament and will be discussed in conjunction with the surgical approaches of the flexor tendons in the wrist.

SURGICAL EXPOSURE TO THE FLEXOR TENDONS IN THE WRIST

The surgical approach of the flexor tendons in the wrist involves release of the carpal tunnel and approach of the flexor tendons in the proximal part of the palm and the distal forearm.

Important landmarks for this approach are the thenar crease, the transverse skin crease of the wrist, and the tendon of palmaris longus whenever it is present. The incision is placed just ulnar to the thenar crease at the level of the Kaplan's cardinal line, curving radially proximally, remaining always on the ulnar side until the level of the wrist crease. At that point, the incision is curved ulnarly in order to avoid crossing the wrist crease transversely and continues along the midline of the forearm **(Fig. 1-30A)**.

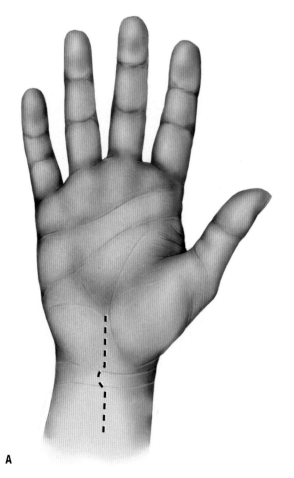
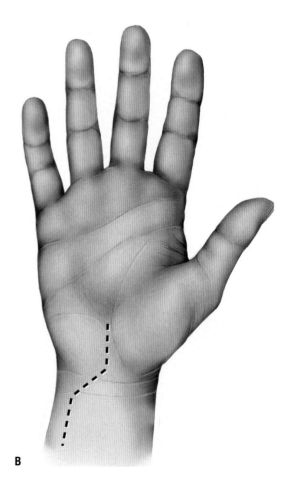

A   B

FIGURE 1-30

Surgical approach of the flexor tendons in the wrist with proximal midline extension in the forearm **(A)** and ulnar proximal forearm extension **(B)**. The diagonal line represents the Kaplan's cardinal line.

The skin incision starts proximally in the palm where the skin flaps should be incised carefully. The palmar cutaneous branch of the median nerve lies superficially between the flexor carpi radialis and the median nerve and enters the palm in a variable course. Dissection of the subcutaneous fat should be performed carefully, trying to identify and protect branches of this nerve. After incision of the subcutaneous fat, the tendon of the palmaris longus is visible proximally and its insertion, the fibers of the palmar fascia, is visible distally. The fibers of the palmar fascia should be incised longitudinally along the line of the skin incision. The tendon of the palmaris longus inserting in these fibers should be retracted ulnarly. The median nerve is located under the tendon of the palmaris longus between the palmaris longus and the tendon of the flexor carpi radialis. The muscle fibers of the palmaris brevis muscle are located under the palmar fascia and are incised longitudinally. The fibers of the transverse carpal ligament are visible with their most proximal part located at the level of the transverse wrist crease. A blunt spatula-like instrument is placed between the median nerve and the transverse carpal ligament. Careful incision of the fibers cutting on the instrument to avoid any injury to the median nerve is performed. It is advisable to transect the fibers on the ulnar side of the median nerve to avoid injury to the motor branch to the thenar muscles. The flexor tendons are visible around the median nerve within the carpal tunnel and in the distal forearm. The tendons of the FDS, FDP, and FPL are directly accessible along this incision. The flexor carpi radialis and the FCU are located at the most ulnar and radial parts of the incision at the level of the distal third of the forearm.

Besides the palmar cutaneous branch of the median nerve, several dangers exist in this extended approach of the flexor tendons in the wrist. The superficial palmar arch lies exactly over the tendons at the exit of the carpal tunnel and proximal extension should be performed cautiously. The motor branch of the median nerve usually emerges from the radial part of the nerve either distal or under to the transverse carpal ligament. There are few cases where the motor branch arises within the carpal tunnel and pierces the transverse carpal ligament posing a possible danger during the release of the carpal tunnel. In the most proximal part of the incision, the ulnar nerve and artery, the median nerve, and the radial artery are located between the flexor tendons and should be protected during dissection.

Several variations exist for the most proximal part of the incision. Instead of a proximal midline extension in the distal forearm, an ulnar longitudinal incision can be performed (**Fig. 1-30B**). An advantage of this alternative approach is that the incision is not performed exactly over the median nerve providing a well vascularized skin flap over the nerve. A similar radial longitudinal incision should be avoided because it places the palmar cutaneous branch of the median nerve at risk.

SURGICAL INCISIONS AND SKIN LACERATIONS

Skin lacerations with flexor tendon lacerations are very common clinical situations. In these cases, the previously mentioned surgical approaches have to be modified in order to incorporate the skin lacerations. As a general principle, the skin laceration can be extended proximally or distally using the Brunner zigzag approach (**Fig. 1-31**). Adequate surgical exposure is needed to identify and expose the tendon ends. Lacerated flexor tendons retract frequently in the palm unless there is intact vinculum or lumbrical muscle preventing further proximal retraction. The proximal end of the tendon may retract so much that a wide exposure is needed. Another alternative is to perform an independent proximal surgical exposure and retrieve the tendon at that point and retract it to the more distal surgical approach under the intact skin bridge. Such incisions can be performed in the palm at the level of the distal palmar crease. In case of FPL laceration at the base of the thumb, the proximal part of the tendon usually retracts under the thenar musculature or even in the palm. An isolated radial longitudinal incision may be necessary to retrieve the tendon in the palm and retract it to the thumb.

The skin wounds should be closed early, but not necessarily immediately, to lessen the chance of a wound infection. Whenever there is tendon, bone, or neurovascular structure exposed immediate coverage is essential. Primary skin closure is preferable if it can be achieved without tension; otherwise some type of skin grafting is preferable.

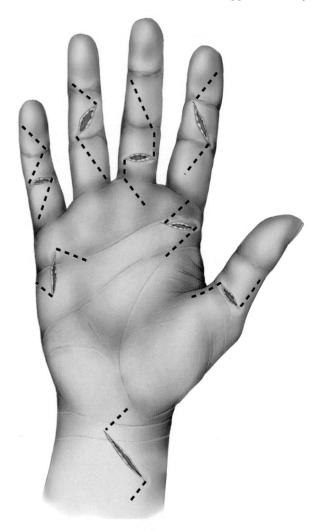

FIGURE 1-31

Incorporation of skin lacerations into the surgical approaches of the flexor tendons.

PART 4. Volar Approach to the Wrist

William P. Cooney, III and David Dennison

There are a variety of approaches to the wrist joint and distal radius. While the most common is the dorsal approach, which allows full exposure of the radiocarpal and midcarpal joints, the volar approach for the treatment of fractures of the scaphoid (1–6) and for internal fixation of distal radius fractures has had increasing clinical application and reported value (7–9).

The volar approach to the wrist is divided into two common surgical approaches: (a) the volar radial approach for fractures of the distal third and waist of the scaphoid and scaphoid nonunions and (b) an extended volar radial forearm approach for the treatment of distal radius fractures. These two surgical approaches will be described.

INDICATIONS

Scaphoid Fractures and Nonunions

The primary indications for use of the volar radial approach is for the treatment of acute displaced fractures of the scaphoid and for the treatment of scaphoid nonunions when there is a volar flex or humpback deformity present (2,5,6,10–13). It has the potential for proximal extension to obtain bone graft from the distal radius in the treatment of comminuted scaphoid fractures or scaphoid nonunions. It has a further advantage of allowing correction of a volar angulation deformity of a scaphoid fracture or scaphoid nonunion (10,14).

Scaphoid Fractures

Acute fractures of the scaphoid with displacement are best managed by closed reduction and percutaneous screw fixation or by open reduction and compression screw fixation (5,12,13,15–17). The volar radial approach extended from the scaphotrapezial joint distally to the distal radius proximally (see Figs. 1-32 and 1-33) provides an excellent view to reduce the displaced scaphoid, bone graft comminuted fractures, and insert a cannulated compression screw from a distal to proximal direction across the fracture site.

Scaphoid Nonunions

The volar radial approach is also ideal for scaphoid nonunions with a humpback deformity. To provide adequate realignment of the scaphoid and correction of carpal collapse associated with scaphoid nonunion, interposition bone graft is often required (10,11,14). A volar radial approach (see Figs. 1-34 and 1-35) allows for direct visualization of the nonunion site, mobilization of the scaphoid fracture nonunion components, and insertion of a volar radial bone graft to correct scaphoid nonunions and internal fixation with compression screws.

Distal Radius Fractures

With this surgical approach, a rigid locked or nonlocked plate can be placed on the tensile side of the radius and is protected by overlying soft tissues (7–9,18–21). The volar approach for treatment of distal radius fractures is basically an approach through the flexor carpi radialis subsheath. The interval between the flexor carpi radialis and radial artery is developed. Exposure of the entire distal radius or displaced extra-articular and occasionally intra-articular fractures of the distal radius can be achieved. This is a different approach than the extended Henry approach in that the latter is lateral to the flexor carpi radialis and includes a carpal tunnel exposure. The volar-radial approach to a distal radius fracture can be combined with arthroscopic reduction of intra-articular fractures of the distal radius or with percutaneous pinning.

CONTRAINDICATIONS

Scaphoid Fractures

A volar radial approach to the scaphoid is contraindicated for proximal pole scaphoid fractures where a dorsal approach is preferred (6,17,22). It is also contraindicated if there is a fracture dislocation of the scaphoid wherein repair of dorsal ligaments is required along with scaphoid fracture fixation through a dorsal surgical approach.

Distal Radius

The volar radial approach to the distal radius is contraindicated when there is severe comminution of the distal radius requiring open reduction and internal fixation of the joint articular surfaces unless it is combined with a dorsal approach to the radiocarpal joint or wrist arthroscopy (18,23–25). Precise anatomic alignment of the distal radius is required that cannot be achieved from a volar approach alone.

PREOPERATIVE PREPARATION

Scaphoid Fractures/Nonunion

In the treatment of the displaced scaphoid fracture and, in particular, scaphoid nonunions, computerized tomography (CT) or magnetic resonant imaging (MRI) is essential. MRI is preferred for acute fractures with displacement and if one suspects vascular damage to the scaphoid (avascular necrosis). CT (AP, lateral, axial) is preferred to determine the degree of scaphoid angulation and displacement and to measure the size of a potential interposition bone graft (26–28).

Distal Radius

In the treatment of fractures of the distal radius, traction posteroanterior and lateral radiographs provide the best preoperative view of the extent of fracture displacement. Alternatively one can use computed tomography (CT scans) (8,29).

SURGICAL TECHNIQUE

Radial Volar Approach to the Scaphoid for Scaphoid Fractures and Nonunion

Landmarks   The key anatomic points for the volar radial approach to the scaphoid are to localize the radial styloid, the tuberosities of the scaphoid and the trapezium, and the flexor carpi radialis tendon and tendon sheath (**Fig. 1-32**).

Technique

1. Incision: a curvilinear incision or straight incision is made along the volar radial aspect of the wrist just over the tuberosity of the scaphoid if palpable and along the flexor carpi radialis tendon sheath (**Fig. 1-33**).
2. Careful dissection is performed to locate branches of the lateral antebrachial cutaneous nerve and the volar branch of the radial artery. The operative approach is then extended proximally and dis-

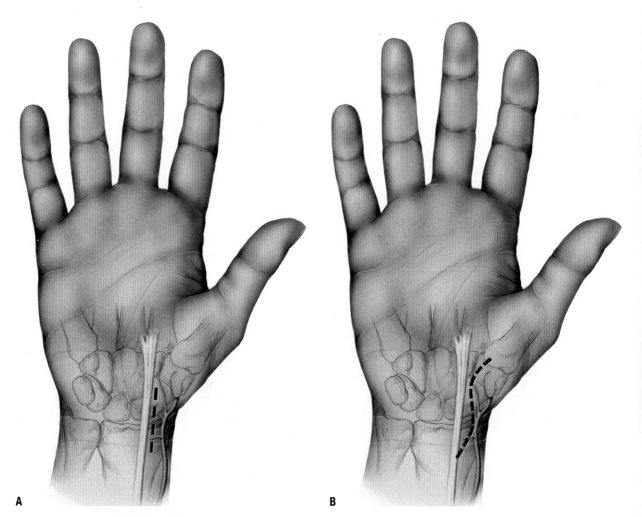

A   B

FIGURE 1-32

Radial volar approach to scaphoid. **A:** Longitudinal incision between the flexor carpi radialis (FCR) and radial styloid and radial artery. **B:** Zigzag incision between radial styloid and flexor carpi radialis.

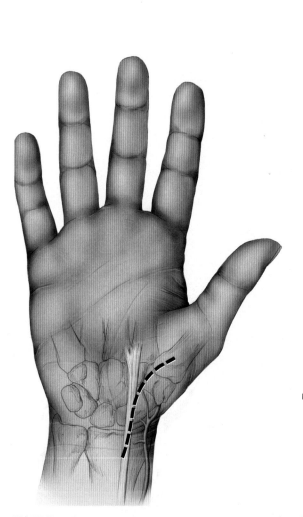

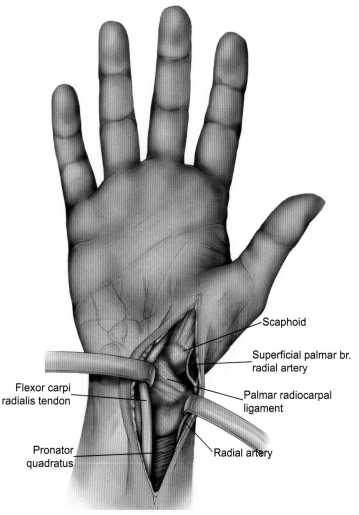

FIGURE 1-33

Extended S-shaped exposure to the scaphoid; note radial artery, flexor carpi radialis tendon, trapezium tubercle, scaphoid, trapezoid. Surgical approach to scaphoid.

FIGURE 1-34

Extended palmar incision to distal scaphoid demonstrating deep palmar radiocarpal ligaments, palmar branch of the radial artery retracted radially or ligated; and distally, trapezium and the scaphotrapezial joint.

tally between the radial artery and the flexor carpi radialis tendon dissecting down to the capsule of the wrist **(Fig. 1-34)**.

3. The anatomic location for the wrist capsule incision is between the radial collateral ligament and the palmar radial scaphocapitate ligament **(Fig. 1-35)**.

4. Occasionally, the incision needs to be extended more ulnarly through the volar long radiolunate ligament. The palmar (superficial) branch of the radial artery may need to be divided.
   * *Note:* With traction of the thumb, the articulation between the distal radius and proximal pole of the scaphoid comes into view.

5. The volar carpal ligaments are reflected from the waist and proximal pole of the scaphoid and the incision is extended distally to the scaphotrapezial joint. With continued traction on the wrist and thumb, one can assess the degree of displacement of an acute scaphoid fracture as well as the amount of comminution present.

Volar Approach to the Distal Radius

Technique

1. Incision: for the volar radial approach to the distal radius, the incision (curvilinear or straight) **(Fig. 1-36)** is performed just radial to the flexor carpi radialis tendon and tendon sheath. This is

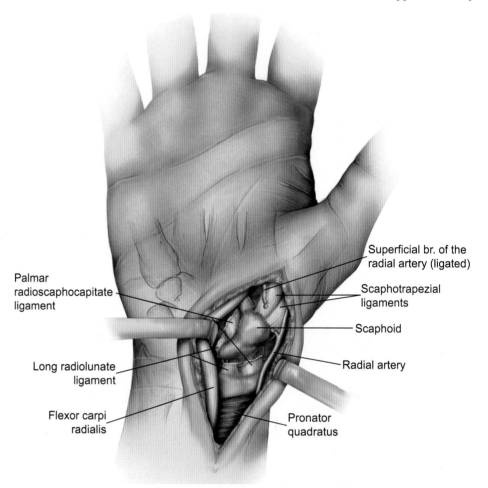

Palmar
radioscaphocapitate
ligament

Long radiolunate
ligament

Flexor carpi
radialis

Superficial br. of the
radial artery (ligated)

Scaphotrapezial
ligaments

Scaphoid

Radial artery

Pronator
quadratus

FIGURE 1-35

Exposure and division of radial
volar carpal ligaments (palmar
radioscaphocapitate and long
radiolunate ligaments); divided
and ligated superficial branch of
radial artery. *Inset*: Divided volar
radiocarpal ligaments (scaphoid
fracture site).

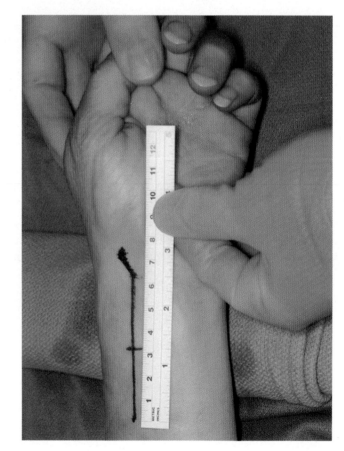

FIGURE 1-36

Exposure core of distal radius fracture. Longitudinal incision 6 to 8
cm in length.

similar to the volar radial approach to the scaphoid. The incision extends deep along the flexor carpi radialis tendon sheath interval between the radial artery and flexor radialis from a distal to proximal direction until the entire view of the distal radius fracture comes about for inspection (8,9).

2. The length of the incision should be 7 to 8 cm to provide for plate insertion.

3. The flexor carpi radial tendon is fully mobilized (**Fig. 1-37**).

4. The flexor carpi radialis is released from the subsheath and retracted radially.

5. The brachioradialis muscle insertion is detached from the lateral (radial) aspect of the distal radius (**Fig. 1-38**) and divided. This reduces supinating force from the brachioradialis.

6. The pronator quadratus is released (**Fig. 1-39**) and reflected from the distal radius from a radial to ulnar direction with attached periosteum (**Fig. 1-40**).

7. With different forms of distraction (finger traps or an occasional external fixator), alignment of the distal radius fracture is obtained and the plate is applied (**Fig. 1-41**). Percutaneous pins are inserted to hold the fracture in alignment.

8. Appropriate x-rays are taken to ensure that the fracture is adequately reduced and then one of a variety of volar fixation plates is applied (**Fig. 1-42**).

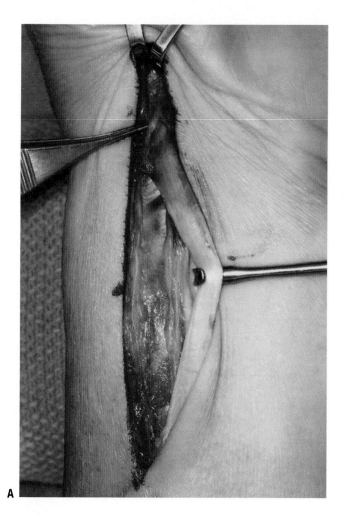

A

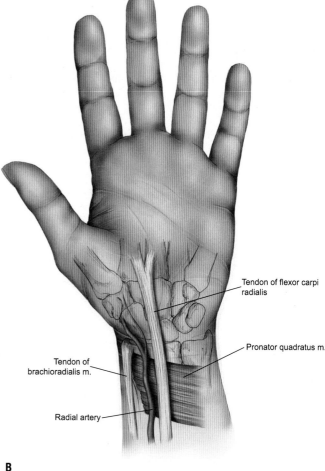

Tendon of flexor carpi radialis

Pronator quadratus m.

Tendon of brachioradialis m.

Radial artery

B

FIGURE 1-37

A,B: Release and mobilization of flexor carpi radialis.

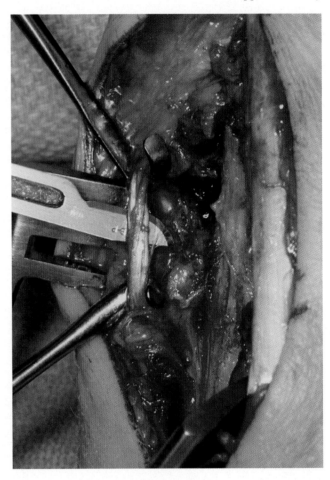

FIGURE 1-38
Release and division of brachioradialis tendon.

PEARLS AND PITFALLS

Pearls

Volar Radial Approach to the Scaphoid

- It is important to extend the volar radial approach distal enough to the scaphotrapezial joint and to remove the lateral border of the trapezium if one is going to use a Heune jig for compression of the scaphoid (6,10,14,30,31).
- A mini C-arm imaging of the wrist can help to determine central position of a guidewire for cannulated screws as well as proper placement of the proximal tip of the Heune jig against the proximal pole of the scaphoid.
- Occasionally a radial styloidectomy may be helpful to provide improved exposure of the scaphoid and to allow ease of insertion of a volar radial interposition bone graft.
- To expedite volar capsular closure and prevent late carpal instability, it is best to suture tag the radial collateral and the radioscaphocapitate ligament and the long radioscapholunate ligament and to carefully repair the volar wrist capsule (3).

Volar Radial Approach to the Distal Radius

- To allow for closure of the pronator quadratus, it is important to incise the volar periosteum of the distal radius as far radially as possible or to do a step cut detachment of the pronator quadratus so that closure of the pronator over the volar plate can be achieved (9).

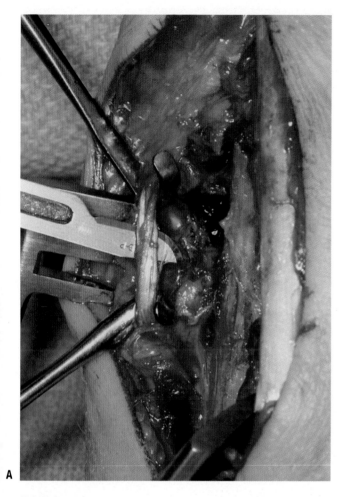 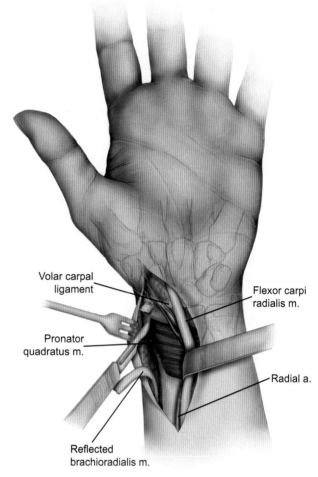

FIGURE 1-39

A,B: Release of the radial border (insertion) of the pronator quadratus.

- Often there are two main distal radius fracture fragments when there is an intra-articular fracture of the distal radius: the radial styloid component and the lunate fracture component (7,23,32). We recommend beginning ulnarly, reducing the lunate fossa fracture components with intra-articular K-wire placed either dorsal to volar or volar to dorsal, and then transfix the lunate fossa to the distal radius.
- In wound closure, it is not necessary to reattach the brachioradialis (deforming supinating force on the distal radius). It is important as noted previously to reattach the pronator quadratus and then allow the FCR subsheath to fall naturally back into place and reapproximate, if possible, the deep and superficial fascia of the forearm.

Pitfalls

Scaphoid Fractures and Nonunions

- Avoid overcompression of the scaphoid.
- Always leave a temporary K-wire in place before screw insertion to prevent rotational displacement of the scaphoid.
- Remove the lateral portion of the trapezium when using a Heune jig or K-wire to ensure central position of any compression screw.

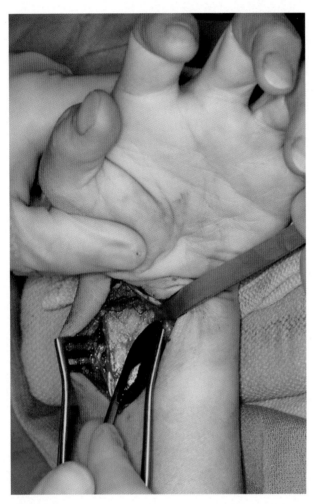

FIGURE 1-40

Reflection of pronator quadratus to expose the distal radius–volar surface.

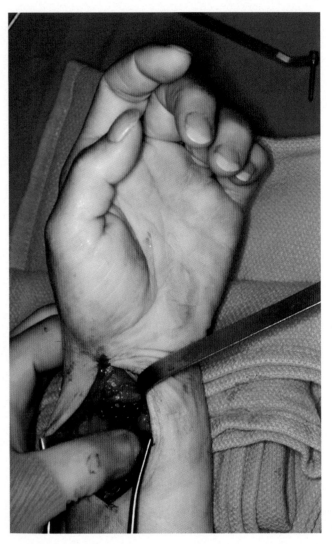

FIGURE 1-41

Plate application to the distal radius.

- Realign the lunate and proximal scaphoid (correcting any dorsal angulation) before fracture or nonunion reduction.
- Avoid excessive lateral (radial) dissection with risk of injury to the scaphoid blood supply.
- Tag and later repair the volar carpal ligaments.
- Choose appropriate length internal fixation screws and then subtract back 2 mm.

Distal Radius Fractures

- Obtain anatomic reduction with K-wires before plate fixation.
- Use traction to assist with reduction (manual traction or external fixation).
- Operate early (within the first 12 hours) or late (>36 hours) to avoid wound closure problems.
- Consider step-cut lengthening the pronator quadratus to allow re-attachment during closure.
- Consider reduction with external fixation for the very unstable, comminuted fractures.
- Bone graft (autograft or allograft) for comminuted fractures, especially in the elderly.

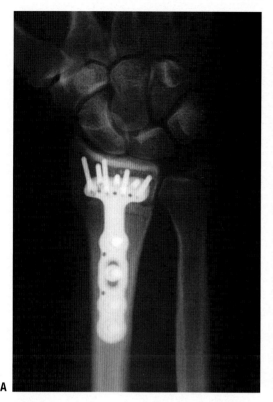
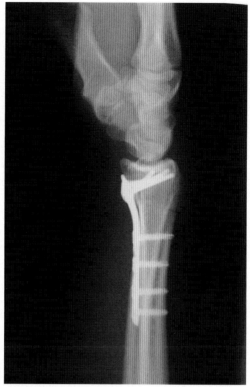

A   **B**

FIGURE 1-42

Posteroanterior **(A)** and lateral **(B)** x-rays of the distal radius after plate fixation. Note lateral view position of screws proximal to the radiocarpal joint articular surface.

PART 5. Dorsal Radial Exposure of the Scaphoid

Steven L. Moran

INDICATIONS

The use of the dorsal radial exposure of the scaphoid is most commonly employed in the setting of an acute proximal pole scaphoid fracture; however, surgical exposure and internal fixation of the scaphoid may also be indicated for (a) any displaced scaphoid fracture; (b) scaphoid fractures with significant bone loss; (c) fractures with angulation or rotation; or (d) scaphoid fractures resulting in loss of the lateral intrascaphoid angle, fracture dislocations of the scaphoid and greater arc injuries (1–7). In addition, any scaphoid fracture which results in loss of carpal alignment or which cannot be satisfactorily corrected or maintained by manipulation and casting should be treated by operative reduction and internal fixation (8).

The scaphoid may be exposed through a palmar or dorsal approach. The palmar approach has been classically used for the treatment of waist fractures and for the repair of nonunions (9). A dorsal longitudinal approach to the wrist may also be used for scaphoid exposure in cases of pan-carpal injury or in cases involving concomitant distal radius fractures. When the scaphoid alone is fractured one may utilize a *dorsal radial exposure*. The dorsal radial approach to the scaphoid allows for exposure of the proximal pole of the scaphoid, the dorsal mid waist, the scapho-trapezial-trapezoid joint as well as the dorsal portion of scapholunate interosseous ligament. The dorsal radial approach may be used for cases of scaphoid non-union and allows for the utilization of vascularized bone grafts from the dorsal distal radius (**Fig. 1-43**). The dorsal radial exposure has the benefits of not violating the palmar supporting ligaments of the wrist and preserves the palmar blood supply to the scaphoid (1,10,11). The dorsal radial exposure may place the superficial branch of the radial nerve at risk (**Fig. 1-44**). This approach provides only minimal exposure of the lunate and allows for no visualization of the ulnar aspect of the wrist, because of this the dorsal radial approach should not be used for the evaluation or treatment of lesser or greater arc injury patterns, or in cases where significant collapse is present within the scaphoid.

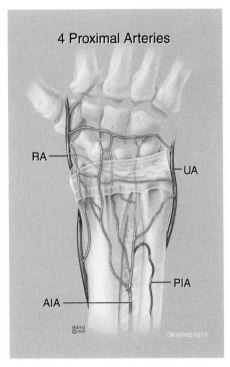

FIGURE 1-43

Arterial supply to the distal radius and scaphoid. The properly placed dorsal radial exposure protects the critical vascular supply to the scaphoid.

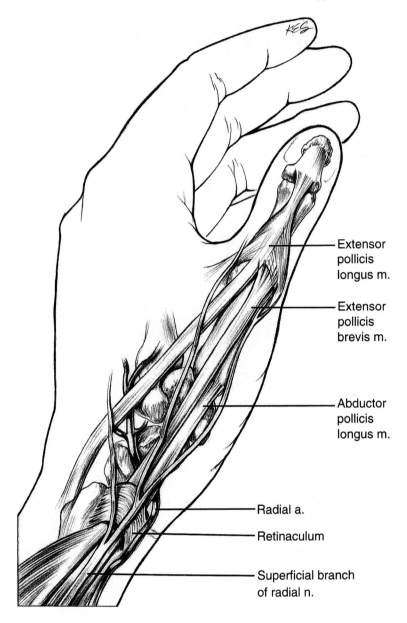

FIGURE 1-44

The superficial branch of the radial nerve although at risk can be avoided with the properly placed dorsal radial incision to expose the scaphoid.

TECHNIQUE (12)

1. Incision: the exposure begins with a 3 to 4 cm incision beginning over Lister's tubercle and extending distally along the line of extensor pollicis longus (EPL) **(Fig. 1-45)**.
2. A dorsal longitudinal approach to the wrist may also be used for scaphoid exposure in cases of pan-carpal injury or with concomitant distal radius fractures and intercarpal or radiocarpal arthrodesis. Subcutaneous dissection is carried out to identify the branches of the radial nerve, passing over the 2nd compartment, which are retracted radially.
3. The 2nd and 3rd extensor compartments are opened and the EPL is mobilized towards the base of the thumb **(Fig. 1-46)**.
4. The ECRL and ECRB and EPL are the retracted radially **(Fig. 1-47)**. If necessary the EPL may be released entirely from its compartment and transposed radial to Lister's tubercle to facilitate retraction. Mobilization of the EPL also allows for identification of the posterior interosseus

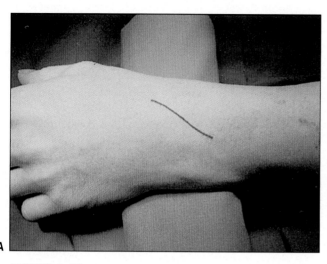
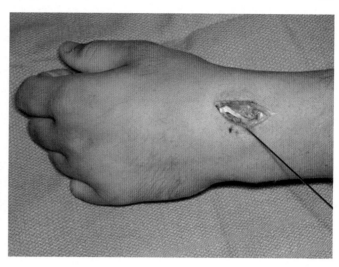

FIGURE 1-45

Standard skin incision used for the dorsal radial approach to the scaphoid **(A)**. K-wire marks the position of the central scaphoid axis. The EPL can be seen in the base of the wound **(B)**.

nerve running on the ulnar side of Lister's tubercle which may be excised for partial wrist denervation.

5. The wrist capsule is incised in line with the fibers of the dorsal intercarpal ligament, with a straight axial cut, or a "T" shaped incision **(Fig. 1-48)** (13).

- *Pearl:* The scapholunate joint is usually directly in line with Lister's tubercle and, the tubercle provides a useful anatomic landmark for the initiation of the capsulotomy.

6. Following capsulotomy, the scaphoid and the dorsal portion of the scapholunate ligament is inspected. Loose fragments of articular cartilage, loose bodies, synovitis, and hemarthrosis may need to be removed to improve visualization. The proximal pole may be further evaluated by flexing and radially deviating the wrist.

- *Pearl:* It is important to remember that even in the presence of an acute scaphoid fracture the scapholunate ligament may be injured and should be examined for the possibility of instability or concomitant rupture.

Bone Graft Harvesting

7. If a vascularized graft is required, the initial skin incision can be extended in a curvilinear fashion over the 1st dorsal compartment **(Fig. 1-49)**. The vascularized bone graft may then be harvested from the 1, 2 intercompartmental supra-retinacular vessels (ICSRA).

8. Subcutaneous tissues are gently retracted, and the 1, 2 ICSRA and venae comitantes are visualized on the surface of the retinaculum between the 1st and 2nd extensor tendon compartments **(Fig. 1-50)**.

9. The vessels are dissected towards their distal anastomosis with the radial artery (towards the anatomic snuff box). The 1st and 2nd dorsal extensor compartments are opened at the level of the bone graft site to create a cuff of retinaculum containing the vessels and their nutrient arteries to bone.

10. Prior to elevation of the bone graft, a transverse dorsal-radial capsulotomy is made to expose the scaphoid non-union site and create the trough at the non-union site (Fig. 1-51).

- *Pearl:* With the thumb held in 45 degrees of palmar and radial abduction the EPL tends to follow the long axis of the scaphoid. If there is an uncertainty about fracture location, K-wires may be placed into the scaphoid, prior to capsulotomy, to verify position prior to creating the dorsal capsulotomy.

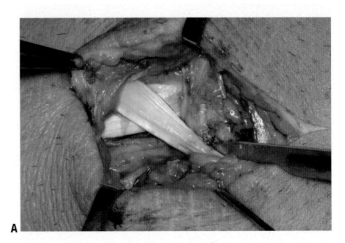

A

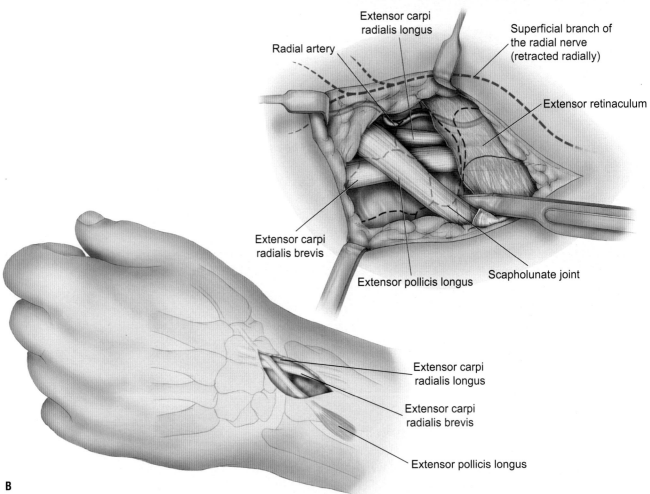

Extensor carpi
radialis longus

Radial artery

Superficial branch of
the radial nerve
(retracted radially)

Extensor retinaculum

Extensor carpi
radialis brevis

Extensor pollicis longus

Scapholunate joint

Extensor carpi
radialis longus

Extensor carpi
radialis brevis

Extensor pollicis longus

B

FIGURE 1-46

A,B: The EPL is mobilized by releasing the distal portion of the 3rd compartment retinaculum. This maneuver facilitates retraction of the EPL.

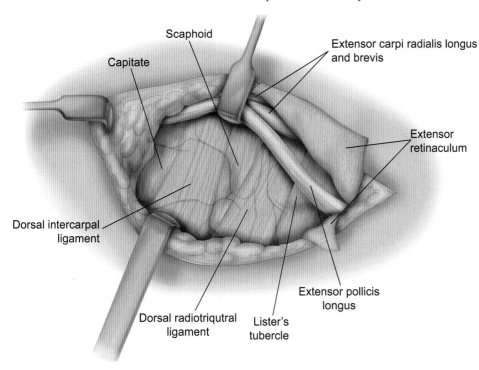

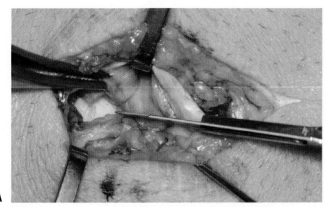

FIGURE 1-47

The dorsal radial capsule is exposed by retracting the extensor carpi radialis longus brevis and the extensor pollicis longus radially. In some instances the extensor pollicis longus will need to be released from its compartment in order to provide adequate visualization.

FIGURE 1-48

A,B: With the EPL and 2nd compartment tendons retracted radially the dorsal wrist capsule is opened through a short vertical incision.

A

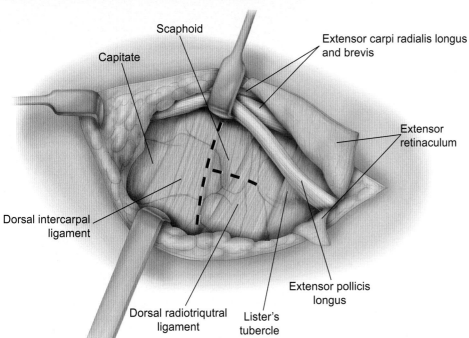

B

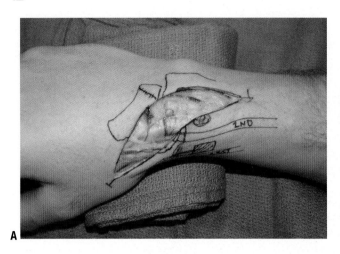

A

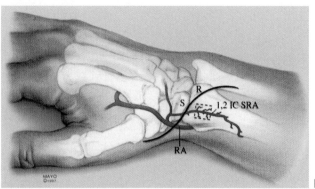

B

FIGURE 1-49

A,B: A modification of dorsal radial incision is made to increase exposure in cases requiring a vascularized graft from the dorsal distal radius. The incision is carried in a lazy S fashion over the first dorsal compartment to allow for exposure of the 1, 2 ICSRA vessels.

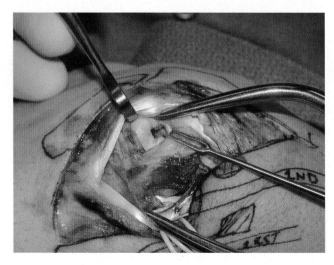

FIGURE 1-50

Identification of the 1, 2 ICSRA vessels, seen at tip of probe.

FIGURE 1-51

A transverse capsulotomy has been made in the dorsal wrist capsule. In cases of vascularized grafting from the 1st and 2nd compartment, the 2nd and 3rd compartment tendons are retracted ulnarly to allow for mobilization and placement of the vascularized graft. Here a trough has been created in the scaphoid at the non-union site to accept the vascularized graft.

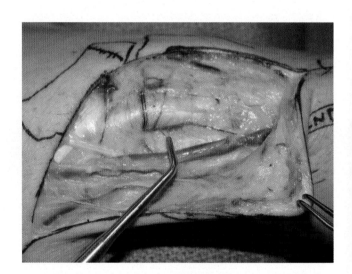

PITFALLS AND COMPLICATIONS

Potential complications from the surgical exposure are few and may include injury to the radial sensory nerve branch, tendon injury to the 2nd or 3rd compartment tendons, and post-operative extensor tendon adhesions. Hypertrophic scarring and wound infection may also occur. The dorsal radial exposure is not ideal for scapholunate or perilunate fracture dislocations, where exposure of the lunate is important for adequate reduction. In addition, this exposure limits access to the dorsal capsule if formal dorsal capsulodesis is to be performed for cases of static scapholunate instability. Also this approach may be inadequate for restoring scaphoid height in cases of scaphoid malunion or nonunions exhibiting significant humpback deformity. In such cases we have found that the volar approach allows for easier cortical graft placement and facilitates correction of scaphoid alignment.

The blood supply to the scaphoid is theoretically at risk with the dorsal radial approach and one must be wary not to injury the vessels entering at the radial dorsal crest during fracture exposure. Overall, however, the dorsal radial approach provides ample and easy access to the scaphoid for most cases of acute fracture and non-union.

PART 1: DORSAL APPROACH TO THE WRIST JOINT REFERENCES

1. Biyani A, Ebraheim NA, Lu J, et al. A modified dorsal approach to the wrist for arthrodesis of the non-rheumatoid wrist. An anatomical study. *J Hand Surg* 1996:21B:434–436.
2. Berger RA, Bishop AT. A fiber-splitting capsulotomy technique for dorsal exposure of the wrist. *Tech Hand Up Extrem Surg* 1997;1:2–10.
3. Jupiter JB. Open reduction and internal fixation. In: Gelberman RH, ed. *Masters Techniques in Orthopaedic Surgery: The Wrist.* New York: Raven Press Ltd, 1994.
4. Dellon AL, Seif SS. Anatomic dissections relating the posterior interosseous nerve to the carpus, and the etiology of dorsal wrist ganglion pain. *J Hand Surg* 1978;3A:326–332.
5. Spinner EB. *Kaplan's Functional and Surgical Anatomy of the Hand.* Philadelphia: Lippincott, Williams & Wilkins, 1984.
6. Mackinnon SE, Dellon AL. The overlap pattern of the lateral antebrachial cutaneous nerve and the superficial branch of the radial nerve. *J Hand Surg* 1985;10A: 522–526.
7. Hollinshead WH, ed. *Anatomy for Surgeons.* New York: Harper and Row, 1966.
8. Palmer AK, Skahen JR, Werner FW, et al. The extensor retinaculum of the wrist: an anatomical and biomechanical study. *J Hand Surg* 1985;10B:11–16.
9. Hoppenfeld S. *Physical Examination of the Spine and Extremities.* Norwalk, CT: Prentice Hall, 1976.
10. Weil C, Ruby LK. The dorsal approach to the wrist revisited. *J Hand Surg* 1986;11A: 911–912.
11. Dellon AL. Partial dorsal wrist denervation: resection of the distal posterior interosseous nerve. *J Hand Surg* 1985;10A:527–533.

PART 2: SURGICAL APPROACH OF THE ULNAR NERVE AT THE LEVEL OF THE WRIST REFERENCES

1. Guyon F. Note sur une disposition anatomique propre à la face antérieure de la région du poignet et non encore décrite par le docteur. *Bull Soc Anat Paris* 1861;6:184–186.
2. Engber WD, Gmeiner JG. Palmar cutaneous branch of the ulnar nerve. *J Hand Surg* 1980;5A:26–29.
3. Lindsey JT, Watumull D. Anatomic study of the ulnar nerve and related vascular anatomy at Guyon's canal: A practical classification. *J Hand Surg* 1996;21A:626–633.
4. Gross MS, Gelberman RH. The anatomy of the distal ulnar tunnel. *Clin Orthop* 1985;196:238–247.

PART 3: SURGICAL APPROACHES OF FLEXOR TENDONS IN WRIST AND HAND REFERENCES

1. Doyle JR, Blythe W. The finger flexor tendon sheath and pulleys: Anatomy and reconstruction. In: AAOS Symposium on Tendon Surgery in the Hand. St. Louis: CV Mosby, 1975:81–87.
2. Doyle JR, Blythe WF. Anatomy of the flexor tendon sheath and pulleys of the tendon sheath and pulleys of the thumb. *J Hand Surg* 1977; 2A:149–151.
3. Kleinert HE, Verdan CE. Report of the Committee on Tendon Injuries (International Federation of Societies for Surgery of the Hand). *J Hand Surg* 1983;8A:794–798.
4. Bunnell S. *Surgery of the Hand*, 2nd ed. Philadelphia: JB Lipincott, 1948:627.
5. Wilgis EFS. Observations on the effects of tourniquet ischemia. *J Bone Joint Surg* 1971;53A:1343.
6. Brunner JM. The zigzag volar digital incision for flexor tendon surgery. *Plast Reconstr Surg* 1967;40:571.

PART 4: VOLAR APPROACH TO THE WRIST REFERENCES

1. Botte MJ, Gelberman RH. Modified technique for Herbert screw insertion in fractures of the scaphoid. *J Hand Surg* 1987;12A:149–150.
2. Cooney WP, Dobyns JH, Linscheid RL. Fractures of the scaphoid: A rational approach to management. *Clin Orthop* 1980;149:90–97.
3. Garcia-Elias M, Vall A, Salo JM, et al. Carpal alignment after different surgical approaches to the scaphoid: A comparative study. *J Hand Surg* 1988;13A:604–612.
4. Huene DR, Huene DS. Treatment of nonunions of the scaphoid with the Ender compression blade plate system. *J Hand Surg* 1991;16A:913–922.
5. Puopolo SM, Rettig ME. Management of acute scaphoid fractures. *Bull Hosp Joint Dis* 2003;61(3–4):160–163.
6. Cooney WP III. Scaphoid fractures: Current treatments and techniques. *AAOS Instruc Course Lect* 2003;52:197–208.
7. Rikli DA, Regazzoni P. Fractures of the distal end of the radius treated by internal fixation and early function. *J Bone Joint Surg* 1996;78B:588–592.
8. Nana AD, Joshi A, Lichtman D. Plating of the distal radius. *J Am Acad Orthop Surg* 2005;13(3):159–191.
9. Orbay JL. The treatment of unstable distal radius fractures with volar fixation. *Hand Surg* 2000;5:103–112.
10. Fernandez DL. A technique for anterior wedge-shaped grafts for scaphoid nonunions with carpal instability. *J Hand Surg* 1984;9A:733–737.
11. Inoue G, Miura T. Treatment of ununited fractures of the carpal scaphoid by iliac bone grafts and Herbert screw fixation. *Int Orthop* 1991;15:279–282.
12. Ring D, Jupiter JB, Herndon JH. Acute fractures of the scaphoid. *J Am Acad Orthop Surg* 2000;8(4):225–231.
13. Trumble TE, Gilbert M, Murray LW, et al. Displaced scaphoid fractures treated with open reduction and internal fixation with a cannulated screw. *J Bone Joint Surg* 2000;82A(5):633–641.
14. Cooney WP, Linscheid RL, Dobyns JH, et al. Scaphoid nonunion: Role of anterior interpositional bone grafts. *J Hand Surg* 1988;13A:635–650.
15. Herbert TJ, Fisher WE, Leicester AW. The Herbert bone screw: A ten year perspective. *J Hand Surg* 1992;17B:415–419.
16. Jeon IH, Oh CW, Park BC, et al. Minimal invasive percutaneous Herbert screw fixation in acute unstable scaphoid fracture. *Hand Surg* 2003;8(2):213–218.
17. Raskin KB, Parisi D, Baker J, et al. Dorsal open repair of proximal pole scaphoid fractures. *Hand Clinics* 2001;17(4):601–610, ix.
18. Sanders WE. Distal radius fractures. In: Manske PR, ed. *Hand Surgery Update*. Rosemont IL: American Academy of Orthopaedic Surgeons, 1996:117–123.
19. Fernandez DL, Geissler WB. Treatment of displaced articular fractures of the radius. *J Hand Surg* 1999;24A:102–107.
20. Fitoussi F, Ip WY, Chow SP. Treatment of displaced intra-articular fractures of the distal end of the radius with plates. *J Bone Joint Surg* 1997;79A:1303–1312.
21. Orbay JL, Fernandez DL. Volar fixation for dorsally displaced fractures of the distal radius: A preliminary report. *J Hand Surg* 2002;27A:205–215.
22. DeMaagd RL, Engber WD. Retrograde Herbert screw fixation for treatment of proximal pole scaphoid nonunions. *J Hand Surg* 1989;14A:996–1003.
23. Melone CP Jr. Articular fractures of the distal radius. *Orthop Clin North Am* 1984;15:217–236.
24. Richards RS, Bennett JD, Roth JH, et al. Arthroscopic diagnosis of intra-articular soft tissue injuries associated with distal radius fractures. *J Hand Surg* 1997;22A:772–776.
25. Wright T, Horodyski M, Smith DW. Functional outcomes of unstable distal radius fractures: ORIF with a volar plate versus external fixation. *J Hand Surg* 2005;30A(2):89–99.
26. Amrami K. Radiology corner: Review of plain radiographs. *J Assoc Soc Surg Hand* 2005;5:4–7.
27. Perlik PC, Guilford WB. Magnetic resonance imaging to assess vascularity of scaphoid nonunions. *J Hand Surg* 1991;16A:479–484.
28. Sanders WE. Evaluation of the humpback scaphoid by computed tomography in the longitudinal axial plane of the scaphoid. *J Hand Surg* 1988;13A:182–187.
29. Jakob M, Rikli DA, Regazzoni P. Fractures of the distal radius treated by internal fixation and early function. *J Bone Joint Surg* 2000;82B:340–344.
30. Chan KW, McAdams TR. Central screw placement in percutaneous screw scaphoid fixation: A cadaveric comparison of proximal and distal techniques. *J Hand Surg* 2004;29A(1):74–79.
31. Menapace KA, Larabee L, Arnoczky SP, et al. Anatomic placement of the Herbert-Whipple screw in scaphoid fractures: A cadaver study. *J Hand Surg* 2001;26A(5):883–892.
32. Putnam MD, Fischer MD. Treatment of unstable distal radius fractures: Methods and comparison of external distraction and ORIF versus external distraction-ORIF neutralization. *J Hand Surg* 1997;22A:238–251.

PART 5: DORSAL RADIAL EXPOSURE OF THE SCAPHOID
REFERENCES

1. Cooney WP, Dobyns JH, Linscheid RL. Fractures of the scaphoid: A rational approach to management. *Clin Orthop* 1980;149:90–97.
2. Smith DK, Cooney WP III, An KN, et al. The effects of simulated unstable scaphoid fractures on carpal motion. *J Hand Surg* 1989;14A:283–291.
3. Amadio PC, Berquist TH, Smith DK, et al. Scaphoid malunion. *J Hand Surg* 1989;14A:679–687.
4. Cooney III, WP, Dobyns JH, Linscheid RL. Nonunion of the scaphoid: Analysis of the results from bone grafting. *J Hand Surg* 1980;5:343–354.
5. Eddeland A, Eiken O, Hellgren E, et al. Fractures of the scaphoid. *Scand J Plast Reconstr Surg* 1975;9:234–239.
6. Viegas SF, Bean JW, Schram RA. Transcaphoid fracture dislocations treated with open reduction and Herbert screw internal fixation. *J Hand Surg* 1987;12:992–999.
7. Cooney WP, Bussey R, Dobyns JH, et al. Difficult wrist fractures. Perilunate fracture-dislocations of the wrist. *Clin Orthop* 1987;214:136–147.
8. Rettig AC, Kozin SH, Cooney WP. Open reduction and internal fixation of acute displaced scaphoid wrist fractures. *J Hand Surg* 2001;26:271–276.
9. Garcia-Elias M, Vall A, Salo JM, et al. Carpal alignment after different surgical approaches to the scaphoid: A comparative study. *J Hand Surg* 1988;13A:604–612.
10. Russe O. Fracture of the carpal navicular. Diagnosis, non-operative treatment and operative treatment. *J Bone Joint Surg* 1960;42A:759–768.
11. Herbert TJ, Fisher WE. Management of the fractured scaphoid using a new bone screw. *J Bone Joint Surg* 1984;66B:114–123.
12. Shin AY, Bishop AT. Vascularized bone grafts for scaphoid nonunion and Kienböck's disease. *Ortho Clin North Am* 2001;30(2):263–277.
13. Tubiana T, Gilbert A, Masuelet AC. Bones and joints. In: *An Atlas of Surgical Techniques of the Hand and Wrist*. London: Martin Dunitz, Ltd, 1999:63–73.

2 Forearm

Bernard F. Morrey

Clinically, there are only three relevant exposures of the forearm. These expose the radius from a posterior (Thompson) and from an anterior (Henry) perspective and the ulna from a dorsal perspective. All three are readily extended depending on the pathology being treated.

POSTERIOR APPROACH TO THE RADIUS (THOMPSON)

Indications

Fracture, tumor, and infection when access to posterior radius desired.

Note

This approach is not commonly employed but may be used to expose either the proximal, mid or distal radius but is most effective for the proximal and middle thirds.

Position

The patient is supine with arm across the chest or on arm/elbow table.

Landmarks

Lateral epicondyle to radial styloid.

Technique

1. Incision: straight from the lateral epicondyle to the radial styloid. With the forearm pronated the line of the incision is a straight line. Use all or any portion (**Fig. 2-1A**).
2. Expose the interval between the anterior border of the extensor digitorum communis and the posterior or radial border of the extensor carpi radialis brevis.
3. Distally palpate the bare portion of the radius distally that superficially demarcates the natural interval between these two muscle groups (**Fig. 2-1B**). Deep to these muscles the bare area identifies the distal aspect of the supinator and proximal attachment of the pronator teres tendon.
4. The forearm fascia is split proximally and distally allowing the extensor digitorum communis to be retracted posteriorly and extensor carpi radialis brevis to be retracted anteriorly to the ulnar side of the radius (**Fig. 2-1C**). The bare shaft of the radius between the supinator and pronator attachments is well defined (**Fig. 2-1D**).
5. Proximally with the forearm in supination, the supinator muscle is noted and the posterior interosseous nerve observed and may or may not be exposed.
6. The supinator muscle is then released either in its mid-portion exposing the posterior interosseous nerve or, more commonly, is released from the shaft of the radius (**Fig. 2-1E**).

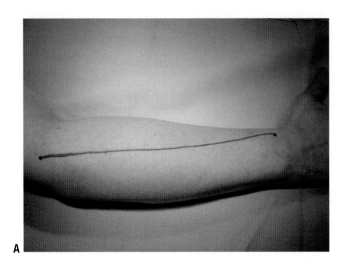

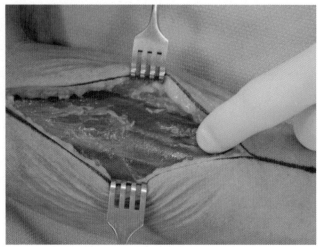

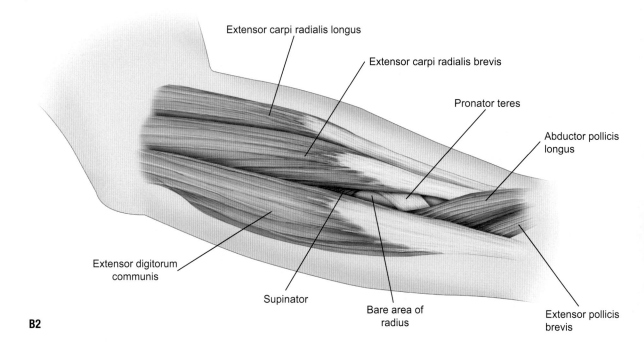

Extensor carpi radialis longus

Extensor carpi radialis brevis

Pronator teres

Abductor pollicis longus

Extensor digitorum communis

Supinator

Bare area of radius

Extensor pollicis brevis

B2

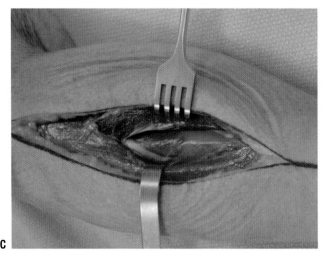

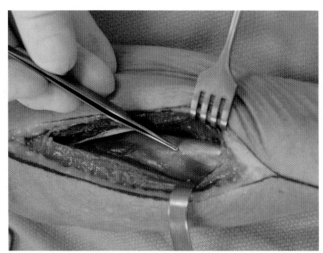

FIGURE 2-1

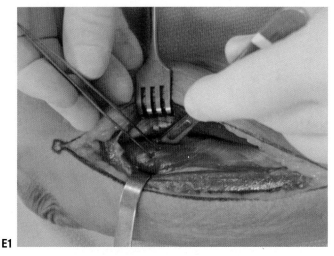

E1

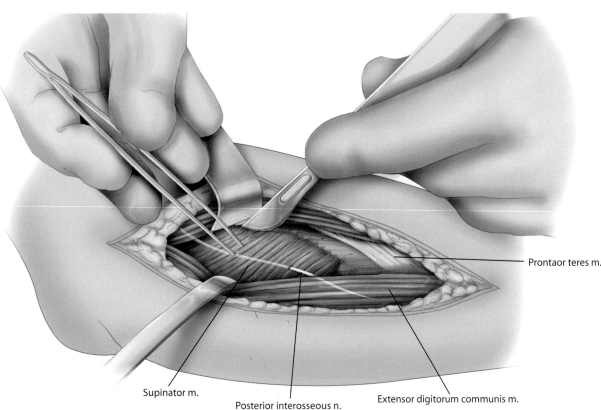

Prontaor teres m.

Supinator m.

Posterior interosseous n.

Extensor digitorum communis m.

E2

FIGURE 2-1 *(Continued)*

● *Pearls*

    ● This is facilitated by fully supinating the forearm which brings the supinator attachment of the radius easily within the wound allowing excellent visualization for the release of its origin.

    ● It is not necessary to identify the posterior interosseous nerve during this procedure but one should be gentle to avoid nerve injury.

7. The supinator muscle is reflected towards its ulnar attachment and the proximal portion of the radius is exposed (**Fig. 2-1F**).

8. After splitting the forearm fascia distally, the common extensor is reflected posteriorly and the tendinous portion of the brevis and longus is isolated in the midforearm (**Fig. 2-1G**). The radial attachment of the pronator teres muscle is in the mid-portion of the exposure.

9. Distally, by retracting the extensor digitorum communis posteriorly and extensor carpi radialis brevis anteriorly, the abductor pollicis longus and extensor polis brevis are observed to course obliquely superficial to the extensor carpi radialis brevis tendon at the distal aspect of the incision (**Fig. 2-1H**). The middle 80% of the radius is exposed.

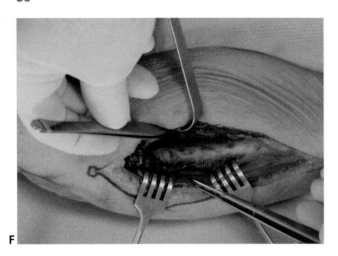

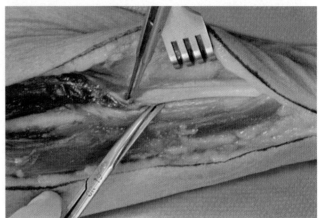

F   G1

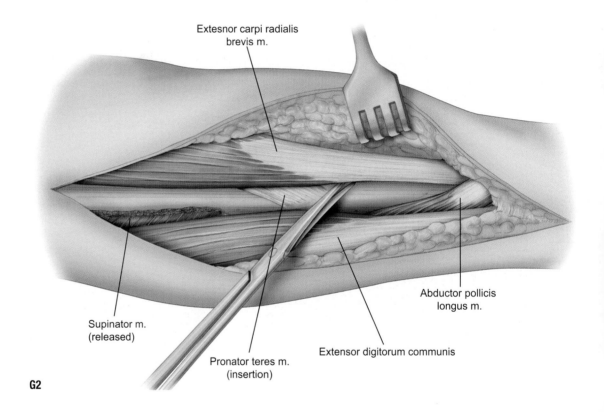

Extesnor carpi radialis
brevis m.

Supinator m.
(released)

Pronator teres m.
(insertion)

Extensor digitorum communis

Abductor pollicis
longus m.

G2

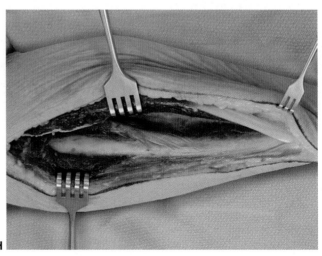

FIGURE 2-1   *(Continued)*   H

ANTERIOR (HENRY) SURGICAL EXPOSURE TO THE PROXIMAL RADIUS

Indications

Fracture, malignancy, and osteomyelitis.

Position

The patient is supine with the arm on an elbow table.

Landmarks

1. The mobile wad is identified and palpated, the lateral aspect of the distal fourth of the biceps, the cubital crease proximally, and the radial styloid distally are identified (**Fig. 2-2A**).
2. Skin incision: After splitting the brachial fascia, the lateral margin of the biceps muscle is identified in the proximal aspect of the wound (**Fig. 2-2B**).
3. The interval between the biceps and brachialis is developed by blunt and sharp dissection.
4. The terminal branch of the musculocutaneous nerve is identified and protected as the skin incision extends distally (**Fig. 2-2C**).
5. The recurrent branch of the radial artery is identified and ligated (**Fig. 2-2D**).

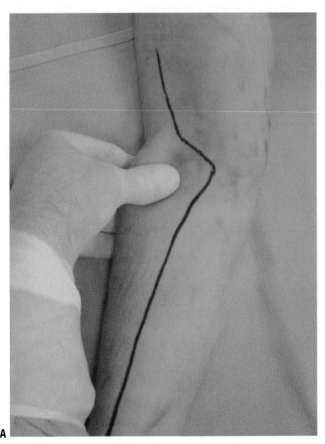

A

FIGURE 2-2

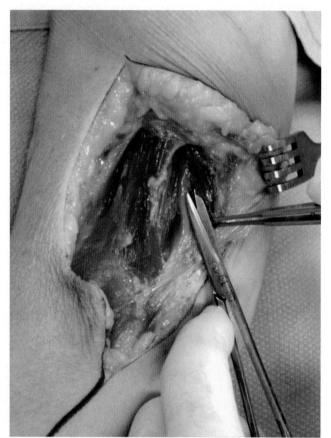

B1

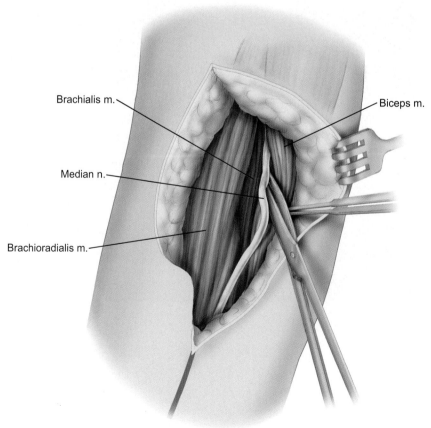

Brachialis m.

Biceps m.

Median n.

Brachioradialis m.

FIGURE 2-2 *(Continued)*   **B2**

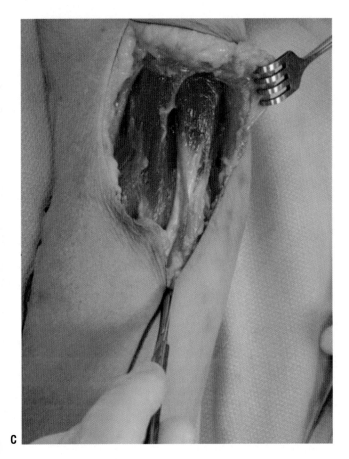

C

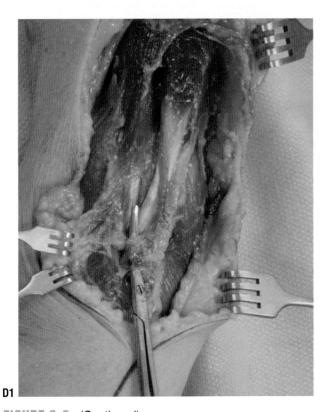

D1

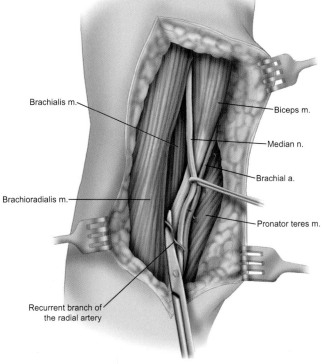

D2

Brachialis m.

Biceps m.

Median n.

Brachial a.

Brachioradialis m.

Pronator teres m.

Recurrent branch of
the radial artery

FIGURE 2-2 *(Continued)*

- ***Pearl:*** This is the key step that allows distal expansion of this exposure.

6. The origin of the biceps on the radial tuberosity is identified medially. Laterally the brachioradialis muscle is observed along with the radial nerve **(Fig. 2-2E)** that travels in the interval between the brachioradialis and brachialis muscles proximally.

- ***Note:*** Observe proximacy of posterior interosseous nerve to the anterior capsule over the radial head.

7. The forearm fascia is split distally between the pronator teres medially and the brachioradialis muscle laterally **(Fig. 2-2F)**. The pronator teres muscle belly is followed distally and is retracted exposing the supinator muscle and the pronator attachment.
8. By supinating the forearm, the radial origin of the supinator muscle is identified. The posterior interosseous nerve is observed entering under the arcade of Froche **(Fig. 2-2G)**. The superficial radial nerve is identified on the undersurface of the brachioradialis and protected.
9. The supinator muscle is released from the proximal radius, exposing the anterior aspect of the proximal radius **(Fig. 2-2H,I)**.
10. The fascia between the brachioradialis and the pronator teres and flexor carpi radialis is split distally **(Fig. 2-2J)**.
11. The brachioradialis along with the radial nerve is retracted laterally, the pronator teres and flexor carpi radialis muscles are retracted medially. The insertion of the pronator teres is identified at the proximal aspect of the dissection **(Fig. 2-2K)**.
12. Pronation of the forearm allows visualization of the attachment of the pronator teres and flexor pollicis longus. Distally the pronator quadratus is elevated from the medial aspect of the radius **(Fig. 2-2L)**.
13. By supinating the forearm, sharp periosteal elevation of all remaining muscular attachments of the radial shaft allows complete exposure of the radius **(Fig. 2-2M)**.

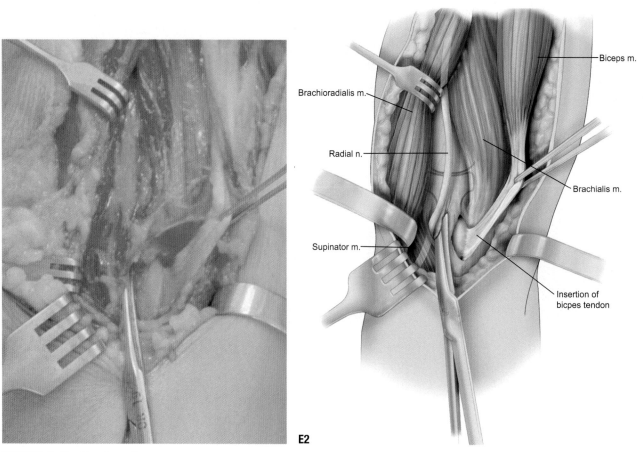

FIGURE 2-2 *(Continued)*

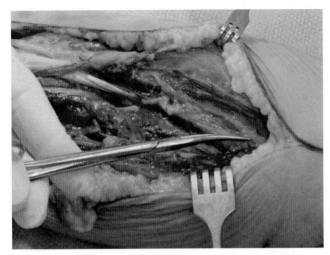

F

FIGURE 2-2F

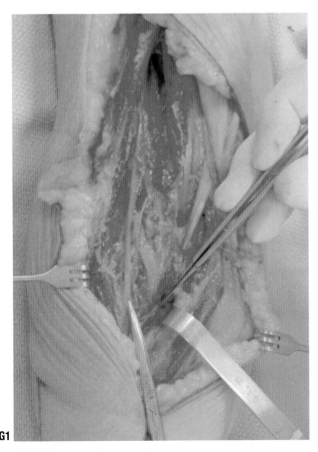

G1

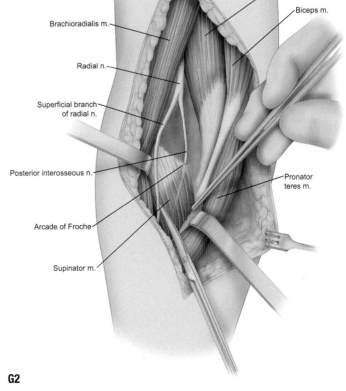

G2

Brachialis m.

Biceps m.

Brachioradialis m.

Radial n.

Superficial branch
of radial n.

Posterior interosseous n.

Arcade of Froche

Supinator m.

Pronator
teres m.

FIGURE 2-2   (Continued)

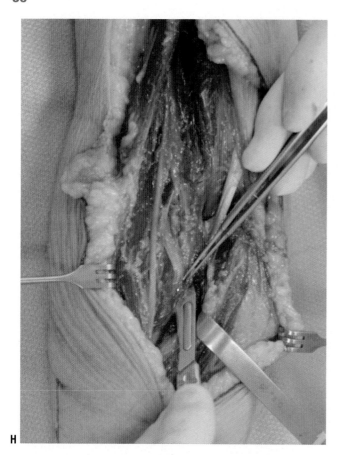

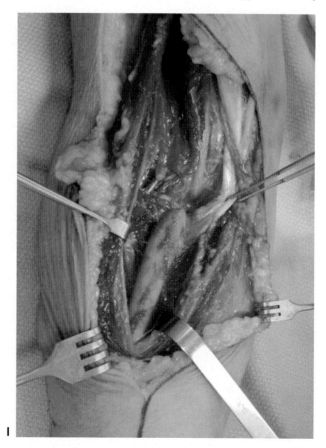

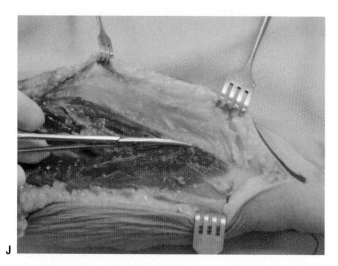

FIGURE 2-2 *(Continued)*

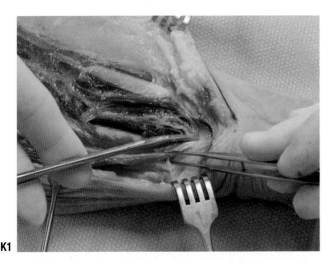

K1

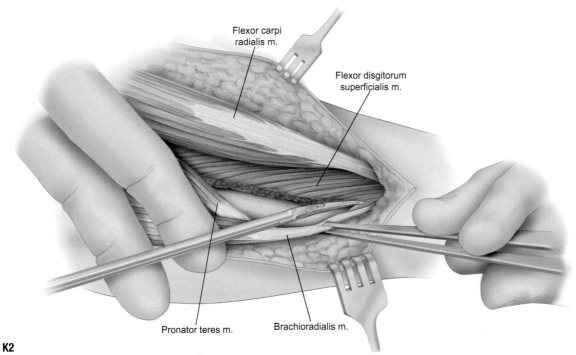

Flexor carpi
radialis m.

Flexor disgitorum
superficialis m.

Pronator teres m.   Brachioradialis m.

K2

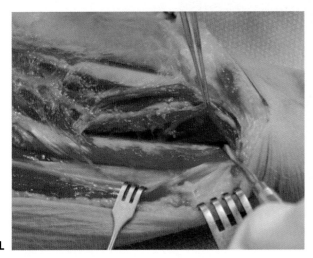

L

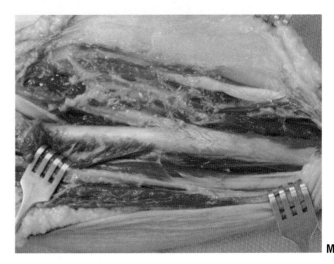

M

FIGURE 2-2   *(Continued)*

EXPOSURE OF THE SHAFT OF THE ULNA

This is probably the easiest exposure of the entire musculoskeletal system as the ulna lies in a subcutaneous position throughout its course and there are no neurovascular structures at risk (**Fig. 2-3A**).

Indication

Fracture and revision of ulnar component.

Position

The patient is prone with forearm across the chest.

Landmarks

Tip of olecranon, subcutaneous border of ulna, and ulnar styloid.

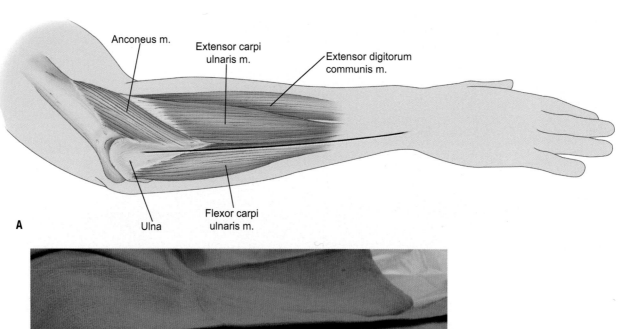

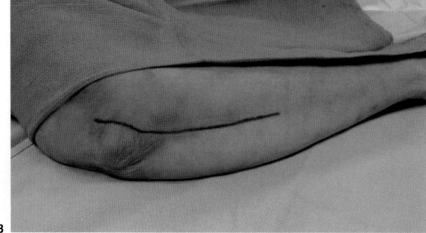

FIGURE 2-3

Technique

1. Incision: A straight incision from the medial or lateral aspects of the olecranon or originating directly over the olecranon, proceeds distally to the ulnar styloid, as needed (**Fig. 2-3B**).
2. The subcutaneous border of the ulna is easily palpated (**Fig. 2-3C**).
3. Elevating the anconeus and the extensor carpi ulnaris muscles allows exposure of the radial side of the ulna (**Fig. 2-3D**).
4. The flexor carpi ulnaris and flexor digitorum profundus muscles attach to the medial aspect of the ulna and are freed subperiosteally (**Fig. 2-3E**).
5. The dissection extends distally as far as is needed (**Fig. 2-3F**).

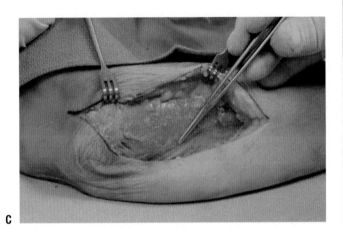

C

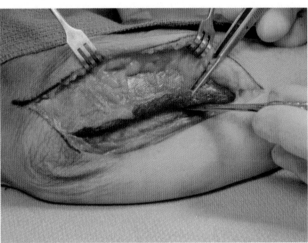

D

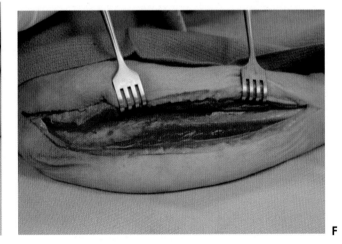

E

F

FIGURE 2-3 *(Continued)*

RECOMMENDED READING

Anson BJ, Maddock WG. *Callander's Surgical Anatomy*, 4th ed. Philadelphia: W.B. Saunders, 1958.

Banks S, Laufman H. *An Atlas of Surgical Exposures of the Extremities*. Philadelphia: W.B. Saunders, 1953.

Campbell WC. Incision for exposure of the elbow joint. *Am J Surg* 1932;15:65–67.

Grant JCB. *An Atlas of Anatomy*, 6th ed. Baltimore: Williams & Wilkins, 1972.

Gray H. *The Anatomy of the Human Body*, 29th ed. Philadelphia: Lea & Febiger, 1975.

Henry AK. *Extensile Exposure*, 2nd ed. New York: Churchill-Livingstone, Inc., 1963.

Hollinshead WH. *Anatomy for Surgeons: The Back and Limbs*, 3rd ed. Philadelphia: Harper & Row, 1982.

Hoppenfeld S, deBoer P. *Surgical Exposures in Orthopaedics: The Anatomical Approach*, 1st ed. Philadelphia: JB Lippincott Co., 1984.

Kaplan EB. Surgical approach to the proximal end of the radius and its use in fractures of the head and neck of the radius. *J Bone Joint Surg* 1941;23:86–92.

Kocher T. *Textbook of Operative Surgery* [translated from 4th German edition by HJ Stiles]. London: Adam & Charles Black, 1903.

Morrey BF. *Master Techniques in Orthopaedic Surgery: The Elbow*, 2nd ed. Philadelphia: Lippincott Williams & Wilkins, 2002.

Reckling FW, Reckling JB, Mohr MC. *Orthopedic Anatomy and Surgical Approaches*. St. Louis: Mosby Yearbook, 1990.

Thompson JE. Anatomical methods of approach in operations on the long bones of the extremities. *Ann Surg* 1918;68:309–329.

Tubiana R, McCullough CJ, Masquelet AC. *An Atlas of Surgical Exposures of the Upper Extremity*. London: Martin Dunitz Publisher, 1990.

3 Elbow

Bernard F. Morrey

Facility with exposures to the elbow characterized by flexibility and extensibility is an essential prerequisite to the execution of the full spectrum of elbow surgery which is discussed in detail in *Master Techniques in Orthopedic Surgery: The Elbow* (1). In this chapter we emphasize how limited exposures to the elbow can be expanded to address broadened pathology and perform more complex procedures. Specific details of exposure and technique are found in the above cited volume.

There are two conceptual incision types: an extensile posterior or posterior/lateral or a limited, specific for-purpose exposure **(Fig. 3-1)**. For extensile exposures, a straight posterior or posterior lateral incision is used. We term the posterior exposure the "universal" incision since both medial and lateral elbow pathology can be addressed through a posterior skin incision by elevating skin flaps **(Fig. 3-2)**. For fear of injuring the ulnar nerve, a posterior incision of variable length (12 to 18 cm) is placed just medial or lateral to the tip of the olecranon and not directly over the cubital tunnel.

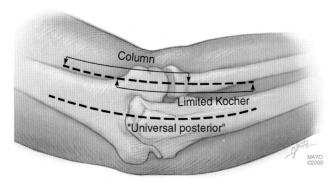

FIGURE 3-1

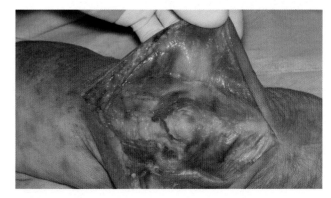

FIGURE 3-2

OLECRANON OSTEOTOMY

Indications

Reduction and fixation, distal humeral, and comminuted fractures (C3).

Landmarks

Tip of olecranon, medial epicondyle, ulnar nerve in cubital tunnel, nonarticular portion of olecranon.

Position

The patient is supine with arm across the chest.

Technique

1. Skin incision: direct posterior from 6 to 8 cm proximal to the tip of the olecranon, over subcutaneous border of ulna; distal as required **(Fig. 3-3A)**.
2. Elevate skin flaps medially and laterally to the epicondyles **(Fig. 3-3B)**.
3. Identify ulnar nerve and incise medial ulnohumeral capsule.
4. The anconeus is released from the triceps, the ulnohumeral capsule is incised, and the nonarticular portion of the greater sigmoid notch is identified **(Fig. 3-3C)**.

   - *Alternate:* Laterally, we prefer to protect and elevate the anconeus distal to proximal thereby protecting its origin from the triceps fascia (see later).

5. A Chevron osteotomy is performed, apex distal with a depth of 5 to 10 mm **(Fig. 3-3D)**. Protect the ulnar nerve medially. Use osteotome to crack last few millimeters to assure accurate subsequent reduction.

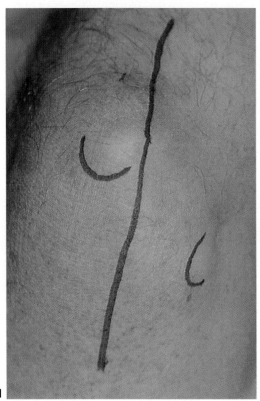

A1

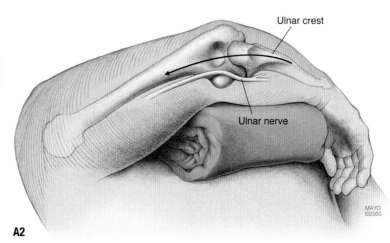

A2

FIGURE 3-3

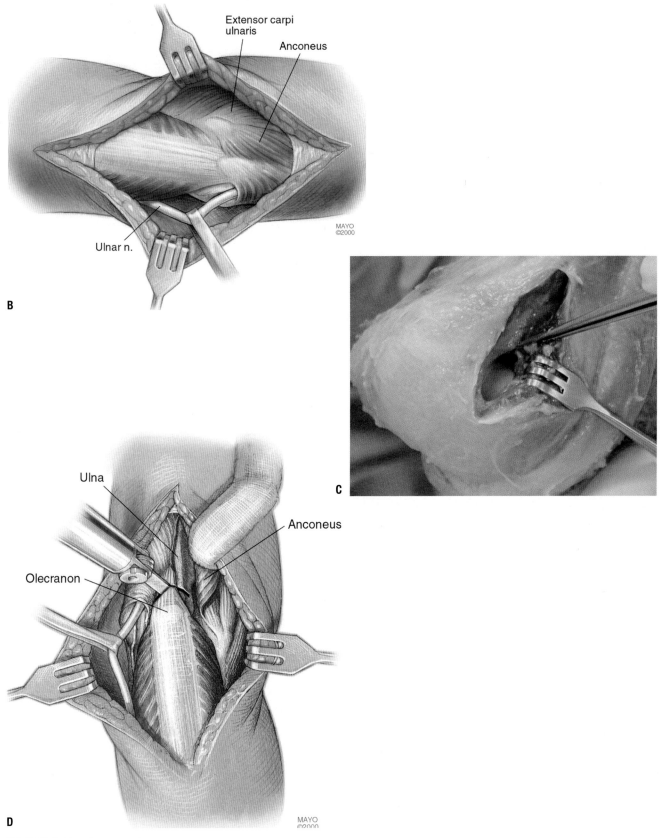

FIGURE 3-3 *(Continued)*

6. The olecranon fragment is reflected proximally exposing the distal humerus (**Fig. 3-3E**).
7. Repair uses the AO-K-wire, tension band technique with the wires in the anterior cortex, not down the canal (**Fig. 3-3F**).

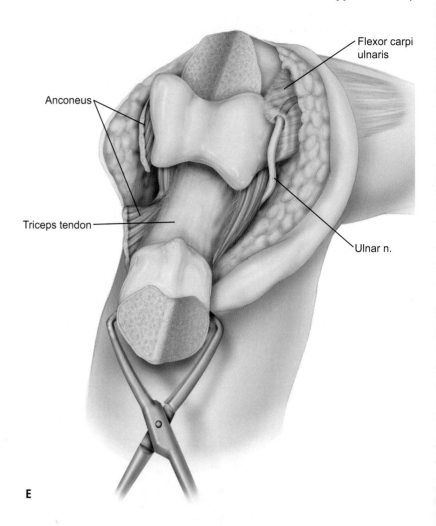

Flexor carpi
ulnaris

Anconeus

Triceps tendon

Ulnar n.

E

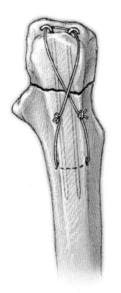

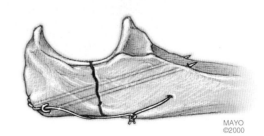

Pins oblique, cortex engaged

F

MAYO
©2000

FIGURE 3-3 *(Continued)*

Mayo Olecranon Osteotomy of the Elbow—Anconeus Preserving

Concern with regard to transecting the anconeus attachment to the triceps has prompted the development of an olecranon osteotomy that preserves the anconeus origin and viability.

Position   The patient is supine with the arm across the chest.

Technique

1. The exposure is as required by the pathology. Deep exposure is at the Kocher's interval between the extensor carpi ulnaris and anconeus **(Fig. 3-4A)**.
2. The interval is entered and the anconeus is identified and isolated **(Fig. 3-4B)**.
3. The anconeus is elevated from its bed by sharp dissection leaving the attachment of its origin at the fascial expansion of the triceps and the mid-portion of the sigmoid notch is identified laterally **(Fig. 3-4C)**.
4. Medially the ulnar nerve is identified **(Fig. 3-4D)** and the mid-portion of the articulation is exposed **(Fig. 3-4E)**.
5. A V-shaped osteotomy is carried out as above with an oscillating saw **(Fig. 3-4F)**. The osteotomy is completed with an osteotome **(Fig. 3-4G)**.
6. The osteotomized olecranon along with the attached anconeus is elevated proximally **(Fig. 3-4H)**.
7. Closure consists of the standard AO reattachment of the olecranon. The anconeus is brought back to its insertion on the ulna. The fascia over the anconeus is closed with a running 2-0 absorbable suture **(Fig. 3-4I)**.

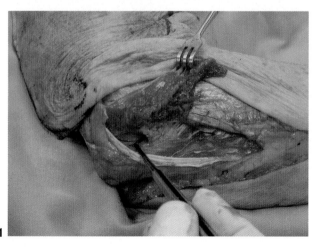
A

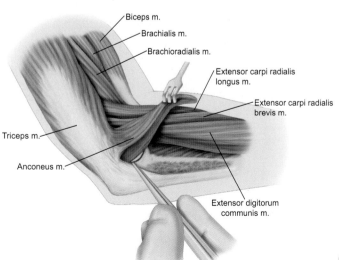
B

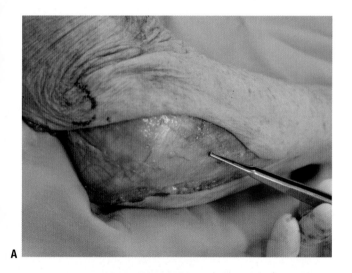
C1

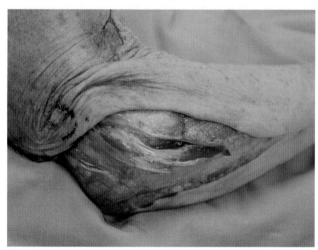

C2

FIGURE 3-4

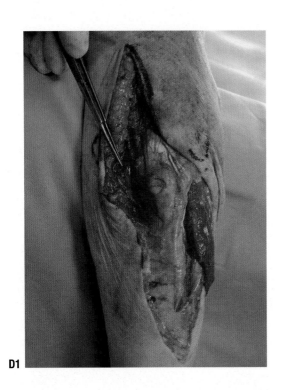

D1

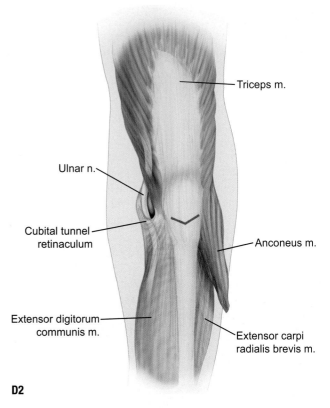

Triceps m.

Ulnar n.

Cubital tunnel
retinaculum

Anconeus m.

Extensor digitorum
communis m.

Extensor carpi
radialis brevis m.

D2

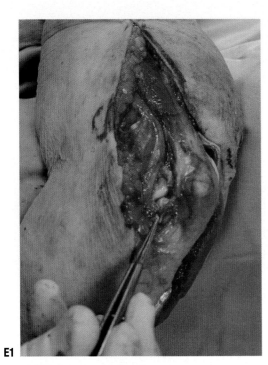

E1

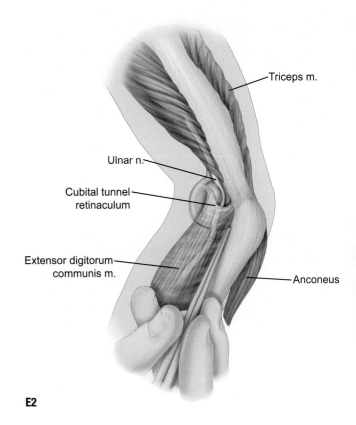

Triceps m.

Ulnar n.

Cubital tunnel
retinaculum

Extensor digitorum
communis m.

Anconeus

E2

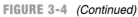

FIGURE 3-4 *(Continued)*

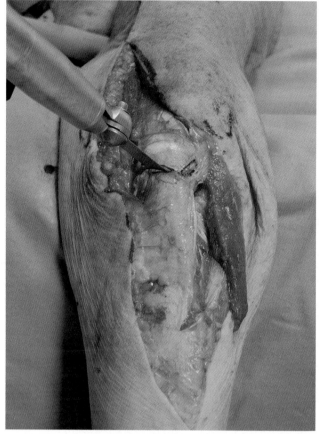

F

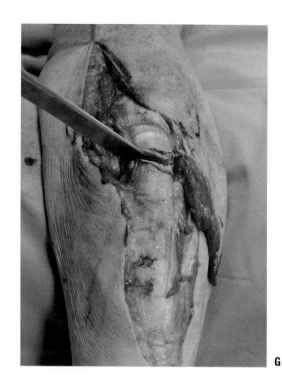

G

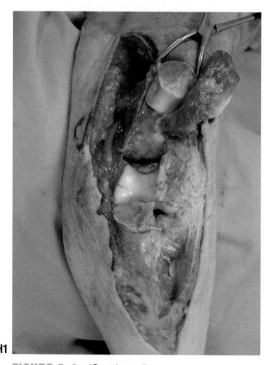

H1

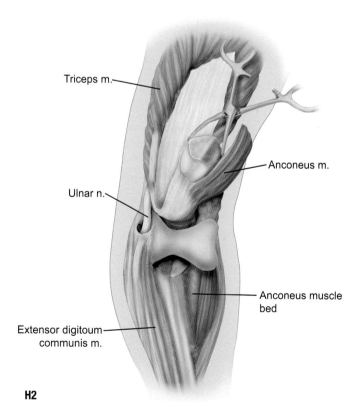

Triceps m.

Anconeus m.

Ulnar n.

Anconeus muscle bed

Extensor digitoum communis m.

H2

FIGURE 3-4 *(Continued)*

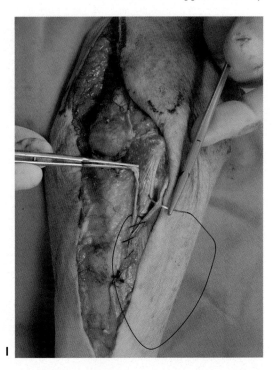

FIGURE 3-4 *(Continued)*   **I**

Pearls/Pitfalls/Comments

- *Pearl:* The ulnar nerve does not need to be mobilized unless dictated by the pathology.
- *Comments:* The attractiveness of this exposure is that the anconeus dissection can be done very safely and quickly. This does preserve the anconeus triceps continuity in the event that a later reconstructive procedure may be necessary that uses the anconeus.
- *Pitfalls:* Avoid osteotomy in rheumatoid arthritis as the thin olecranon compromises healing if an osteotomy is carried out (2). The transverse osteotomy of McAusland is associated with an approximately 5% nonunion rate (2). Although for fractures the Chevron osteotomy may improve these results and decrease the nonunion rate, I personally have not had the clinical need to osteotomize the olecranon in the last 14 years, and osteotomy should be avoided if the olecranon is resorbed.

LATERAL EXPOSURES

The central concept is predicated on raising subcutaneous flaps both medially and laterally. This in turn is strongly dependent on recognizing the flexibility of extending limited incisions as needed.

A limited proximal lateral approach exposes the supracondylar column. A limited distal approach enters Kocher's interval and exposes the radial head and the lateral collateral ligament. Connecting the two defines the extensile Kocher exposure **(Fig. 3-5)**.

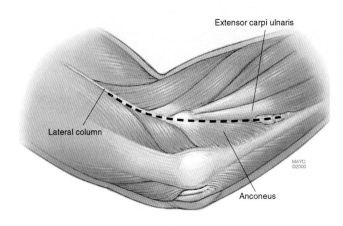

FIGURE 3-5

The Column Exposure (3)

Indications   Anterior-posterior capsular release for stiff elbow.

Landmarks   Lateral epicondyle, the common extensor tendon, the extensor carpi radialis longus, and the anterior capsule.

Position   The patient is supine with arm across the chest.

Technique

1. Incision: the skin incision starts over the lateral column 5 cm proximal to the lateral epicondyle and extends distally 2 cm past the epicondyle (**Fig. 3-6A**).
2. The extensor carpi radialis longus is identified and elevated from the lateral column and epicondyle and the anterior capsule is visualized (**Fig. 3-6B**).
3. An incision is made in the capsule just superior to the collateral ligament (**Fig. 3-6C**).
4. If the posterior joint needs to be exposed the triceps is easily elevated (**Fig. 3-6D**).

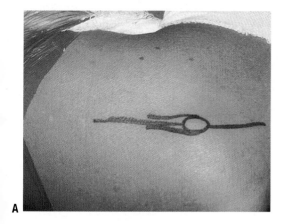

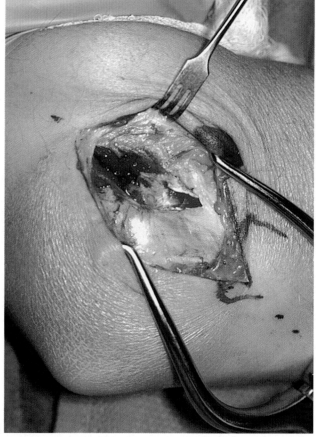

FIGURE 3-6

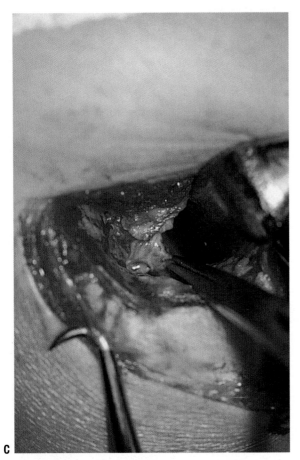

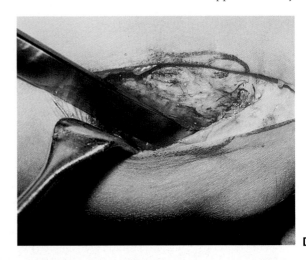

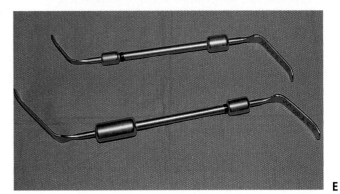

FIGURE 3-6 *(Continued)*

Pearls/Pitfalls/Comments

- A periosteal elevator is used to elevate the brachialis muscle off the anterior capsule which can be safely performed since the arthrotomy provides accurate spatial orientation from lateral to medial across the joint.
- Special contoured retractors have been designed making the soft tissue retractor easier (**Fig. 3-6E**).
- If an extensile exposure is anticipated, a posterior incision is made. The same deep exposure can be accomplished by extending the posterior lateral skin incision and elevating the lateral skin cutaneous flap.

Limited Kocher Exposure of the Elbow

Indications   Simple excision of the radial head and repair of lateral ulnar collateral ligament.

Landmarks   Lateral epicondyle, radial head, and interval between anconeus and extensor carpi ulnaris.

Position   The patient is supine with arm across the chest.

Technique

1. Incision: from the subcutaneous border of the ulna obliquely across the posterolateral aspect of the elbow ending just proximal to the lateral epicondyle (**Fig. 3-7A**).
   - *Note:* This follows Kocher's interval.
2. The interval between the anconeus and extensor carpi ulnaris is identified and entered (**Fig. 3-7B**).
3. For excision of the radial head, the extensor carpi ulnaris and a small portion of the supinator muscle are dissected free of the capsule and retracted anteriorly (**Fig. 3-7C**).

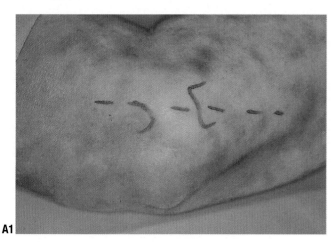

A1

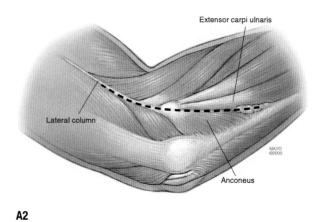

A2

Extensor carpi ulnaris

Lateral column

Anconeus

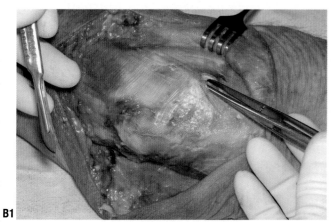

B1

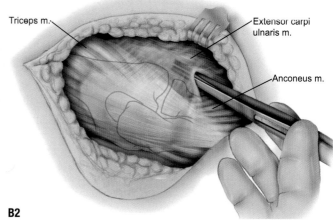

B2

Triceps m.

Extensor carpi ulnaris m.

Anconeus m.

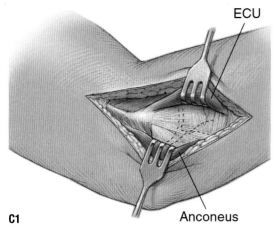

C1

ECU

Anconeus

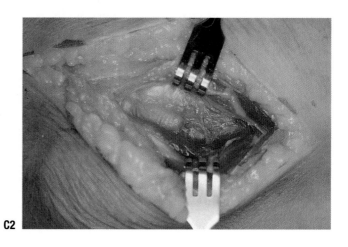

C2

FIGURE 3-7

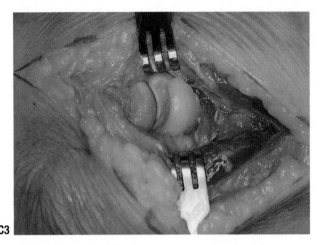

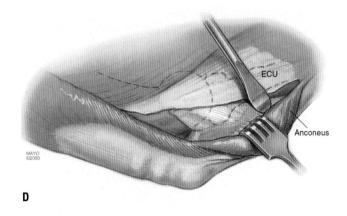

C3

FIGURE 3-7 *(Continued)*

Distal Extension

Landmarks

- The lateral epicondyle, posterior border of the extensor carpi ulnaris, anterior edge of the anconeus, and the crista supinatoris.
- The anconeus is elevated from the ulna and the tubercle of the supinator is palpated (**Fig. 3-7D**).

Extensile Posterior Lateral Exposure (Kocher)

We have found that the described surgical exposures to the elbow sufficient for virtually all reconstructive procedures and all may be executed with a posterior skin incision. The classic extensile approach described by Kocher implies that the anterior capsule has been incised and the lateral collateral ligament has been released (4).

Indications   Reconstructive procedures, including open reduction internal fixation, total elbow arthroplasty (unlinked), and interposition arthroplasty.

Landmarks   The proximal lateral column and the distal Kocher interval.

Position   The patient is supine with arm across the chest.

Technique   The basic interval is the connection of the above two exposures, the column, and the distal limited Kocher. The lateral collateral ligament is released and the triceps may be elevated from the posterior aspect of the humerus by extending the skin incision 6 to 7 cm proximal to the lateral epicondyle (see Fig. 3-1).

1. Enter Kocher's interval and elevate the extensor carpi ulnaris.
2. The common extensor tendon is identified and reflected anteriorly exposing the capsule (**Fig. 3-8A,B**).
3. The insertion of the extensor carpi radialis longus and the distal fibers of the brachioradialis muscle are released from the lateral column of the distal humerus (**Fig. 3-8C**).
4. The anterior capsule is entered (**Fig. 3-8D**) and released to the extent necessary to expose the anterior joint.
5. Proceed as shown in Figure 3-8B completely elevating the anconeus from the ulna and from its humeral attachment (**Fig. 3-8E**).
6. The triceps is easily elevated from the posterior humerus in the normal situation and even in posttraumatic contractures it can be elevated with a periosteal elevator without much additional difficulty (**Fig. 3-8F**).
7. The lateral collateral ligament is released from the humeral origin as a separate structure or, if prior surgery has caused scarring, it is released with the common extensor tendon complex (**Fig. 3-8G**).

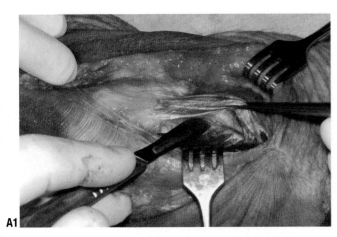

A1

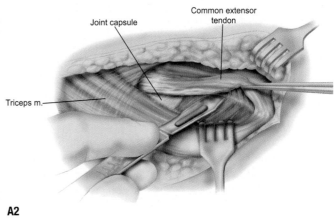

A2

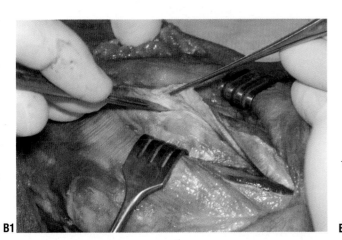

B1

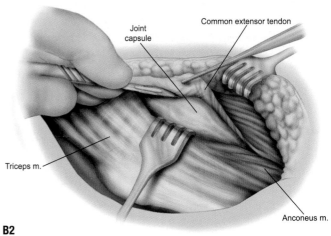

B2

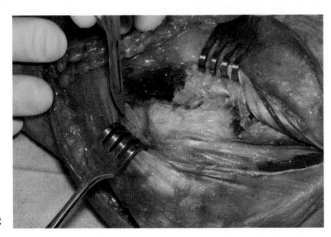

C

FIGURE 3-8

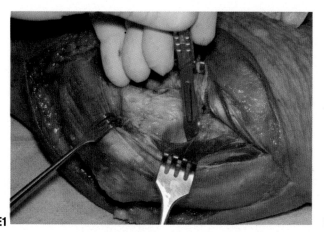

D1

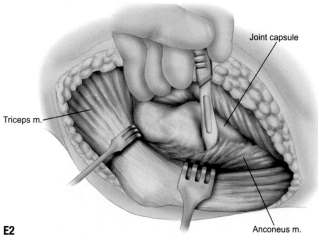

D2

Common extensor tendon

Capsule

Triceps m.

Anconeus m.

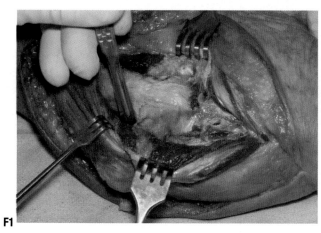

E1

Joint capsule

Triceps m.

Anconeus m.

E2

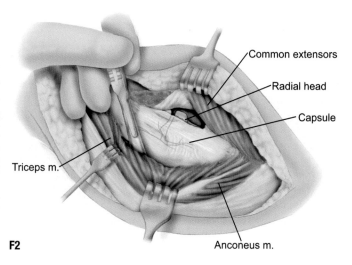

F1

Common extensors

Radial head

Capsule

Triceps m.

Anconeus m.

F2

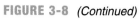

FIGURE 3-8 (Continued)

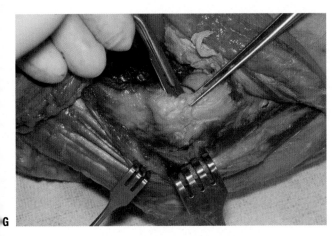
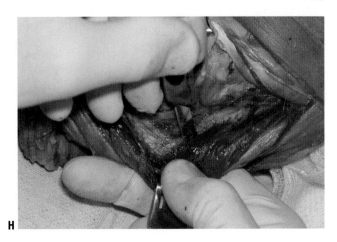

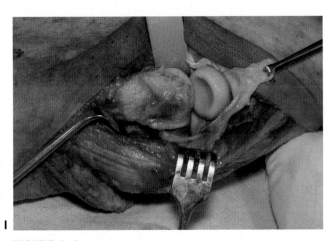

FIGURE 3-8 *(Continued)*

8. The anterior and posterior capsules are then completely incised. We have found it necessary to release approximately 25% of lateral triceps attachment to the ulna to allow the triceps to invert with the maneuver **(Fig. 3-8H)**.
9. A varus supinatory stress is applied to the elbow, which then opens like a book hinging on the medial ulnar collateral ligament and common flexor muscles **(Fig. 3-8I)**. The triceps remains attached to the ulna. Inspect the ulnar nerve to be sure it is not being compressed. If it is, release it from the cubital tunnel.

Mayo Modified Extensile Kocher Posterior-Lateral Exposure

The Mayo (R.S. Bryan) modification of the Kocher approach consists of reflection and release of the extensor mechanism from the tip of the olecranon in a fashion similar to that described for the Mayo approach (5). If reflected, the triceps must be securely reattached to bone. Further, when the Mayo modified Kocher release has been performed, the ulnar nerve must be exposed and released as necessary to avoid compression with varus angular forearm manipulation.

Indictions   More extensile exposure is required than has been obtained with the previous steps.

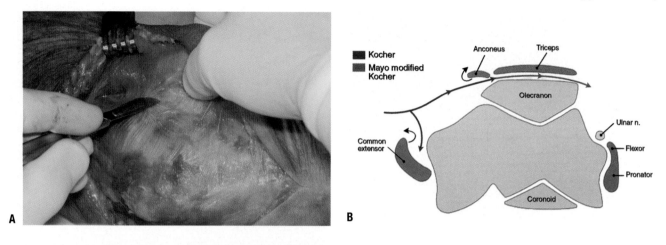

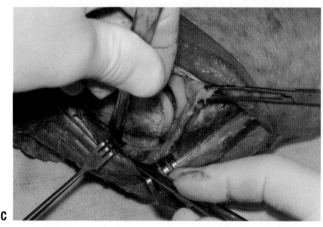

A

C

FIGURE 3-9

B

Technique

1. Incision: medial and lateral skin flaps are elevated using the knife in a flattened disposition to avoid cutting through the skin **(Fig. 3-9A,B)** and is protected or translocated according to the merits of the case.
2. The triceps muscle is elevated laterally and the humeral attachment of the triceps muscle is released **(Fig. 3-9C)**.
3. The triceps-anconeus muscle sleeve is sharply reflected from the tip of the olecranon **(Fig. 3-9D)**.
4. The entire extensor mechanism, including anconeus, is thus reflected from lateral to medial **(Fig. 3-9E)**.
   - *Note:* Lateral collateral ligament detachment from the humerus is optional depending on the pathology **(Fig. 3-9F)**.
5. Flexing the elbow rotating the ulna and removing the tip of the olecranon exposes the articular surface and the posterior humerus **(Fig. 3-9G)**.

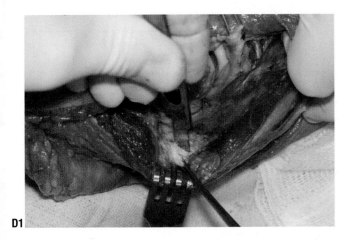

D1

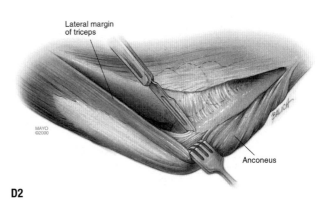

Lateral margin of triceps

Anconeus

MAYO ©2000

D2

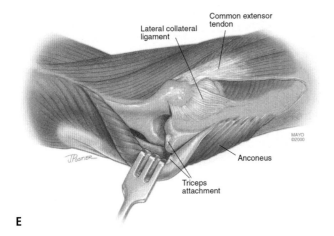

Lateral collateral ligament

Common extensor tendon

Anconeus

Triceps attachment

MAYO ©2000

E

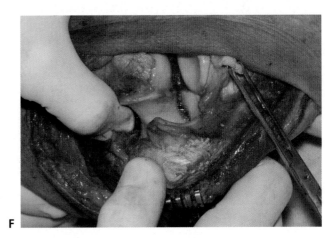

F

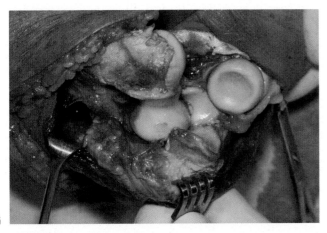

G

FIGURE 3-9 *(Continued)*

POSTERIOR-MEDIAL EXPOSURE

The Mayo Approach (Bryan-Morrey).

Indications

Ankylosis release, total elbow arthroplasty, open reduction internal fixation (ORIF) medial column, and distal humeral fractures.

Position

The patient is supine with arm across the chest.

Landmarks

Medial epicondyle, olecranon, and subcutaneous borer of ulna.

Technique

1. Incision: 7 cm proximal and 7 cm distal and just medial to the tip of the olecranon.
2. The ulnar nerve is released from the margin of the triceps and elevated from its bed **(Fig. 3-10A)**. The cubital tunnel retinaculum is split and the nerve is released to the first motor branch. A subcutaneous pocket is developed, the intermuscular septum is removed **(Fig. 3-10B)**, and the nerve is translated anteriorly.
3. A sleeve of tissue consisting of the forearm fascia and ulnar periosteum is elevated from the medial margin of the ulna.
4. The attachment of the triceps to the olecranon is released by sharp dissection **(Fig. 3-10C)**.
5. The distal forearm fascia and ulnar periosteum are elevated from the ulna.
6. The extensor mechanism and capsule continue to be reflected from the lateral epicondyle and the anconeus is released from the ulna **(Fig. 3-10D)**.

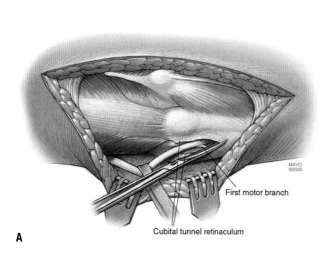

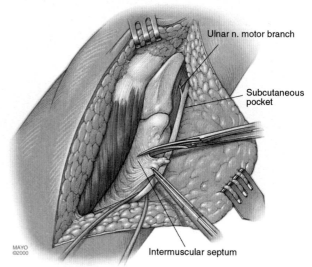

A

B

FIGURE 3-10

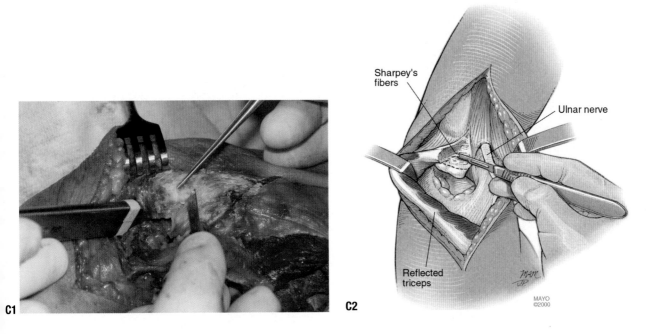

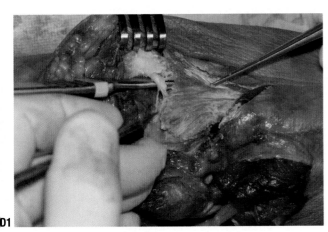

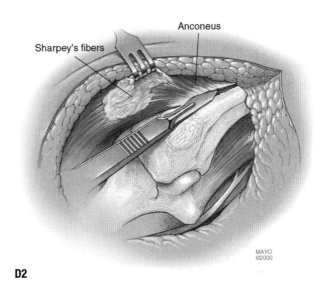

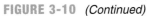

FIGURE 3-10 *(Continued)*

● ***Pearls/Pitfalls:*** For linked total elbow arthroplasty, the lateral and medial collateral ligaments are released and the extensor mechanism is reflected lateral to the epicondyle (**Fig. 3-10E**). The elbow is flexed and the tip of the olecranon is removed to expose the joint (**Fig. 3-10F**).

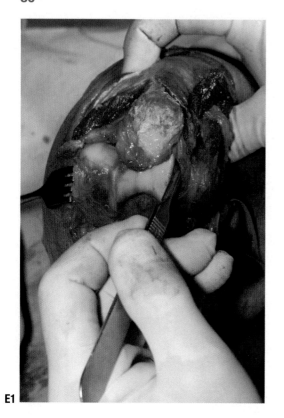

E1

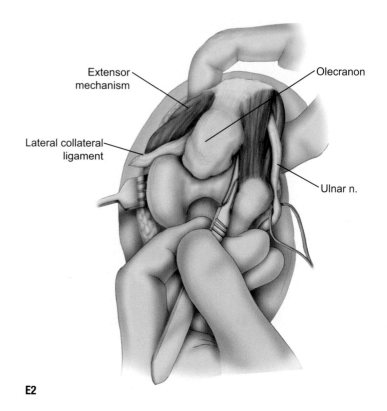

E2

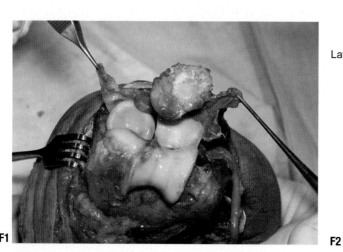

F1

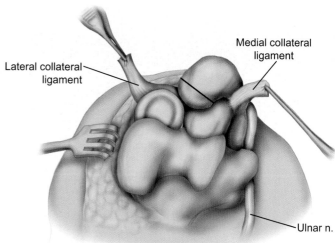

F2

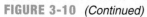

FIGURE 3-10   *(Continued)*

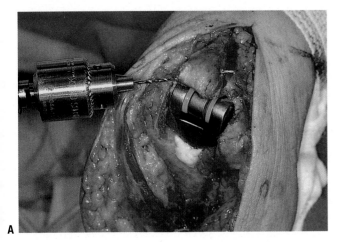

A

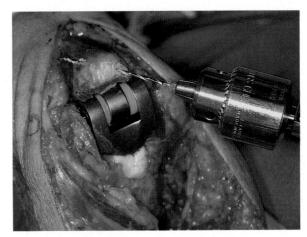

B

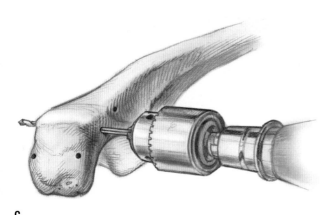

C

FIGURE 3-11 *(Continued)*

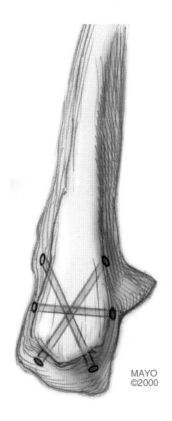

MAYO
©2000

Comment

In every instance in which the triceps has been completely reflected, it is necessary to securely reattach the insertion site to the olecranon with a crisscross type of suture.

1. Drill holes about 3 cm in length are placed in a cruciate fashion in the olecranon from proximal to distal (**Fig. 3-11A,B**).
2. A third transverse hole is drilled through the olecranon to secure a second stabilizing suture (**Fig. 3-11C**).
3. The margin of the triceps is first grasped with an Alis clamp and brought over the olecranon.
4. A no. 5 nonabsorbable suture is introduced with a straight needle from distal lateral to proximal medial.
5. The suture is first brought through the tip of the olecranon and passes through the triceps tissue at its anatomic attachment site with the elbow in 90 degrees (**Fig. 3-11D**).

- *Note:* We prefer to displace the tendon somewhat medially at the time of reattachment after the Bryan-Morrey reflection and somewhat laterally after the modified Kocher release.

6. A locked suture is first placed in the tendon followed by a second locked suture placed more proximally in the contoured portion of the tendon. The suture passes through the triceps tendon opposite its locked attachment site **(Fig. 3-11E)**.

7. The suture then enters the opposite hole in the olecranon now being passed from proximal to distal **(Fig. 3-11F)**. After the suture has emerged from the second hole in the olecranon, it is brought back over the top of the ulna through the soft tissue distal expansion of the extensor sleeve **(Fig. 3-11G)**.

- *Note:* Care is taken to tie this stitch off to the side of the subcutaneous border of the ulna to avoid irritation or skin erosion.

8. To snugly stabilize the triceps insertion against the olecranon, a second suture is placed transversely across the ulna; again, beginning on the side from which the triceps reflection began **(Fig. 3-11H)**. It is brought back across the triceps tendon in a transverse fashion with a locked stitch in the mid/lateral portion of the tendon **(Fig. 3-11I)**. The suture then passes through the lateral margin of the triceps of flexion, again with the knots off the subcutaneous border.

All sutures are tied with the elbow in 90 degrees of flexion, again with the knots off the subcutaneous border.

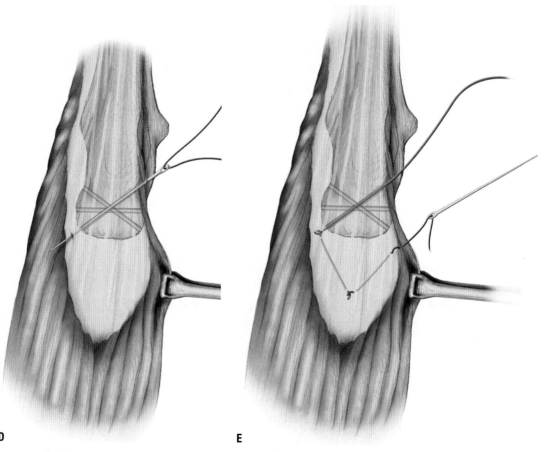

D   E

FIGURE 3-11 *(Continued)*

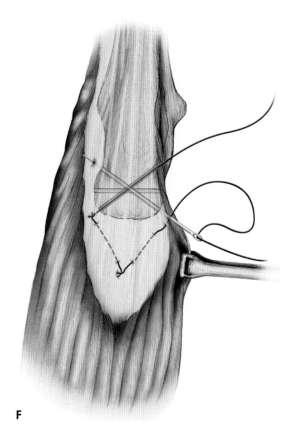

F

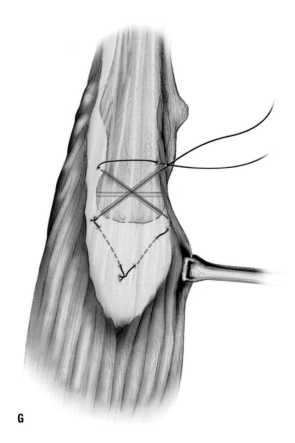

G

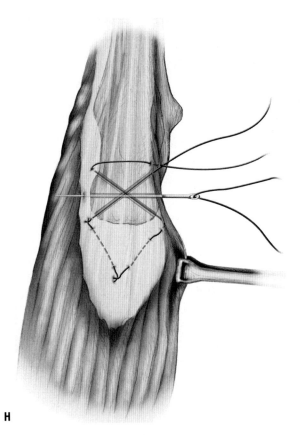

H

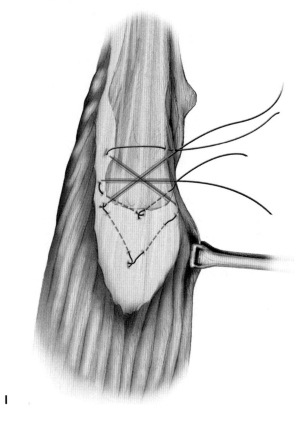

I

FIGURE 3-11 *(Continued)*

MEDIAL EXPOSURES

There are two relevant exposures to the medial aspect of the elbow. The first is a focused exposure to allow identity and management of coronoid fractures. The second is a more extensile medial approach which affords an opportunity to release the anterior and posterior elbow capsules as well as manage fractures and a broader spectrum of pathology.

Focused Medial Exposure of the Coronoid

While this is a limited exposure, it can be modified to a more extensile exposure as described below.

Indications   Coronoid fracture, specifically application of a buttress plate.

Landmark   Medial epicondyle, ulnar nerve, and flexor carpi ulnaris.

Position   The patient is supine with arm on an elbow board.

Technique

1. Skin incision proceeds from 5 cm proximal to 7 cm distal to the medial epicondyle passing posterior to the epicondyle near the midline.
2. The medial epicondyle is identified along with the ulnar nerve. The ulnar nerve is mobilized from its bed, the cubital tunnel retinaculum is released (**Fig. 3-12A**).
3. The flexor carpi ulnaris is split allowing the ulnar nerve to be further mobilized. The sublime tubercle is palpated in the depths of the wound (**Fig. 3-12B**).
4. Sharp dissection frees the muscle mass from the anterior (**Fig. 3-12C**) and posterior (**Fig. 3-12D**) aspects of the capsule.

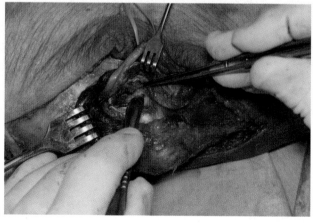

A

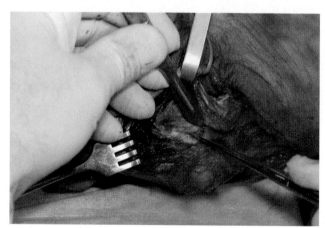

B

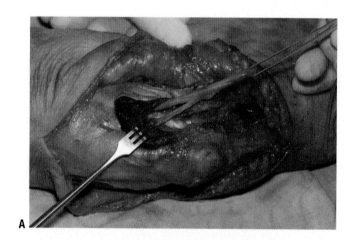

C

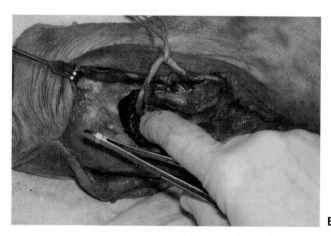

D

FIGURE 3-12

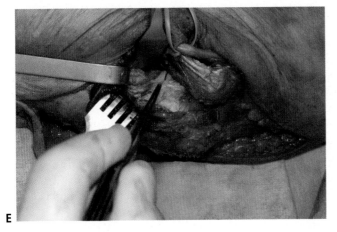
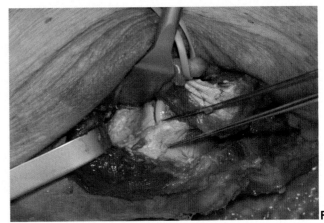

FIGURE 3-12 *(Continued)*

5. The capsule is further identified with a periosteal elevator. The sublime tubercle is identified and the capsule is entered.
6. Releasing the capsule allows clear identity of the coronoid just anterior to the medial collateral ligament (**Fig. 3-12E**).
7. The dissection may be extended distally as necessary to apply the buttress plate or otherwise provide internal fixation for the coronoid.
8. Extension proximally allows adequate exposure to reconstruct the collateral ligament (**Fig. 3-12F**).

Medial Column ("Over the Top," "Hotchkiss") (6)

Indications   Access to the coronoid with an intact radial head, anterior capsule release if ulnar nerve pathology is also to be addressed, anterior and posterior medial ectopic bone excision, and anterior, posterior capsule excision.

- *Note*
  - It is not a good approach if there is need of excision of heterotopic bone from the lateral elbow joint or if access to the radial head is needed.
  - Conversion or extension between the Bryan-Morrey, Mayo, and the Hotchkiss approach is readily accomplished but rarely indicated.

Landmarks   The medial supracondylar ridge of the humerus, the medial intermuscular septum, the origin of the flexor pronator muscle mass, and the ulnar nerve.

Position   The patient is supine with extremity supported by a hand or elbow table (**Fig. 3-13A**).

Technique

1. Skin incision 5 cm distal and proximal to medial epicondyle.
2. The medial intermuscular septum is identified. Anterior to the septum superficial to the fascia (and not in the subdermal tissue), the medial antebrachial cutaneous nerve is identified and protected **(Fig. 3-13B)**. The line of reflection is identified distally at the raphe between the flexor carpi ulnaris and the pronator teres. The intermuscular septum is identified proximally.
   - *Note:* If the patient has had previous surgery, the ulnar nerve is usually most easily identified proximally before proceeding distally.
3. The ulnar nerve is mobilized. The medial intermuscular septum is exposed anteriorly and posterior and then released for a distance of about 5 cm proximally **(Fig. 3-13C)**.
4. Locate the medial supracondylar ridge and begin elevating the anterior brachialis muscle with a periosteal elevator.
5. Subperiosteally elevate enough of the anterior structures of the distal humeral region to allow the placement of a wide retractor. The median nerve, brachial artery, and vein are superficial to the brachialis muscle and need not be identified.
6. The flexor pronator muscle mass is divided in line with its fibers along the raphe which separates the pronator and flexor carpi ulnaris muscles, leaving a portion of the flexor carpi ulnaris tendon attached to the epicondyle **(Fig. 3-13D)**.
   - *Note:* A small cuff of fibrous origin can be left on the supracondylar ridge as the muscle is elevated to facilitate reattachment when closing.
7. The pronator muscle is elevated from the capsule encountering the brachialis muscle which has been mobilized and retracted laterally **(Fig. 3-13E)**.

FIGURE 3-13   **A**

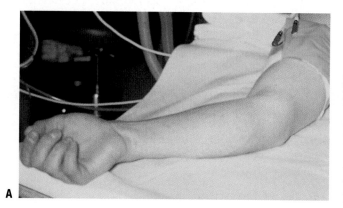

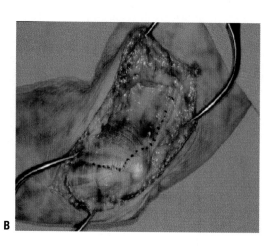

B

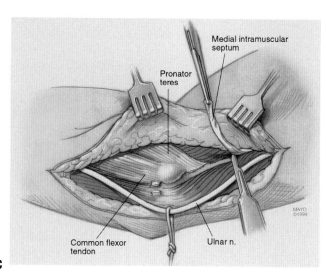

C

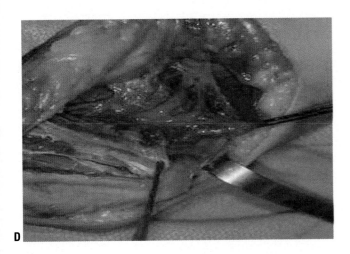

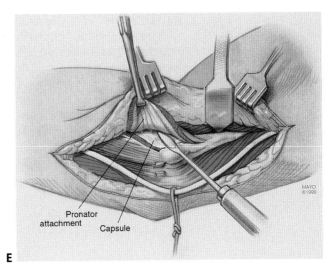

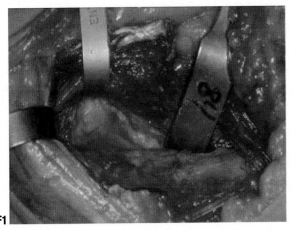

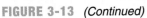

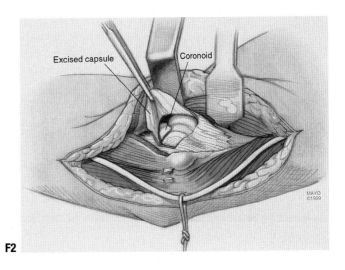

FIGURE 3-13   (Continued)

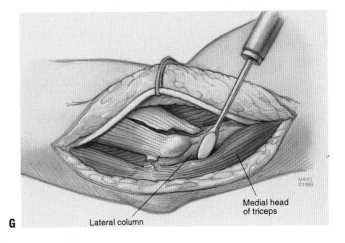

- *Note:* A proximal, transverse incision in the lacertus fibrosis may also be needed to adequately mobilize the brachialis muscle.

8. As the pronator muscle is elevated from the capsule, the entire anterior capsule is exposed (**Fig. 3-13F**).
9. If necessary, the posterior capsule may be exposed by elevating the triceps from its lateral distal humeral attachment (**Fig. 3-13G**).

RESULTS

There have been limited attempts to document the efficacy of one or the other of the various types of triceps-sparing approaches. In the original description we compared the clinical result of the Mayo approach to that of the triceps splitting or transverse release of the triceps attachment (5). There were no triceps disruptions after approximately 75 procedures done with the triceps being released in continuity (Mayo approach) compared with an approximately 20% complication rate when the triceps was released transversely. Wolfe and Ranawat (7) have also observed no instances of triceps insufficiency with their modification of this approach. The use of the Mayo medial exposure was also shown to have improved triceps strength after total elbow arthroplasty (8). This manner of exposing the elbow was found to be associated with approximately 20% greater extension strength than with the Campbell fascial turn-down (Van Gorder) type of exposure.

COMPLICATIONS

One beauty of the previously described exposures is that they are relatively free of complication. Today most problems are related to the pathology rather than to the surgical approach.

Difficult ankylosis release procedures are associated with a significant amount of swelling as often occurs in patients undergoing total elbow arthroplasty. Wound healing is generally not a problem, however, and is related to the presence of prior incisions and the magnitude of the dissection, as is typical for release of the stiff elbow. The elevation of the large medial and lateral flaps does not retard healing but occasionally can give rise to subcutaneous seroma. Rarely does this need to be addressed or drained.

The infection rate after total elbow arthroplasty has been reduced at our institution from a high of 11% in 1970 to approximately 3% over the last 10 years (9). This reduction is coincident with adopting the Mayo approach to the elbow, but other technique changes have occurred in this period, including using antibiotic-impregnated cement and splinting the elbow in extension.

Injury to the ulnar nerve appears to be more common in those instances in which the ulnar nerve is not exposed and the elbow is flexed on the medial collateral ligament, as with the classical extensile Kocher approach (9,10). Simply exposing the ulnar nerve, although it decreases the complication, does not completely obviate it. The theoretical disadvantage of the Mayo approach, which allows translocation of the ulnar nerve, is that this maneuver devascularizes the nerve and the dissection itself may cause ulnar nerve irritation. Having used this particular exposure in more than 500 cases, the incidence of permanent ulnar nerve injury with motor dysfunction is less than 1%. I am, therefore, comfortable exposing and moving the ulnar nerve in a subcutaneous pocket as an essential and integral part of the Mayo triceps-sparing approach.

Although posterior interosseous nerve palsy is known to occur with some approaches to the radial head (11–13), the complication is virtually unheard of when the joint is exposed through Kocher's interval.

Triceps disruption is very uncommon with either the Mayo modified extensile Kocher exposure or the Mayo medial-to-lateral type of approach. The incidence of triceps disruption after total elbow replacement, therefore, is less than 1% in our experience (14). If, however, the triceps should become disrupted after either of the procedures described earlier, if adequate tissue is present, it may be reattached as described for the primary procedure (14). If the remaining tissue is inadequate, triceps power is restored by either an anconeus slide or an Achilles tendon allograft reconstruction (15).

REFERENCES

1. Morrey BF. Surgical exposures. In: Morrey BF, ed. *Master Techniques in Orthopedic Surgery: The Elbow*, 2nd ed. Philadelphia: Lippincott Williams & Wilkins, 2002.
2. Morrey BF. Surgical exposures of the elbow. In: Morrey BF, ed. *The Elbow and Its Disorders*, 3rd ed. Philadelphia: WB Saunders, 2000:109–134.
3. Mansat P, Morrey BF. The column procedure: A limited lateral approach for extrinsic contracture of the elbow. *J Bone Joint Surg* 1998;80A(11):1603–1615.
4. Kocher T. *Text-book of Operative Surgery*, 3rd ed. London: A and C Black, 1911.
5. Bryan RS, Morrey BF. Extensive posterior exposure of the elbow: a triceps-sparing approach. *Clin Orthop* 1982;166:188.

6. Kasparyan NG, Hotchkiss RN. Dynamic skeletal fixation in the upper extremity. *Hand Clin* 1997;13:643–663.
7. Wolfe SW, Ranawat CS. The osteo-anconeus flap: an approach for total elbow arthroplasty. *J Bone Joint Surg* 1990;72A:684.
8. Morrey BF, Askew LJ, An KN. Strength function after elbow arthroplasty. *Clin Orthop* 1988;234:43–50.
9. Morrey BF, Bryan RS. Complications of total elbow arthroplasty. *Clin Orthop* 1982;170:204–212.
10. Ewald FC, Jacobs MA. Total elbow arthroplasty. *Clin Orthop* 1984;182:137.
11. Hoppenfield S, deBoer P. *Surgical Exposures in Orthopaedics: The Anatomic Approach*. Philadelphia: J.B. Lippincott Co., 1984.
12. Kaplan EB. Surgical approaches to the proximal end of the radius and its use in fractures of the head and neck of the radius. *J Bone Joint Surg* 1941;23:86.
13. Strachan JH, Ellis BW. Vulnerability of the posterior interosseous nerve during radial head resection. *J Bone Joint Surg* 1971;53B:320.
14. Celli A, Arash A, Adams RA, et al. Triceps insufficiency following total elbow arthroplasty. *J Bone Joint Surg Am* 2005;87(9):1957–1964.
15. Sanchez-Sotelo J, Morrey BF. Surgical techniques for reconstruction of chronic insufficiency of the triceps—Rotation flap using anconeus and tendo Achillis allograft. *J Bone Joint Surg* 2002;84B(8):1116–1120.

4 Humerus

Bernard F. Morrey

I n this chapter the theme is extensile type of exposure to the anterior and posterior aspects of the humerus. Limited portions of these exposures, of course, may be employed depending on the pathology being addressed. The flexibility, expressed in this chapter, is quite effective in addressing the majority of pathology encountered in the brachium.

EXTENSILE ANTERIOR LATERAL APPROACH TO THE HUMERUS

The most common and useful approach to the anterior aspect of the humerus is through the antero-lateral interval. The value of this exposure is that it can be extended through the deltopectoral interval to expose the proximal humerus and extension distally allows adequate access even to the anterior aspect of the elbow joint.

Indications

Fracture of the proximal mid and midshafts of the humerus, malignancy, osteomyelitis, access to shift for periprosthetic fracture, and revision.

Position

The patient is placed in the semi-sitting, barber chair position or supine on the table with the arm resting to the side and the forearm across the abdomen.

- *Note:* By tilting the table 10 degrees to the contralateral direction easier access is provided.

Preparation

For the proximal exposures, the shoulder and arm is draped free sufficiently proximally to allow extension to the clavicle and to expose the shoulder joint if necessary.

Landmarks

The deltopectoral groove proximally, the lateral margin of the biceps, and the mobile wad distally.

Technique

Proximal Portion

1. Skin incision: beginning at, or just distal to, the coracoid proceed distal and lateral in the del-topectoral groove curving distally at the insertion of the deltoid following the lateral margin of the biceps (**Fig. 4-1A**).
2. The deltopectoral groove is identified and is entered. Proximally the medial margin of the deltoid is defined along with the cephalic vein. This is done by blunt and sharp dissection (**Fig. 4-1B**). The insertion of the pectoralis major muscle is identified.

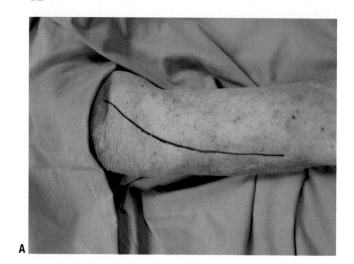

A

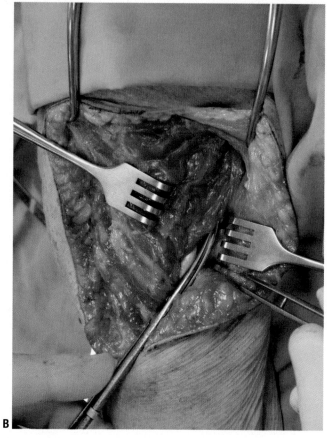

B

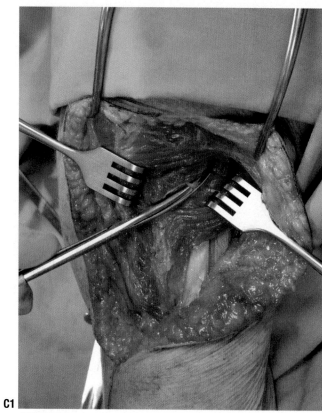

C1

FIGURE 4-1

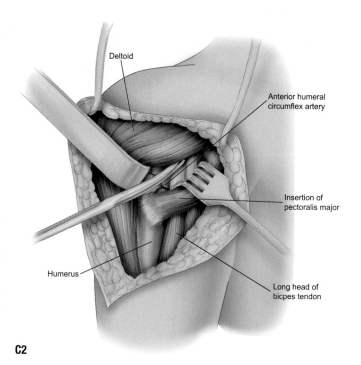

Deltoid

Anterior humeral
circumflex artery

Insertion of
pectoralis major

Humerus

Long head of
bicpes tendon

C2

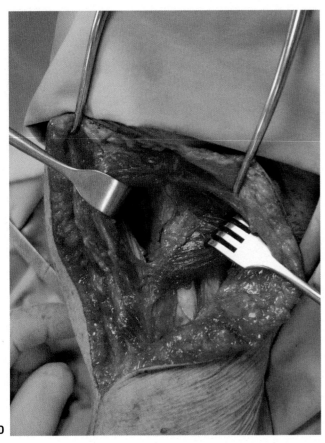

D   FIGURE 4-1 *(Continued)*

3. The proximal humerus is exposed medially by incising the humeral insertion of the pectoralis insertion and laterally by mobilizing and elevating the medial margin of the deltoid. This allows exposure of the humerus proximal to the deltoid insertion. The long head of the biceps tendon is identified in the medial aspect of the exposure (**Fig. 4-1C**). The anterior circumflex humeral artery is present at the proximal aspect of the pectoralis insertion on the humerus.
4. Retracting the deltoid laterally and the pectoralis major medially allows ready access to the proximal humeral shaft distal to the subscapularis muscle and lateral to the long head of the biceps tendon (**Fig. 4-1D**).

   - *Pearls/Pitfalls:* If a greater medial/lateral exposure is required, the pectoralis tendinous attachment may be released from the humerus and the deltoid insertion may be elevated from the lateral aspect of the humerus. Care must be taken to avoid injury to the axillary nerve with reflection and retraction of the deltoid.

Distal Extension—Anterior/Lateral Humeral Shaft

1. For a distal expansion the skin incision is carried distally over the lateral margin of the biceps muscle to the extent needed (see Fig. 4-1A).
2. The brachial fascia is split distally exposing the lateral margin of the biceps. The lateral brachial cutaneous nerve is identified and protected as it crosses anterolaterally to the biceps muscle near the tendinous junction (**Fig. 4-2A**).
3. The interval between the biceps and the brachialis muscles is identified and developed by blunt and sharp dissection. The biceps is retracted medially and, in so doing, the musculocutaneous nerve is identified between the two muscles and is retracted medially with the biceps muscle (**Fig. 4-2B**).
4. Exposure of the humeral shaft is accomplished by either splitting the brachialis muscles longitudinally or elevating its lateral attachment from the intermuscular septum of the humerus. The dis-

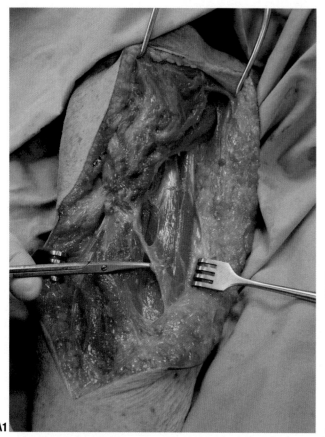

A1

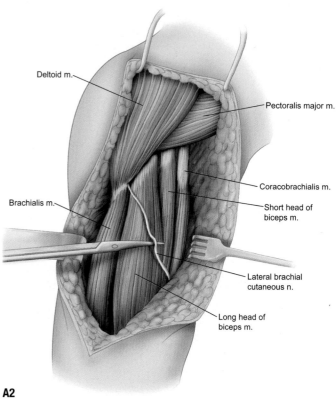

A2

Deltoid m.

Pectoralis major m.

Coracobrachialis m.

Short head of
biceps m.

Brachialis m.

Lateral brachial
cutaneous n.

Long head of
biceps m.

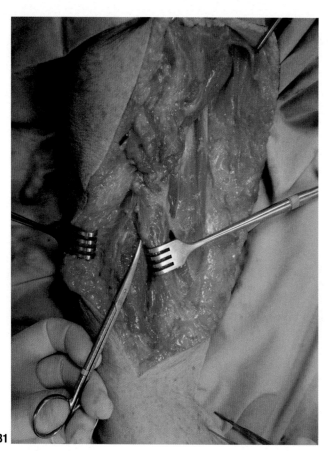

B1

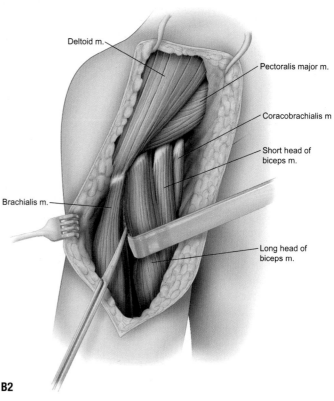

B2

Deltoid m.

Pectoralis major m.

Coracobrachialis m

Short head of
biceps m.

Brachialis m.

Long head of
biceps m.

FIGURE 4-2

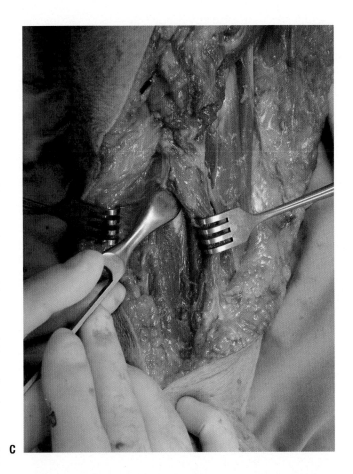

C

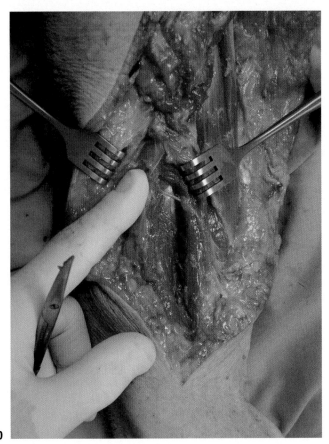

D

FIGURE 4-2 (Continued)

section continues with subperiosteal elevation of muscle medially and laterally thus exposing the proximal half of the humerus **(Fig. 4-2C)**.

- *Pearls/Pitfalls:* The site of the radial nerve perforation of the intermuscular septum should be noted and excessive traction at this locus should be avoided by palpation **(Fig. 4-2D)**. The safest exposure of the shaft is brachialis muscle splitting as this protects the radial nerve from injury.

More Distal Extension

5. If a more distal or extensive exposure is required, the interval between the brachialis and the brachioradialis is further developed at the site of the radial nerve as it emerges from the intermuscular septum.
6. The radial nerve is palpated or observed on the undersurface of the brachioradialis and is exposed by sharp dissection **(Fig. 4-3A)**.
7. The brachialis muscle is retracted medially protecting the cutaneous branch of the musculocutaneous nerve and the humeral shaft is exposed with a periosteal elevator. The radial nerve is protected and retracted laterally **(Fig. 4-3B)**.
8. The humeral shaft may be further exposed by sharp dissection proximally to the lateral origin of the brachialis muscle on the humerus which is confluent with the deltoid attachment distally **(Fig. 4-3C)**. Both attachments may be released to afford complete access to the entire proximal two-thirds of the humeral shaft **(Fig. 4-3D)**.

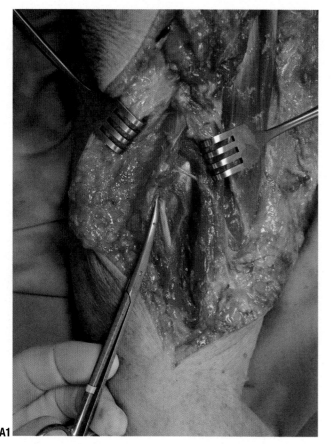

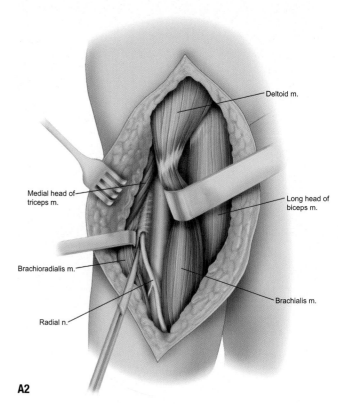

A1

A2

Deltoid m.

Medial head of triceps m.

Long head of biceps m.

Brachioradialis m.

Brachialis m.

Radial n.

FIGURE 4-3

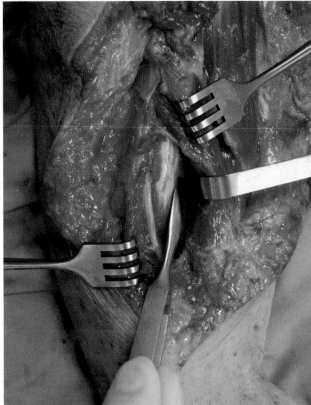

B

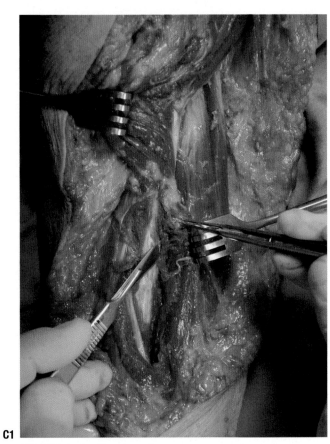

C1

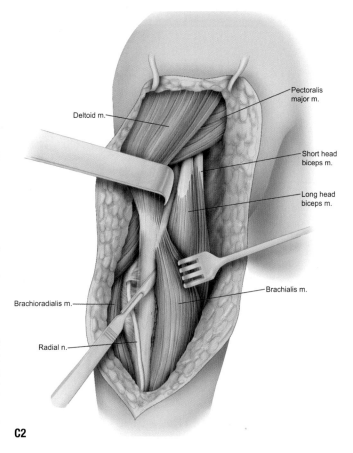

C2

FIGURE 4-3 *(Continued)*

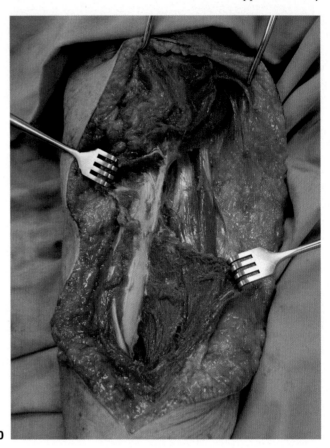

FIGURE 4-3 *(Continued)*   **D**

POSTERIOR EXPOSURES

The Extensile Posterior Medial Exposure of the Humerus (Mayo Exposure)

We have found this approach extremely valuable for exposing the posterior aspect of the humerus since it allows extension distally by employing the triceps reflexion exposure from the olecranon. The unique (Mayo) feature is to the manner of exposing and protecting the radial nerve.

Indications   Fractures of the posterior aspect of the humerus, extensile exposure for revision of total elbow, and humeral and ulnar components.

Position   The patient is supine and the arm is brought across the chest. The surgical table is tilted 10 degrees to the contralateral side.

Landmarks   Olecranon, medial epicondyle distally.

Technique

1. Skin incision: proximally from the posterior medial aspect of the triceps in line with the long head, distally between the medial epicondyle and tip of the olecranon **(Fig. 4-4A)**.
   - *Note:* The skin excision can be extended distally over the subcutaneous border of the ulna if required. This provides an extensile exposure that can include the elbow joint and entire humeral shaft.
2. The skin and subcutaneous tissue is entered. The ulnar nerve is identified distally at the cubital tunnel and skin flaps are raised medially and distally **(Fig. 4-4B)**.

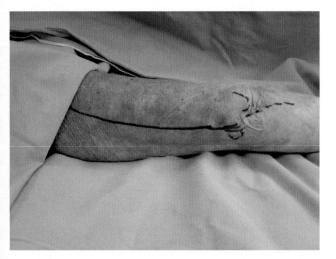

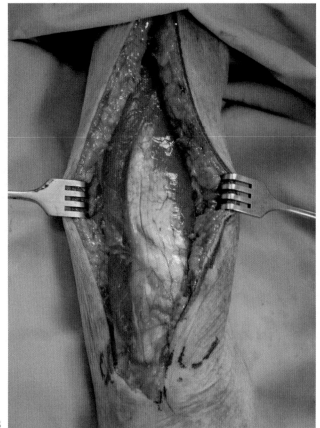

B

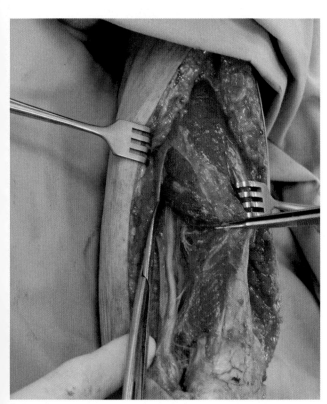

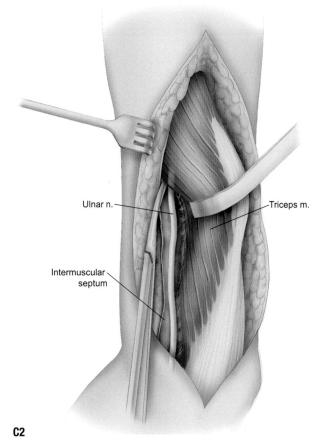

Ulnar n.

Triceps m.

Intermuscular
septum

C2

FIGURE 4-4

3. The ulnar nerve is released as it lies on the anterior surface of the intermuscular septum. The nerve is mobilized including release of the ligament of Struthers proximally. The nerve is identified distally to the level of the cubital tunnel but the cubital tunnel retinaculum is not released unless an extensile exposure is performed distally (**Fig. 4-4C**).

4. With sharp dissection, the medial head of the triceps is freed from the distal aspect of the humerus (**Fig. 4-4D**). The triceps muscle is elevated and retracted laterally.

5. The muscle is then easily elevated from the entire posterior medial aspect of the humerus with a periosteal elevator (**Fig. 4-4E**).

   ● *Note:* The critical departure of this exposure is that laterally elevating the radial nerve subperiosteally provides more proximal exposure of the humerus.

6. At this point the triceps position is restored and is retracted medially. A subcutaneous flap is elevated laterally. The location of the radial nerve is identified by palpation as it penetrates the intermuscular septum (**Fig. 4-4F**).

7. The triceps muscle is then again elevated and further reflected from medial to lateral. The radial nerve is identified at the site of penetration of the intermuscular septum laterally which is then elevated from the lateral aspect of the humerus (**Fig. 4-4G**). This affords greater access to the proximal aspect of the humerus (**Fig. 4-4H**).

8. The radial nerve is protected and retracted laterally for greater exposure of the posterior proximal aspect of the humerus (**Fig. 4-4I**).

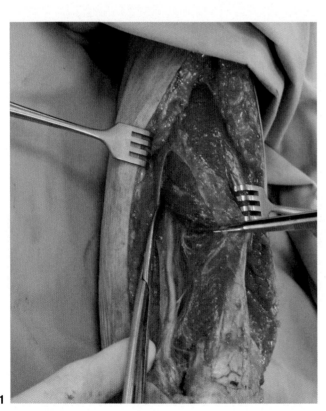

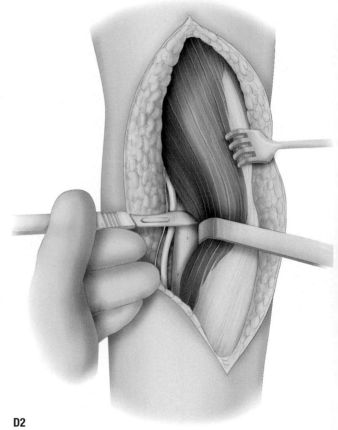

D1

D2

FIGURE 4-4 *(Continued)*

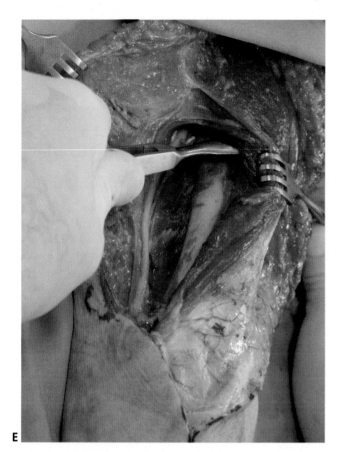

E

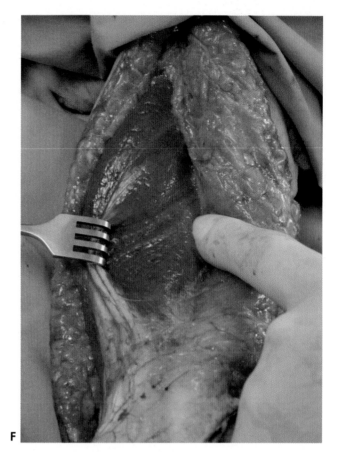

F

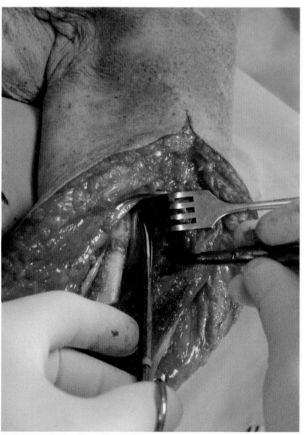

G1

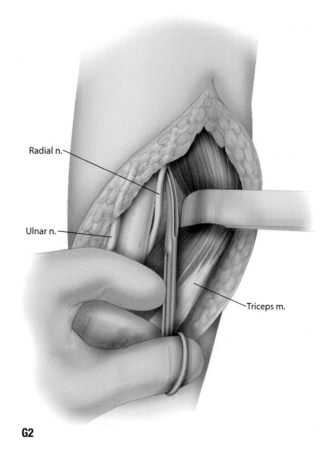

G2

Radial n.

Ulnar n.

Triceps m.

FIGURE 4-4 *(Continued)*

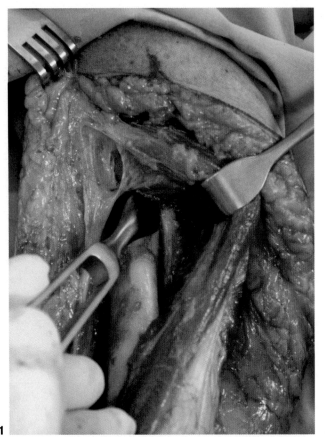

H1

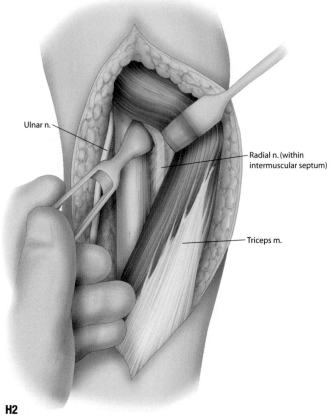

Ulnar n.

Radial n. (within intermuscular septum)

Triceps m.

H2

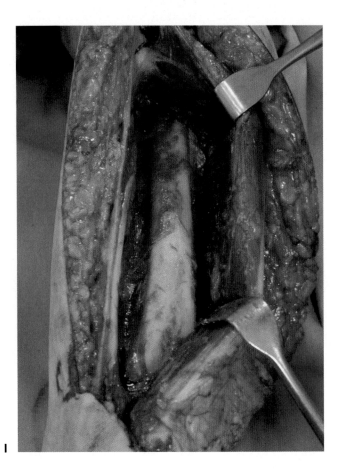

I

FIGURE 4-4 *(Continued)*

- *Pearls/Pitfalls:* If concern regarding impingement or pressure on the radial nerve exists the nerve is exposed and decompressed by incising the intermuscular septum. Further, since the radial nerve has been freed from the intermuscular septum, it is safely protected and is retracted medially with the brachioradialis muscle distally.

9. Closure: The muscle is allowed to return to its anatomic position. If the triceps has been reflected, the recommended reattachment is described in the elbow exposure chapter (see Fig. 3-11). Otherwise, only a subcutaneous and skin closure is required.

Distal Extension   If more distal exposure is necessary, the triceps may be reflected from the tip of the olecranon using the Bryan-Morrey technique. This allows complete exposure of the entire posterior humerus, elbow joint, and proximal ulna.

Posterior Triceps Splitting Approach

This along with exposure of the ulna is the easiest and safest exposure of the upper extremity.

Indications   Mid and distal shaft fractures, when extended distally, can be used for exposure for total elbow arthroplasty and fracture of the midshaft of the humerus.

Position   The patient is supine and the arm brought across the chest. The table is tilted 10 degrees away from the involved extremity.

Landmarks   Tip of olecranon, ulnar nerve, and medial and lateral epicondyle.

Technique

1. Skin incision: a longitudinal skin incision is made from the tip of the olecranon distally to the posterior aspect of the deltoid proximally. The length is dictated by the pathology (**Fig. 4-5A**).
2. Flaps are elevated medially and laterally and the tendon of the triceps distally and the muscle fibers proximally are identified (**Fig. 4-5B**).
3. A longitudinal incision is made in the tendinous portion of the triceps exposing the posterior aspect of the humerus (**Fig. 4-5C**).

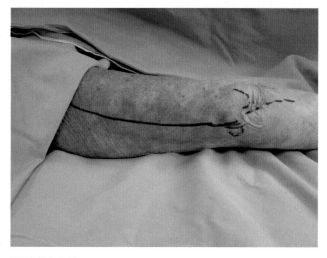
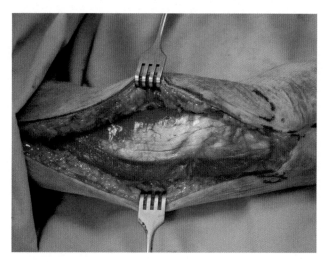

B

FIGURE 4-5

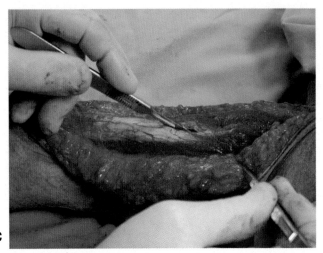

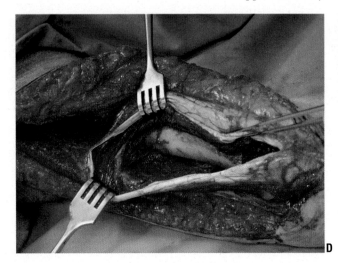

FIGURE 4-5 *(Continued)*

4. The triceps muscle is split proximally and distally. The tendon is incised to the level of its attachment on the olecranon. Subperiosteal dissection medially and laterally exposes the posterior aspect of the humerus **(Fig. 4-5D).**

RECOMMENDED READING

Banks S, Laufman H. *An Atlas of Surgical Exposures of the Extremities*. Philadelphia: W.B. Saunders Co., 1953.

Campbell WC. Incision for exposure of the elbow joint. *Am J Surg* 1932;15:65–67.

Grant JCB. *An Atlas of Anatomy*, 6th ed. Baltimore: Williams & Wilkins Co., 1972.

Gray H. *The Anatomy of the Human Body*, 29th ed. Philadelphia: Lea & Febiger, 1975.

Henry AK. *Extensile Exposure*, 2nd ed. New York: Churchill-Livingstone, Inc., 1963.

Hollinshead WH. *Anatomy for Surgeons: The Back and Limbs*, 3rd ed. Philadelphia: Harper & Row, 1982.

Hoppenfeld S, deBoer P. *Surgical Exposures in Orthopaedics: The Anatomical Approach*, 1st ed. Philadelphia: JB Lippincott Co., 1984.

Reckling FW, Reckling JB, Mohr MC. *Orthopedic Anatomy and Surgical Approaches*. St. Louis: Mosby Year-book, 1990.

Tubiana R, McCullough CJ, Masquelet AC. *An Atlas of Surgical Exposures of the Upper Extremity*. London: Martin Dunitz Publisher, 1990.

5 Shoulder

John William Sperling

ANTERIOR SUPERIOR APPROACH FOR ROTATOR CUFF REPAIR

Indications

- Acromioplasty
- Rotator cuff repair

Position

The patient is carefully positioned in the beach chair position. The waist should be in approximately 45 degrees of flexion and the knees in 30 degrees of flexion. The table may be slightly rolled away from the surgical shoulder.

Landmarks

One should palpate the posterior scapular spine, the lateral border of the acromion, the anterior border of the acromion, and the anterior portion of the clavicle and coracoid. These should be marked out with a marking pen (**Fig. 5-1**). If one is performing arthroscopy prior to an open procedure, one may wish to mark out the standard anterior incision and attempt to place the anterior portal in line with this future incision.

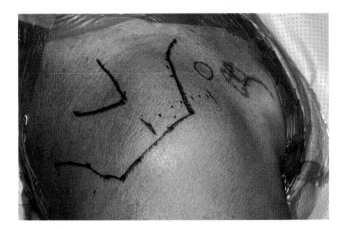

FIGURE 5-1

The landmarks on the shoulder are carefully identified and outlined. A 4 to 5 cm incision is marked out on the shoulder parallel to the lateral border of the acromion.

TECHNIQUE

1. Incision: there is significant variability in the skin incision used for an anterior superior approach to the shoulder including oblique incisions, horizontal incisions, as well as vertical incisions. It is based on the individual preference of the surgeon which incision to use.

2. An incision is made over the superior aspect of the shoulder parallel with the lateral border of the acromion in line with Langer's lines. The length of the skin incision is typically about 4 to 5 cm in length. The skin is incised as well as the fat. Skin flaps are carefully created and mobilized.

3. The deltoid muscle is clearly identified. There is significant variability among surgeons in regard to the manner with which they prefer to take down the deltoid (**Fig. 5-2**). In this example, the deltoid is taken down off the anterior aspect of the acromion with full thickness sleeves (**Fig. 5-3**). It is critical to carefully include both the deep and superficial fascia of the deltoid when this is performed. The surgeon then has the option of splitting the deltoid in line with the fibers starting from the acromioclavicular (AC) joint anteriorly for approximately 3 to 4 cm, or the surgeon has the option of extending the deltoid detachment posteriorly over the lateral border of the acromion. The extent of the deltoid detachment over the lateral border of the acromion can be modified based on the size of the rotator cuff tear. One must be careful to avoid splitting the deltoid more than several centimeters from the acromial border to protect the axillary nerve. The area where the proximal deltoid split is made can be marked with a retention stitch (**Fig. 5-4**). An additional stitch is placed distally in the deltoid split to prevent propagation (**Fig. 5-5**).

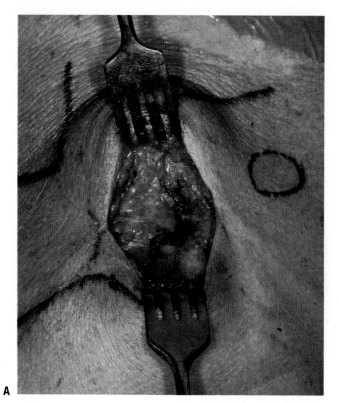

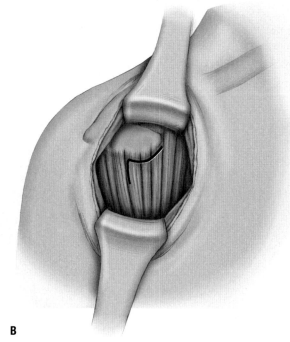

A   B

FIGURE 5-2

A,B: The area of deltoid to be taken off of the acromion is outlined.

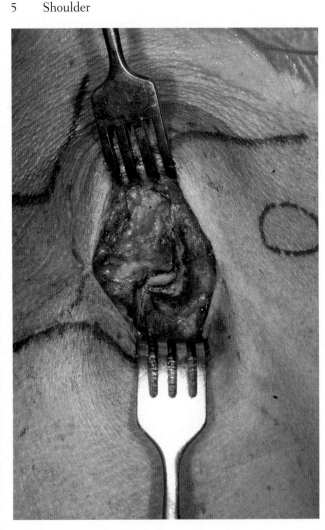

FIGURE 5-3
Full thickness flaps of the deltoid are taken down.

4. An acromioplasty may then be performed based on surgeon preference **(Fig. 5-6)**. Retention stitches are then placed in the rotator cuff tear **(Fig. 5-7)**. The rotator cuff repair can then be performed **(Fig. 5-8)**.

5. For closure, a meticulous repair of the deltoid is required. At the end of the procedure, the deltoid is repaired back in a tendon-to-tendon as well as a tendon-to-bone manner **(Figs. 5-9 to 5-11)**. Drill holes are placed through the acromion with tendon-to-bone stitches. Additionally, the split within the deltoid itself is repaired with side-to-side stitches. Complications in this approach may be related to deltoid dehiscence postoperatively.

- *Pearls/Pitfalls:* A meticulous and strong repair of the deltoid is essential to avoid postoperative dehiscence. It is critical to carefully identify both the deep and superficial deltoid fascia layers during the exposure and repair.

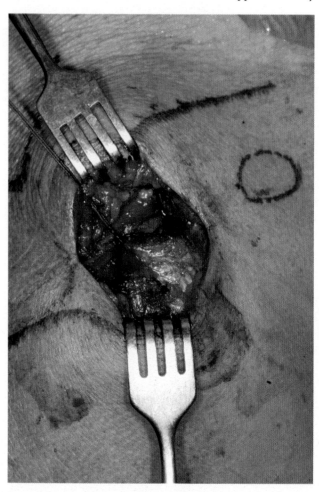

FIGURE 5-4

A marking stitch is placed in the corner of the deltoid to assist in later repair and ensure proper alignment of the deltoid at the time of repair.

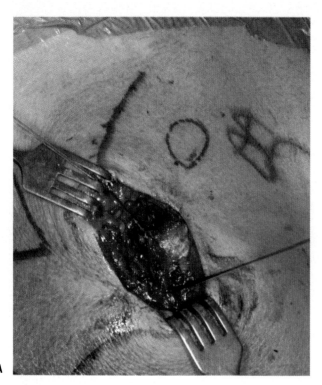

A

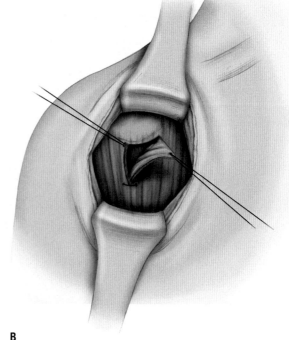

B

FIGURE 5-5

A stitch is placed in the deltoid split distally to prevent propagation.

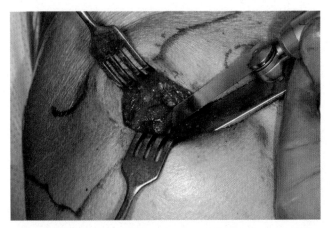

FIGURE 5-6
An acromioplasty may be performed.

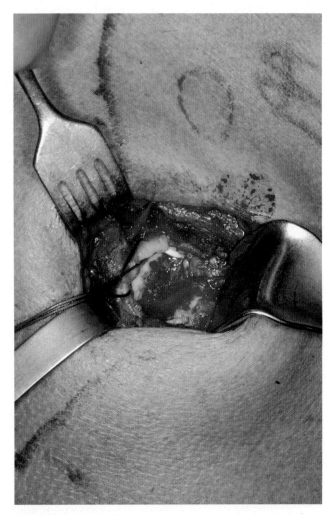

FIGURE 5-7
The rotator cuff tear is identified and retention stitches are placed.

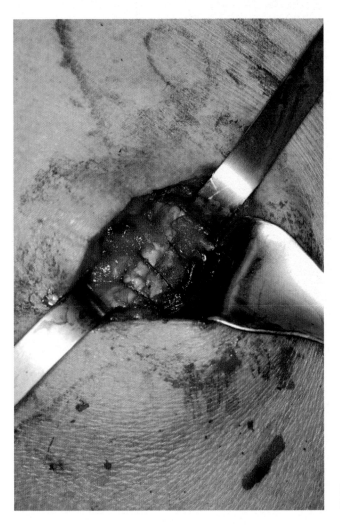

FIGURE 5-8
Rotator cuff repair is performed.

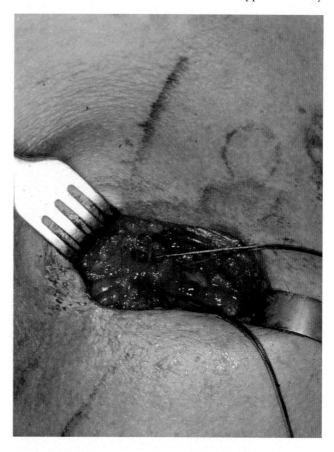

FIGURE 5-9
Drill holes can be placed in the acromion for deltoid repair.

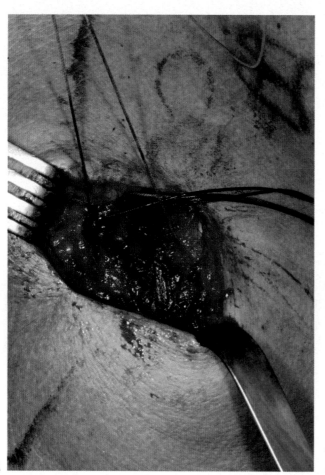

A

B

FIGURE 5-10
The corner of the deltoid is sutured back to its anatomic location.

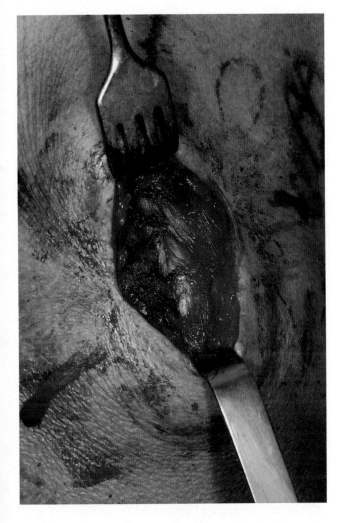

FIGURE 5-11
Final deltoid repair.

HORIZONTAL INCISION FOR CLAVICLE FRACTURES AND NONUNIONS

Indication

Clavicle fracture or nonunion.

Positioning

The patient is placed on the operating room table in the beach chair position. The entire upper extremity is sterilely prepped and draped in the usual manner. The endotracheal tube is positioned to the opposite corner of the mouth. A rolled up towel may also be placed at the medial border of the scapula to make the clavicle more readily accessible.

Technique

1. Incision: the incision runs parallel to Langer's line along the inferior border of the clavicle overlying the fracture nonunion (**Fig. 5-12**). The incision is placed inferiorly so that the scar will not lie directly on top of the instrumentation. The skin is incised as well as the fat. It should be done with great care and caution to carefully identify any supraclavicular nerves (**Fig. 5-13**). These should be carefully preserved. The fascia of the overlying trapezius and the deltoid is carefully identified and incised. Sutures are placed on the fascial ends for later reattachment.
2. Additionally during the course of the procedure, one must be very diligent that the neurovascular structures are present on the undersurface of the clavicle.

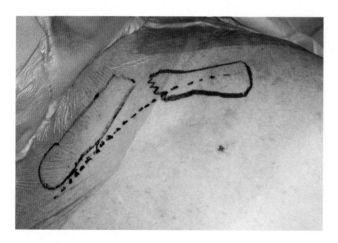

FIGURE 5-12

The skin incision is carefully outlined.

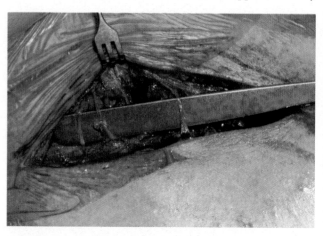

FIGURE 5-13

Great care is taken to preserve the supraclavicular nerves.

3. The fracture is then identified and reduced (**Fig. 5-14**). Internal fixation may be performed based on surgeon preference (**Fig. 5-15**). Closure of the wound is performed (**Fig. 5-16**).

- *Pearls/Pitfalls:* Attention should be made to the identification and preservation of the supraclavicular nerves to avoid potential creation of a neuroma.

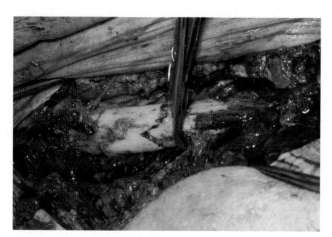

FIGURE 5-14

The fracture ends are reduced and held in place.

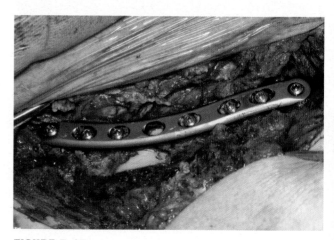

FIGURE 5-15

Open reduction, internal fixation can be performed.

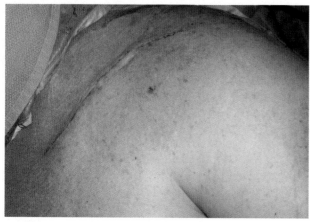

FIGURE 5-16

Closure of the wound.

DELTOPECTORAL APPROACH FOR FRACTURES AND ARTHROPLASTY

Indications

- Total shoulder or hemiarthroplasty
- Open reduction, internal fixation of proximal humerus fractures

Positioning

The patient is carefully padded and positioned in the beach chair position. The waist is flexed approximately 45 degrees and the knees are placed in 30 degrees of flexion. The table may be slightly rolled away from the surgical shoulder. In addition, a rolled up towel under the medial border of the scapula may help with exposure of the shoulder region. It is critically important to have the medial border of the scapula on the operative side free to allow adequate exposure of the upper extremity.

Landmarks

The landmarks of the shoulder are carefully palpated and marked with a marking pen including the posterior spine of the scapula, lateral border of the acromion, anterior border of the acromion, anterior portion of the clavicle, and the coracoid.

Technique

1. Incision: the incision begins at the anterior portion of the clavicle and passes approximately 1 cm lateral to the coracoid and intersects at the arm at the intersection of the medial 40% and the lateral 60% (**Fig. 5-17**). The incision is approximately 15 cm in length. There may be a gentle lateral curve to the incision proximally.
2. The skin is incised as well as the fat. Skin flaps are created medially and laterally.
3. It is easiest for one to find the deltopectoral interval proximally. A small triangle of fat is usually present between the deltoid and the pectoralis major proximally (**Fig. 5-18**). Once the interval is found, one follows the deltopectoral interval distally, usually leaving the cephalic vein medially within its bed (**Fig. 5-19**). It may be advantageous to place the arm on a Mayo stand and abduct the arm approximately 30 degrees to help dissect out the deltopectoral interval. There are multiple crossing branches that are typically present that do need to be cauterized. A retractor is placed under the deltoid and the deltopectoral interval is developed distally.

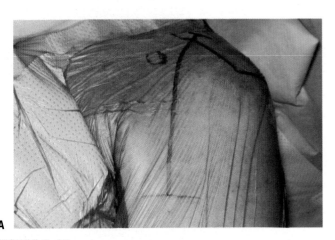

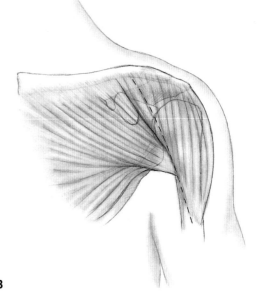

A   **B**

FIGURE 5-17

The landmarks are outlined and the incision is planned.

4. After this, the clavipectoral fascia which lies on the anterior aspect of the subscapularis and conjoined group is carefully incised. One can then place a finger to spread the interval between the conjoint and subscapularis, and a retractor may be placed in this area.

5. One then carefully feels for the axillary nerve. It is felt by using an index finger sweeping under the inferior border of the subscapularis. One may then confirm its presence by performing a "tug test" feeling for the nerve under the undersurface of the deltoid more laterally.

6. The subacromial subdeltoid space is then carefully incised and cleared to allow mobilization of the deltoid and a place for the deltoid retractor. This is started first superiorly under the undersurface of the acromion sweeping the bursa away, then laterally, and then finally anteriorly. A retractor is then placed in the deltoid **(Fig. 5-20)**. One may on occasion need to release the upper 1 cm of the pectoralis major muscle to improve exposure. Next, the overlying bursa of the rotator cuff is carefully débrided and one then clearly identifies the underlying rotator cuff.

   - *Note:* The coracoacromial ligament may be excised for better exposure (see Fig. 5-20B). However, if the cuff is deficient, ligament should be left intact.

7. In cases of shoulder arthroplasty, one then determines how the subscapularis should be taken down. There is significant variability among surgeons in regards to management of the subscapularis in routine shoulder arthroplasty work. There are several options available including incising through the subscapularis tendon for later tendon repair **(Fig 5-21)**. The second option is taking down the subscapularis off of bone. Lastly, there is the option of performing a lesser tuberosity osteotomy.

8. The arm is externally rotated and the head is dislocated **(Fig. 5-22)**.

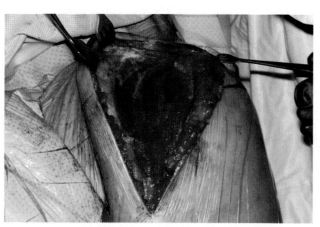

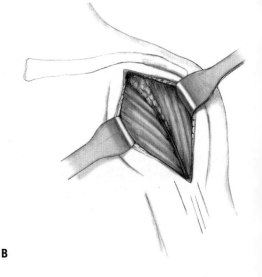

A   B

FIGURE 5-18

The medial border of the deltoid is identified. A triangle of fat is usually present in this location.

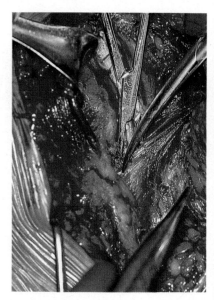

FIGURE 5-19

The superior aspect of the pectoralis major is detached. The cephalic vein is left within its bed medially.

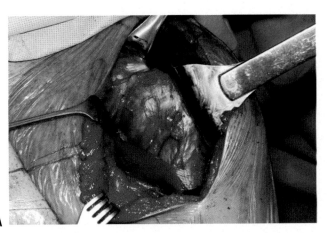
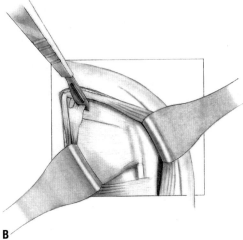

FIGURE 5-20

A retractor is placed medially beneath the pectoralis and laterally under the deltoid. The landmarks are outlined and the incision is planned.

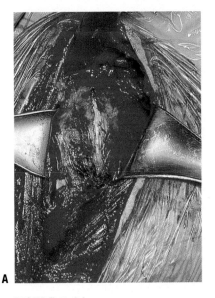
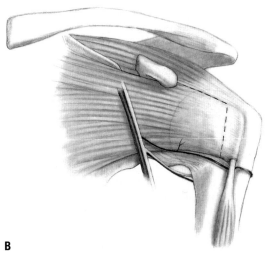

FIGURE 5-21

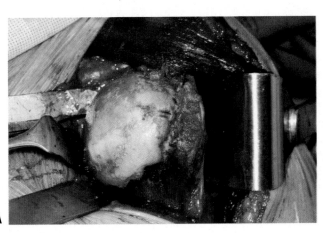
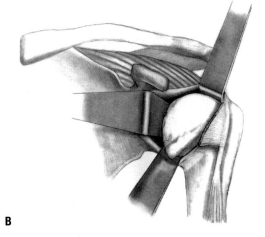

FIGURE 5-22

In this case, the rotator interval and subscapularis were incised and the humeral head was dislocated for a total shoulder arthroplasty.

Pearls and Pitfalls

- Careful deltoid mobilization is critical to exposure for both internal fixation of fractures as well as shoulder arthroplasty.
- One should clearly identify and protect the axillary nerve during the course of all shoulder procedures performed through the deltopectoral interval. The "tug test" is a simple and reproducible manner to clearly confirm the location of the nerve.

POSTERIOR EXPOSURE FOR RECURRENT POSTERIOR SHOULDER INSTABILITY

Indication

The indication for posterior approach to the shoulder is usually treatment of posterior instability that has been refractory to nonoperative treatment.

Positioning

The patient is carefully padded and positioned in the lateral decubitus position with the operative shoulder placed superiorly. Additionally, there are some surgeons that prefer to perform a posterior approach to the shoulder with the patient in the beach chair position. In the beach chair position, however, the patient needs to be sitting at a near 90 degree angle or leaning slightly forward. In the more traditional lateral position, great care is taken to adequately pad the patient including padding the lower extremities to prevent a peroneal nerve palsy.

Landmarks

After the patient is prepped and draped in the usual sterile manner, the anatomical landmarks of the shoulder are carefully palpated and marked including the spine at the scapula, the acromion, clavicle, and coracoid.

Technique

1. Incision: the standard incision for posterior approach of shoulder begins posterior to the acromioclavicular joint and approximately 1 to 2 cm medial to the lateral border of the acromion and extending distally in line with the posterior axillary skin fold (**Fig. 5-23**). An approximately 6 to 8 cm incision is made. The skin is incised as well as the fat. Skin flaps are mobilized medially, laterally, superiorly, and inferiorly. Once the superficial dissection is performed, one visualizes the underlying deltoid muscle.
2. The deltoid muscle is split in line with its fibers approximately 2.5 cm medial to the posterior corner of the acromion. This split should not extend greater than 4 to 5 cm to avoid injury to the underlying axillary nerve (**Fig. 5-24**). The posterior repair itself can be performed without removal of any deltoid from the scapular spine or the underlying acromion. The deltoid flaps are carefully created. A self-retaining retractor may be used to retract the deltoid from the underlying rotator cuff muscles.
3. Once the deltoid is mobilized, one can then expose the underlying infraspinatus and teres minor. Frequently, it is difficult to specifically see the interval between the teres minor and underlying infraspinatus. Therefore, many surgeons have advocated splitting between the two heads in the infraspinatus rather than going through the interval between the teres minor and infraspinatus (**Fig. 5-25**). The infraspinatus does have a specific fat stripe between the two heads. This is a convenient plane to use for the dissection. One, however, needs to take great care that the dissection between the two heads does not proceed more than 1.5 cm medial to the glenoid to avoid injury to the suprascapular nerve.
4. The infraspinatus is carefully freed from the underlying capsule. The capsule is typically more adhered laterally compared to medially. It is critical to obtain full mobility of the plane between the infraspinatus and capsule to allow mobilization of the capsule for later repair. An additional set of self-retaining retractors may be helpful to place between the two heads of the infraspinatus to clearly expose the underlying capsule.

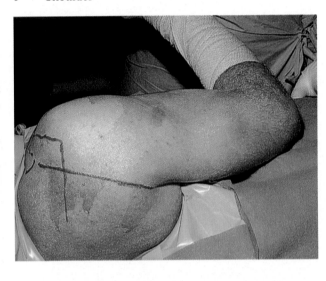

FIGURE 5-23
The patient is positioned in the lateral position and an incision is made 1 to 2 cm medial to the lateral border of the acromion.

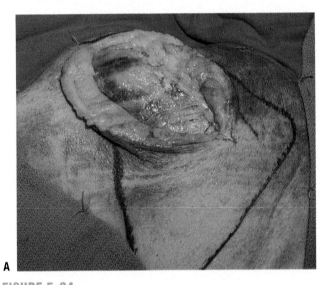

A

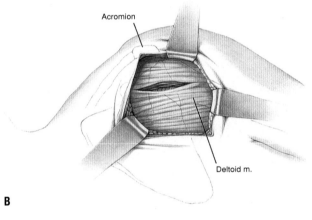

B

FIGURE 5-24

A,B: A split in the deltoid is made approximately 2 to 3 cm medial to the posterior corner of the acromion. The split should not extend more than 4 to 5 cm.

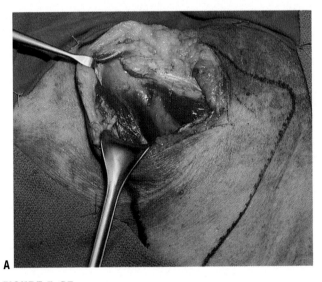

A

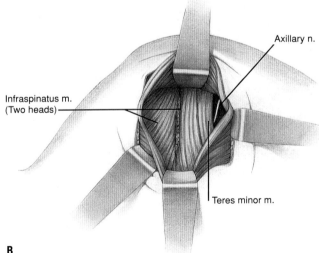

B

FIGURE 5-25

A,B: A split is made between the two heads of the infraspinatus.

5. In regard to the specific capsular repair, there is significant variability in regard to the type of capsular repair that is preferred by the surgeon. Specifically, some surgeons prefer to perform a laterally based capsular repair versus a medially based capsular repair. The procedure then proceeds with performing a capsular application with either a laterally or medially based T-type of split as well as addressing any labral pathology (**Fig. 5-26**).

Pearls and Pitfalls

- One can perform the posterior exposure through the interval between the infraspinatus and teres minor or between the two heads of the infraspinatus. The fatty stripe between the heads of the infraspinatus is a more readily identifiable landmark and may be the easier interval to use for the procedure.

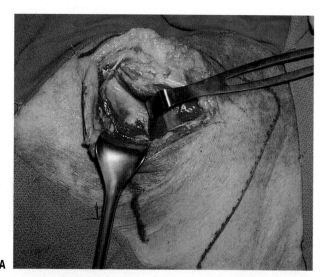

A

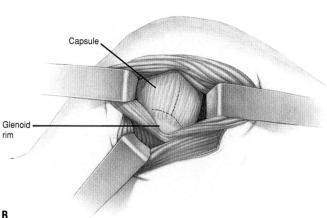

B

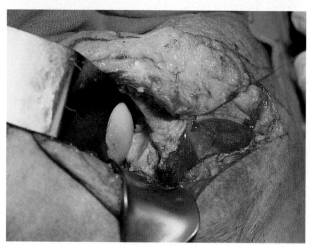

C

FIGURE 5-26

A,B: The infraspinatus is carefully freed from the underlying capsule. A lateral or medial based repair is based on labral pathology and surgeon preference.

ANTERIOR INFERIOR APPROACH FOR SHOULDER INSTABILITY

Indication

Treatment of shoulder instability.

Positioning

The patient is carefully padded and positioned in the beach chair position. The affected upper extremity is sterilely prepped and draped in the usual manner.

Technique

1. Incision: the standard axillary incision begins just inferior to the coracoid process and extends into the axilla in line with the skin folds. This is determined by adducting the arm and seeing the line of the skin fold (**Fig. 5-27**). One may wish to make a more inferior incision in the axilla for improved cosmesis. The more inferior incision, however, does necessitate more extensive subcutaneous dissection.
2. The skin is incised, then the fat, and the deltopectoral interval is identified. It is typically easier to identify the interval more proximally. There is typically a fatty triangle at the most proximal aspect of the deltopectoral interval. The deltopectoral interval is identified and then dissection is continued distally. The cephalic vein is typically retracted laterally (**Fig. 5-28**). The upper 1 cm of the pectoralis major insertion may be released to improve visualization. The deltoid insertion does not need to be detached either from the clavicle or on the humerus. One must take great care when releasing the upper 1 cm of the pectoralis not to injure the long head of the biceps.
3. A Richardson type retractor can be placed laterally under the deltoid. Next, the clavipectoral fascia which overlies the conjoined tendon and subscapularis is carefully incised lateral to the conjoined group. The conjoined group is then freed and mobilized. A retractor can then be placed medially (**Fig. 5-29**). Next, the axillary nerve is carefully identified and can be readily identified by placing a finger along the inferior border of the subscapularis.

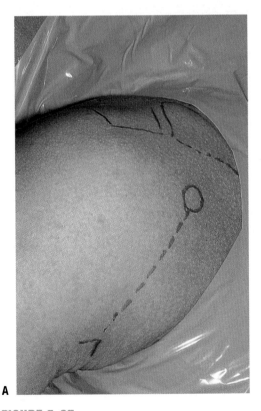

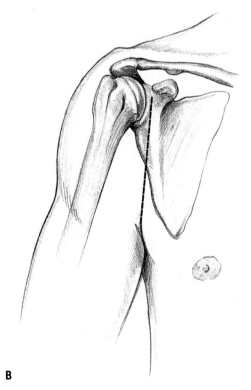

A   B

FIGURE 5-27

Langer skin lines are outlined in the axillary skin crease.

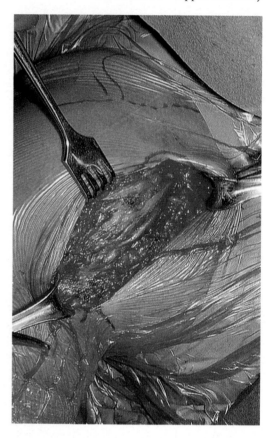

FIGURE 5-28
The cephalic vein is identified and retracted laterally.

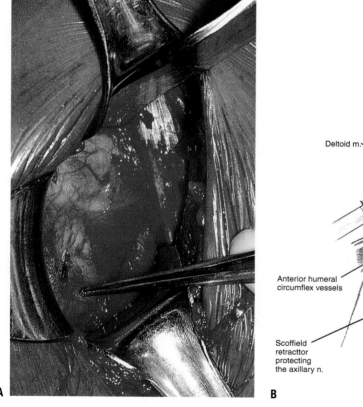

A   B

FIGURE 5-29
The deltoid is retracted laterally and the conjoint group is retracted medially.

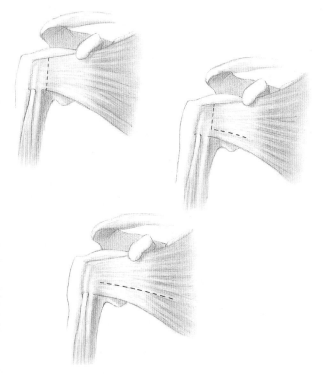

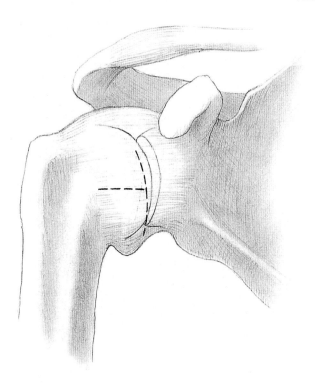

FIGURE 5-30

There are several ways to dissect the subscapularis from the underlying capsule including: **(A)** the entire subscapularis may be reflected off the capsule, **(B)** the lower 25% of the subscapularis may be left intact, and **(C)** the subscapularis may be split horizontally.

FIGURE 5-31

A medial or laterally based T split may be performed. In this example, a medially based shift will be performed.

4. One carefully identifies the borders of the subscapularis. The superior border of the subscapularis is marked by the rotator interval. This is classically a "soft area" present just superior to the subscapularis. This is typically widened in patients with multi-directional instability or may be frankly open. The inferior aspect of the subscapularis is defined by the "three sisters." The three sisters are the anterior humeral circumflex artery and the two accompanying veins.

   - *Note:* There is significant variability in regards to techniques for incising the subscapularis tendon including (**Fig. 5-30**):
   - Incising the subscapularis approximately 1 to 2 cm medial to its insertion off the lesser tuberosity and then elevating this carefully off the underlying capsule.
   - The second is popularized by Rockwood. The lower one-third to one-quarter of the subscapularis may be left intact. Detaching alone the upper portion of the subscapularis.
   - Lastly, the subscapularis muscle may be split horizontally to expose the underlying capsule.

5. Once the underlying capsule is carefully identified, tagging stitches are placed in the subscapularis, and the muscle again is carefully swept off of the underlying capsule. There is significant variability in management of the capsule in regard to either a laterally or medially based split. This is based primarily on the presence of a labral tear as well as surgeon preference (**Fig. 5-31**).

Pearls and Pitfalls

- Careful mobilization of all tissue planes from the deltopectoral interval to the release of the subscapularis off of the capsule is critical to obtain adequate exposure especially when performed through a small incision.
- One must carefully identify and protect the axillary nerve throughout the course of this procedure. The "tug test" is a reproducible way to confirm the exact location of the axillary nerve.

RECOMMENDED READING

Cetik O, Uslu M, Acar HI, et al. Is there a safe area for the axillary nerve in the deltoid muscle? A cadaveric study. *J Bone Joint Surg Am* 2006;88(11):2395–2399.

Cleeman E, Brunelli M, Gothelf T, et al. Releases of subscapularis contracture: an anatomic and clinical study. *J Shoulder Elbow Surg* 2003;12(3):231–236.

Gill DR, Cofield RH, Rowland C. The anteromedial approach for shoulder arthroplasty: the importance of the anterior deltoid. *J Shoulder Elbow Surg* 2004;13(5):532–537.

Gray H. *The Anatomy of the Human Body*, 29th ed. Philadelphia: Lea & Febiger, 1975.

Henry AK. *Extensile Exposure*, 2nd ed. New York: Churchill-Livingstone, Inc., 1963.

Hollinshead WH. *Anatomy for Surgeons: The Back and Limbs*, 3rd ed. Philadelphia: Harper & Row, 1982.

Hoppenfeld S, deBoer P. *Surgical Exposures in Orthopaedics: The Anatomical Approach*, 1st ed. Philadelphia: JB Lippincott Co., 1984.

Reckling FW, Reckling JB, Mohr MC. *Orthopedic Anatomy and Surgical Approaches*. St. Louis: Mosby Year-book, 1990.

Thompson JE. Anatomical methods of approach in operations on the long bones of the extremities. *Ann Surg* 1918;68:309–329.

Tubiana R, McCullough CJ, Masquelet AC. *An Atlas of Surgical Exposures of the Upper Extremity*. London: Martin Dunitz Publisher, 1990.

Uz A, Apaydin N, Bozkurt M, et al. The anatomic branch pattern of the axillary nerve. *J Shoulder Elbow Surg* 2007;16(2):240–244 [Epub Nov 9 2006].

Zlotolow DA, Catalano LW 3rd, Barron OA, et al. Surgical exposures of the humerus. *J Am Acad Orthop Surg* 2006;14(13):754–765.

6 Pelvis

S. Andrew Sems

POSTERIOR APPROACH TO THE SACRUM AND SACROILIAC JOINT

Indications

- Open reduction and internal fixation of sacral fractures.
- Open reduction and internal fixation of sacroiliac fracture-dislocations.
- Open reduction and internal fixation of sacroiliac dislocations.
- Open reduction and internal fixation of sacroiliac dislocations with iliac fractures (crescent fracture).

Position

The patient is placed in the prone position with chest rolls positioned to allow the abdomen to hang free (**Fig. 6-1**). A completely radiolucent table is utilized to allow imaging in multiple planes including Judet views and inlet and outlet views. The chest roll should be placed proximal enough so that the pelvis actually hangs free, as this is helpful in assisting in obtaining reduction of these fractures. By supporting the patient's thorax rather than directly on the anterior pelvis, the axial skeleton will be stabilized proximally, allowing the hemipelvis to hang free and reduce anteriorly.

Landmarks

The posterior-superior iliac spine as well as the entire iliac crest should be palpated. The spinous processes of the sacrum and lumbar vertebrae should be identified.

Technique

1. Incision: the incision is longitudinal in direction (**Fig. 6-2**). It can be translated medially or laterally as appropriate for the particular type of fracture. For sacral fractures, a more medially based incision is appropriate, whereas for crescent type fractures or pure sacroiliac dislocations, the incision can be made based more laterally. For a crescent fracture or sacroiliac dislocation, the in-

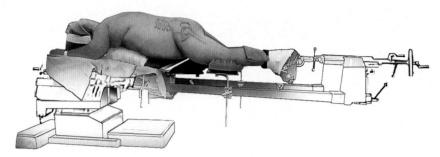

FIGURE 6-1

The prone position allows gravity to assist in reduction of the fracture and hemipelvis.

cision should be just lateral to the posterior-superior iliac spine. It may be curved laterally as it can fall in line with the iliac crest as it travels anteriorly and laterally. However, a vertical incision also can be useful to gain full exposure. In thinner patients, an incision directly over the posterior-superior iliac spine should be avoided, as the subcutaneous location of the bony prominence may cause difficulty with wound healing and breakdown.

- *Note:* Injection of lidocaine and epinephrine mixtures into the surgical site before making the skin incision can assist in controlling bleeding in the area. There is often a large amount of subcutaneous adipose in this region with significant vascularity that can bleed throughout the case and cause exposure and visualization to be difficult, so careful attention to gaining hemostasis throughout the subcutaneous dissection is important.

2. The gluteus maximus is identified as it inserts onto the posterior-superior iliac spine and iliac crest. It is incised in the tendinous portion along the posterior-superior iliac spine, leaving a cuff of tissue on the posterior-superior iliac spine for later repair **(Fig. 6-3)**.

3. As the dissection extends posteriorly, the gluteal tendon is incised toward the midline over the sacrum. This allows complete retraction of the gluteus maximus and exposure of the posterior-superior iliac spine as well as the posterior aspect of the ilium. Care should be taken to not disturb the underlying paraspinal muscles, particularly the multifidus, unless dissection onto the sacrum is necessary. For most sacroiliac dislocations and crescent fractures, these paraspinal muscles can be left undisturbed. For sacral fractures, the injury and initial displacement of the

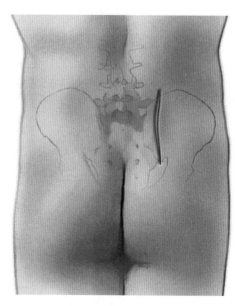

FIGURE 6-2

The posterior incision can be either curved or vertical in nature depending on the exact location of the fracture.

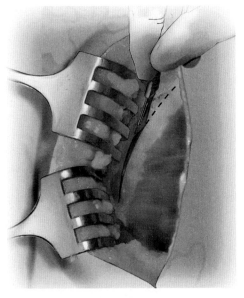

FIGURE 6-3

The gluteus maximus tendon is identified as it inserts on the posterior-superior iliac spine and as it inserts towards the midline distal to the posterior-superior iliac spine. The tendon is incised leaving a cuff of tendon medially for later repair.

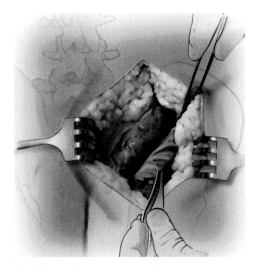

FIGURE 6-4

The gluteus maximus is retracted laterally away from the sacroiliac joint and can be retracted as far as the greater sciatic notch.

fracture has often caused severe injury to the paraspinal muscles and some local debridement during the approach may be all that is necessary in order to fully visualize the fracture.

4. The gluteus maximus is elevated subperiosteally along the posterior aspect of the ilium distally to the greater sciatic notch, giving access to the entire crescent fracture and sacroiliac joint **(Fig. 6-4)**.

5. Finger palpation beneath the greater sciatic notch can be utilized to assess anterior reduction of a sacroiliac dislocation. Exposure of the greater sciatic notch will allow placement of a reduction clamp to correct the vertical displacement of the hemipelvis that occurs in posterior pelvic ring injuries. Care should be taken during dissection into the greater sciatic notch to protect the sciatic nerve as well as the superior gluteal vessels and nerve **(Fig. 6-5)**.

6. Once reduction and fixation of the posterior ring is completed, care should be taken to repair the gluteus maximus insertion in its tendinous portion using a heavy permanent suture such as 0-Ethibon. Subcutaneous tissue should be closed in multiple layers as well, and drain placement is recommended depending on the amount of hemorrhage encountered.

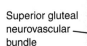

Superior gluteal neurovascular bundle

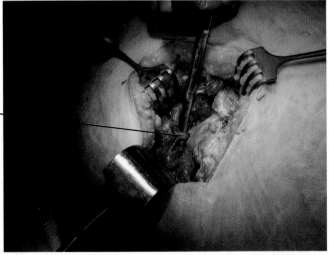

FIGURE 6-5

The superior gluteal neurovascular bundle prevents further lateral retraction of the gluteus maximus.

Pearls and Pitfalls

- Avoid making an incision directly over the most prominent portion of the posterior-superior iliac spine, particularly in thinner patients as this may be very prominent and may break down as the patient lies on their back recovering.
- Subperiosteal dissection along the lateral aspect of the ilium can identify the proximal extent of crescent fractures. Blunt retractors or malleable retractors along the lateral aspect of the ilium can be utilized to visualize these fractures and gain anatomic reduction. Additionally, sacroiliac screws may provide a large amount of stability to a fixation construct for sacroiliac dislocations and crescent fractures. These screws should be placed away from the iliac fracture line so they will not fail by breaking through into the fracture site, and this can be visualized through this approach. However, percutaneous incisions will need to be made over the lateral aspect of the gluteal region in order to place the screws, as the necessary trajectory cannot be obtained through the posterior approach to the sacroiliac joint.

APPROACH TO THE ACETABULUM THROUGH THE ILIOINGUINAL APPROACH

Indications

- Both column fractures of the acetabulum.
- Anterior column posterior hemi-transverse fractures of the acetabulum.
- Anterior column fractures.
- In conjunction with the Kocher-Langenbeck approach for treatment and fixation of transverse, and T-type acetabular fractures.

Position

The patient is positioned supine on a radiolucent table **(Fig. 6-6)**. Traction is often utilized before reduction of these cases and a table such as a Judet-Tasserit table or Pro FX fracture table which is radiolucent and allows the use of traction in multiple directions is optimal.

Landmarks

One should palpate the entire iliac crest as well as paying attention to the anterior-superior iliac spine. The pubic tubercles and symphysis should be identified.

Technique

1. Incision: the incision follows the contour of the iliac crest from posterior to anterior, and then is directed over the inguinal ligament to a point approximately 2 cm proximal to the pubic symphysis **(Fig. 6-7)**.

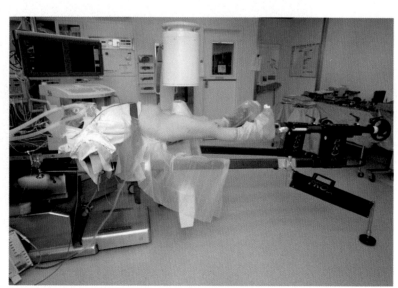

FIGURE 6-6

Patient is positioned supine on a radiolucent fracture table allowing bilateral skin traction with a perineal post in place.

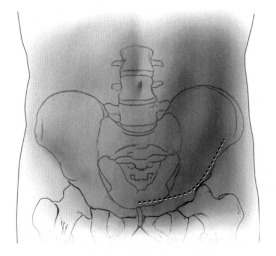

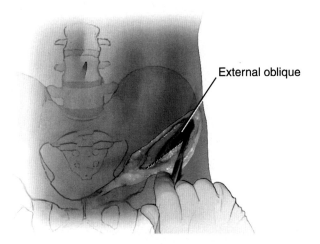

FIGURE 6-7
Incision is made over the iliac crest, anterior-superior iliac spine, and pubic symphysis.

FIGURE 6-8
The abdominal muscles are incised at their aponeurosis and elevated from the iliac crest.

2. The abdominal musculature is identified as it inserts on the iliac crest. The aponeurosis of the abdominal muscles terminates just proximal to an avascular zone between the hip abductors and abdominal musculature. This zone is identified and this interval should be split directly down to the iliac crest **(Fig. 6-8)**.
3. Subperiosteal dissection along the iliac crest with elevation of the abdominal musculature insertion is performed to gain access to the inner table of the pelvis, exposing the lateral window. Once the lateral window has been exposed and the iliopsoas has been elevated off the inner fossa, this area of the wound should be packed with lap sponges and the exposure should continue distally.
4. The skin incision is then extended from the anterior-superior iliac spine to an area approximately 2 cm proximal to the pubic symphysis.
5. The external abdominal oblique musculature and fascia is identified as the fibers course in a direction from superolateral to inferomedial towards the superficial inguinal ring. The spermatic cord should be identified and a Penrose drain should be placed around it to protect it and allow retraction medially and laterally **(Fig. 6-9)**.

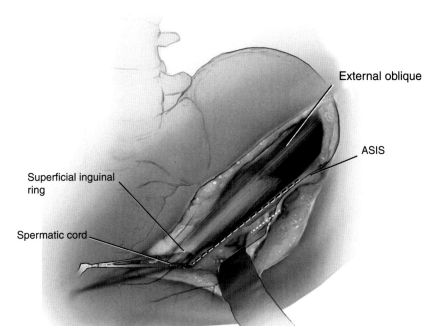

FIGURE 6-9
The external abdominal oblique and spermatic cord are identified and circumferential control of the spermatic cord is gained.

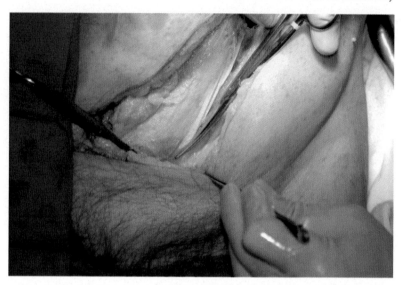

FIGURE 6-10

The external abdominal oblique fascia is identified and split in line with its fibers proximal to the inguinal ligament.

6. The external abdominal oblique is split in line with its fibers just proximal to its insertion on the inguinal ligament (**Fig. 6-10**). Dissection should be continued down towards the inferior aspect of the superficial inguinal ring. If possible the superficial ring should be kept in place so that a later repair is not necessary.

7. At this point the combined tendon of the internal abdominal oblique and transverse abdominus muscle is identified as it inserts on the inguinal ligament. This conjoined tendon should be incised in line with its fibers near its insertion on the inguinal ligament giving ample amount of tendon on both sides of the incision to repair at the end of the case (**Fig. 6-11**).

8. The lateral femoral cutaneous nerve is identified crossing over the psoas muscle near the anterior-superior iliac spine. This nerve may need to be sacrificed for complete exposure of the acetabulum; however, initial attempts should be made to protect and save this nerve.

9. The psoas muscle and femoral nerve should be identified. These structures should be kept together and a Penrose drain should be placed around them in their entirety (**Fig. 6-12**). Care should be taken to elevate the psoas off of the internal fossa of the ilium in its entirety so that trauma to the muscle is minimized.

10. Once the entire psoas muscle and femoral nerve are protected with a Penrose drain, they can be retracted laterally. The iliopectineal fascia is identified and very careful dissection just medial

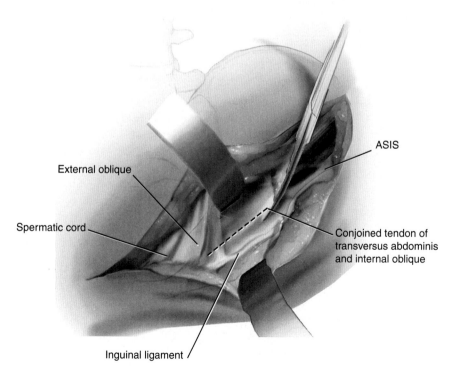

FIGURE 6-11

The combined tendon of the internal abdominal oblique and tranversalis abdominus is identified and incised near its insertion on the inguinal ligament.

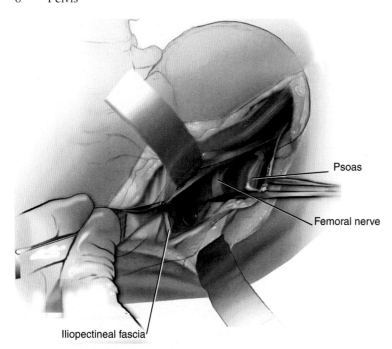

Psoas

Femoral nerve

Iliopectineal fascia

FIGURE 6-12

Circumferential control of the psoas muscle and femoral nerve are obtained with a Penrose drain placed around the structures.

to this should be performed to separate it from the external iliac vessels. Once the iliopectineal fascia is separated from the external iliac vessels, a finger should be placed between the fascia and the vessels to palpate the pulse and confirm the vessels are medial to the finger.

11. Once the external iliac vessels are confirmed to be medial and the fascia is isolated, scissors are used to split the iliopectineal fascia all the way to the pelvic brim **(Fig. 6-13)**.

12. With the combined tendon of the transversalis abdominus and internal abdominal oblique incised near its insertion, dissection should now proceed medially. A small portion of the rectus abdominus muscle will need to be incised transversely as it inserts on the pubic tubercle just medial to the spermatic cord or round ligament **(Fig. 6-14)**. This will allow for exposure of the medial side of the external iliac vessels.

13. Circumferential access to the external iliac vessels can now be gained by placing a Penrose drain around the bundle and it can now be retracted medially and laterally **(Fig. 6-15)**.

14. Once this is performed, all three windows of the ilioinguinal approach have been exposed and reduction and fixation of the acetabular fracture can be performed.

15. Following fixation, care should be taken to tightly repair the structures in the inguinal region to prevent postoperative hernia development. After thorough irritation of the wound, the portion of the transected rectus abdominus is reapproximated using interrupted 0-Ethibon sutures. Next, the internal abdominal oblique and transversalis abdominus conjoined tendon is repaired back to the inguinal ligament using multiple 0-Ethibon sutures.

   ● *Note:* Multiple single sutures are preferred in case one should break or rupture, the remainder of the repair will stay intact.

16. A layered closure is preferred and the external abdominal oblique is then closed using 0-Ethibon sutures. If care has been taken during the dissection to preserve the superficial inguinal ring, the fascia can typically be closed just below this and the ring will be intact.

17. A drain can be placed in the lateral aspect of the wound, resting in the internal iliac fossa. The abdominal aponeurosis can then be reapproximated using multiple 0-Ethibon sutures. The subcutaneous tissue is closed in layers and the skin is closed with either a nonabsorbable monofilament suture or a staple.

Pearls and Pitfalls

● Exposure can be very difficult in obese patients and consideration should be given to adjusting the incision slightly proximal in order to gain the appropriate trajectory for screw and hardware placement. By moving the incision just proximal a few centimeters this amount of soft tissue will not need to be retracted as much during the case and appropriate trajectory of the screw can be obtained.

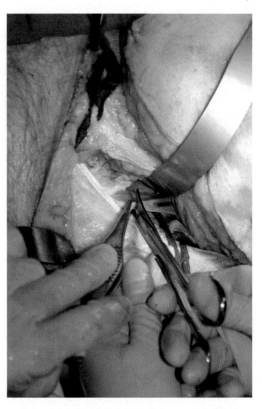

FIGURE 6-13

The iliopectineal fascia is identified and split down to the pelvic rim.

- The femoral nerve should be clearly identified as it sits on the psoas muscle prior to placing a Penrose drain around this neuromuscular group. The femoral nerve may occasionally have multiple branches and care should be taken not to divide them or retract ones without having control of all of them.
- Retraction of the external iliac vessel should be performed carefully. Malleable retractors can be placed in the middle window to retract the vessels medially; however, care should be taken so that the sharp edges of the malleable retractors do not impinge on the external vessels. In patients who are older or who have known atherosclerotic disease, care should be taken to avoid excessive or aggressive retraction of these vessels as plaques may dislodge or intimal damage may occur.

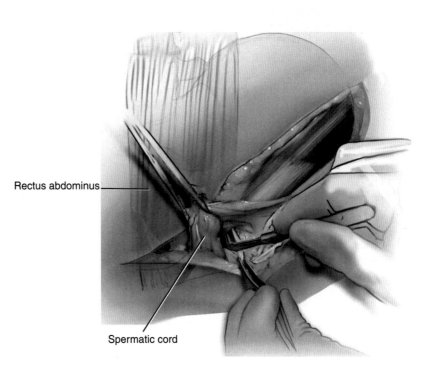

Rectus abdominus

Spermatic cord

FIGURE 6-14

The rectus abdominus is transected just medial to the spermatic cord.

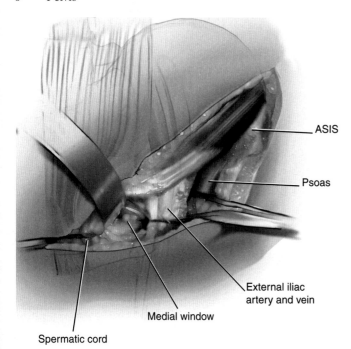

ASIS

Psoas

External iliac
artery and vein

Medial window

Spermatic cord

FIGURE 6-15
Circumferential control of external iliac neurovascular
bundle is obtained.

APPROACH TO THE PUBIC SYMPHYSIS AND STOPPA APPROACH

Indication

- Open reduction and internal fixation of pubic symphyseal diastasis.
- Open reduction and internal fixation of pubic rami fractures and parasymphyseal pubic fractures.
- Open reduction and internal fixation of the quadrilateral surface of the acetabulum and low anterior column fractures.
- Anterior plate fixation of pelvic discontinuity for total hip reconstruction.

Position

The patient is positioned supine on the radiolucent table. Skeletal traction is generally not necessary for this approach and the perineal posts may actually get in the way of exposure and manipulative procedures.

Landmarks

Identify the pubic tubercles and superior edge of the pubic bodies and superior rami.

Technique

1. Incision: identify the midline of the abdomen over the pubic symphysis, and make a transverse Pfannenstiel type incision which is in-line with the skin creases in the suprasymphyseal region **(Fig. 6-16)**. The incision is made 1 to 2 cm proximal to the pubic symphysis. This incision may move further proximal in patients who are more obese to allow appropriate trajectory of screw plates into the pubic bodies.
2. The dissection is carried through the skin and subcutaneous tissues gaining hemostasis along the way. The rectus abdominus muscles are identified. They need to be split in the midline and then elevated off the pubic tubercles leaving a distally based insertion. The pyramidalis muscle may be identified inferiorly in the wound, and oblique fibers of the rectus fascia will tend to point to the midline and can be found crossing in the raphe of the rectus abdominus.
3. Once the midline of the rectus abdominus is identified, a small vertical incision is made just over the pubic symphysis. This incision should go through the rectus fascia and be approximately 5 mm in length, just long enough to allow placement of the right angle clamp through this incision aimed proximally.

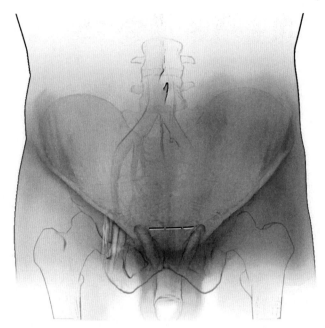

FIGURE 6-16

The incision is based just proximal to the superior aspect of the pubic body and superior pubic rami.

4. With anterior retraction and elevation of this clamp, the rectus is lifted off of the underlying bladder and prevesicular fat. The fascia can then be incised directly onto the right angle clamp as it is translated proximally as the fascia and muscle are split (**Fig. 6-17**).

5. Once the rectus abdominus is split in its midline, access to the space of Retzius is obtained. The rectus should be elevated directly off the tubercles by retracting the rectus anteriorly. The distal insertion of the rectus should be maintained and transection of the rectus abdominus should be avoided for this approach.

6. Once dissection is carried over the pubic tubercles, pointed Holman retractors can be placed over the tubercles to retract the rectus laterally and gain access to the symphysis and anterior aspect of the pubic bodies.

7. Reduction and fixation of pubic symphysis diastasis or parasymphyseal fractures can then be performed.

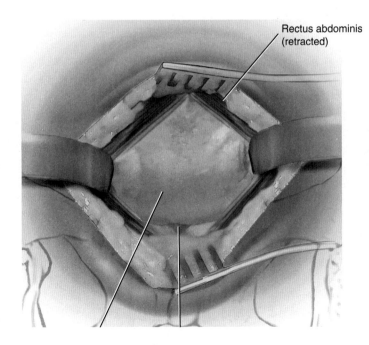

Rectus abdominis (retracted)

FIGURE 6-17

The rectus abdominus is split in line with its fibers and elevated off the pubic tubercles.

Alternate Exposure

8. A Stoppa approach can be performed through this incision by dissection along the pubic ramus to the quadrilateral surface of the acetabulum. Often a headlamp is utilized because of the relatively deep nature of this wound.
9. Dissection is carried along the desired pubic ramus towards the quadrilateral surface. Great care should be taken to observe the corona mortis as it anastomoses between the external iliac vessels and the obturator vessels, crossing the superior pubic ramus 4 to 6 cm lateral to the pubic symphysis **(Fig. 6-18)**.
10. This anastomosis will need to be identified, carefully dissected out, and then ligated prior to full exposure of the quadrilateral surface and pelvic brim. As long as dissection is maintained along the pelvic brim and quadrilateral surface, the soft tissues can be retracted superiorly and inferiorly and access to the spaces can be obtained. Malleable retractors can be utilized to retract the peritoneal cavity medially.
11. Through this approach, access can be gained along the quadrilateral surface all the way to the sacroiliac joint **(Fig. 6-19)**.
12. Following reduction and fixation of the anterior pelvic ring, the rectus abdominus is closed with 0-Ethibon sutures. The subcutaneous tissue is then closed in multiple layers and the skin is closed with either nylon or staples. Care should be taken during closure of the rectus to avoid injury to the bladder and prevesicular fat.

Pearls and Pitfalls

- The incision may be translated proximally in obese patients in order to gain appropriate trajectory for hardware placement. Often the abdominal fat will need to be retracted proximally and compressed in order to be able to place screws down the pubic bodies and into the inferior pubic rami.
- Transection of the rectus should be avoided if at all possible. Dissection can be carried over the pubic tubercles to elevate the rectus abdominus leaving a distally based insertion.
- Retractors can be placed over the pubic tubercles but should not be placed so far laterally as they enter into the obturator foramen due to potential injury to the neurovascular structures in the region.

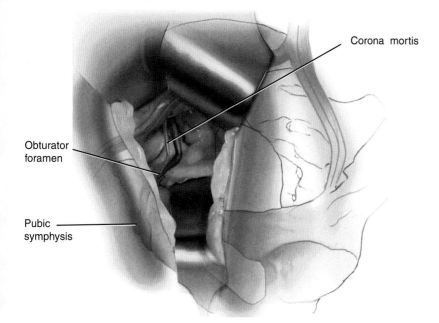

Corona mortis

Obturator foramen

Pubic symphysis

FIGURE 6-18

The exposure is extended along the superior pubic ramus to the quadrilateral surface. The corona mortis is identified and ligated as it crosses the pelvic brim.

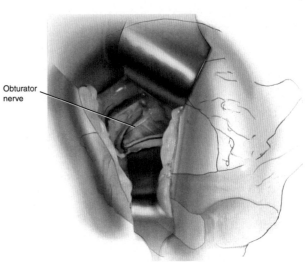

FIGURE 6-19

Access to the entire quadrilateral surface and pelvic brim. The obturator nerve passes across the inferior aspect of the operative field.

APPROACH TO THE POSTERIOR PELVIS (KOCHER-LANGENBECK APPROACH)

Indications

- Open reduction and internal fixation of acetabular fractures.
  - Posterior Wall
  - Posterior Column
  - Transverse Posterior Wall
  - Posterior Column-Posterior Wall
  - T-type
  - Transverse
- Open irrigation and debridement of the hip joint.

Position

The Kocher-Langenbeck approach can be performed either in a lateral or prone position. The patient should be kept with the operative knee flexed 90 degrees at all times to remove tension from the sciatic nerve and to allow for intraoperative retraction. By placing the patient in a prone position on a specialized fracture table, knee flexion can be maintained by a special apparatus holding the traction boot on the operative leg vertically **(Fig. 6-20)**. A distal femoral traction pin can be attached to the traction device to allow precise control of the amount of hip joint distraction. Intraoperative sequential compression devices can also be placed when the patient is in the prone position to help with the deep vein thrombosis (DVT) prophylaxis.

Landmarks

The posterior-superior iliac spine as well as the greater trochanter and lateral aspect of the femur are identified.

Technique

1. Incision: the incision is in a line from the posterior superior iliac spine toward the center of the greater trochanter and then extended distally on the lateral aspect of the femur **(Fig. 6-21)**. The incision can be gently curved at the corner or it can be kept at a sharp angle.
2. The posterior incision over the gluteal region is made first and dissection is carried through the skin and subcutaneous tissue gaining hemostasis through the dissection. The fascia over the gluteus maximus and gluteal muscle fibers are identified.
   - *Note:* In more obese patients, following this portion of the incision, further palpation can be performed to determine the exact location of the greater trochanter. If necessary, the incision can then be extended more anteriorly to reach the center of the greater trochanter.
3. Once the incision has been made to the center of the greater trochanter, it is extended distally along the line of the femur.

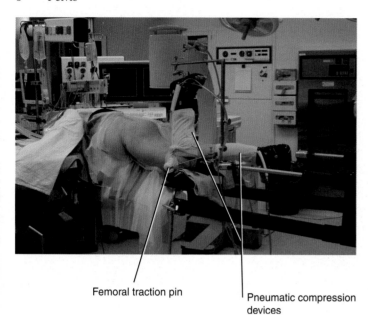

Femoral traction pin   Pneumatic compression
                              devices

FIGURE 6-20

Prone position of the patient on the fracture table with the distal femoral traction pin, knee flexed in 90 degrees, and sequential compression device on the calf to assist in DVT prophylaxis.

4. The iliotibial band and lateral thigh fascia are split in line with their fibers on the lateral aspect of the femur. The fascial incision begins distally at a level equal to the inferior gluteal fold of the skin, as this is the location of the gluteus maximus tendinous sling. This tendon may need to be incised as it inserts on the femur to allow sufficient posterior retraction of the flap.

5. Once this incision reaches the center of the greater trochanter the fascia over gluteus maximus is then split in line with the underlying muscle fibers. The muscle fibers of the gluteus maximus are then split by blunt finger dissection (**Fig. 6-22**).

6. Once the gluteus maximus and iliotibial band have been split, and the posterior flap is created, it can be held in place with large no. 5 Ethibond sutures tacked to the posterior skin. The short external rotators are then identified. The piriformis muscle is tagged approximately 1 cm from its insertion onto the femur and retracted posteriorly.

7. The combined tendon of the gemellae and obturator internus are then identified and tagged, again 1 cm from their insertion on the femur (**Fig. 6-23**).
   - *Note:* Care should be taken not to incise these muscles closer than 1 cm from the insertion on the femur in order to protect the blood supply to the femoral head.

8. Dissection should not be carried into the quadratus femoris as the risk of damage to the femoral head blood supply is encountered. Once the short external rotators are tagged and retracted, subperiosteal dissection along the retroacetabular surface is performed.

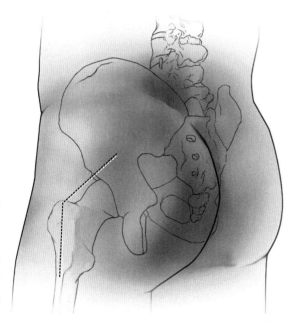

FIGURE 6-21

The incision is based on line from the posterior-superior iliac spine to the center of the greater trochanter and then extending distally in line with the femur.

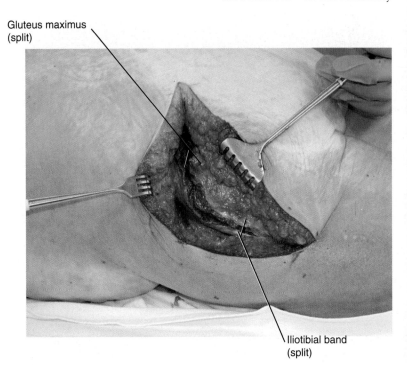

Gluteus maximus
(split)

Iliotibial band
(split)

FIGURE 6-22
The posterior muscular flap is made by incising the iliotibial band fascia in line with its fibers and the gluteus maximus in line with its fibers. The gluteus maximus tendon insertion on the femur may need to be incised for further posterior retraction of the flap.

9. The piriformis muscle is elevated back to the greater sciatic notch and the obturator internus and gemellae muscles are elevated back to their insertions near the lesser sciatic notch (**Fig. 6-24**).
10. Posterior retraction of the obturator internus will provide a sling around the sciatic nerve and protect it during retraction.
11. Once the lesser sciatic notch is then exposed, a retractor may be safely placed into this notch as long as tension is kept on the obturator internus to protect the sciatic nerve at all times.
12. Dissection can be performed beneath the gluteus minimus and the remainder of hip abductor muscle anteriorly.
13. A Homan retractor can be placed beneath the hip abductors to gain access to the superior aspect of the acetabulum and more anteriorly for placement of hardware in this region.
14. Following reduction and fixation of the acetabular fracture, the short external rotators are reapproximated to the greater trochanter. If the patient is in a prone position and the fracture table allows for it, the leg may be externally rotated to allow for a tension-free repair of the short external rotators.
15. Ethibond sutures are utilized through either a drill hole in the trochanter or by suturing them into the tendinous portion of the hip abductors as they insert on the greater trochanter. The posterior flap is then closed using 0-Ethibon sutures both laterally and posteriorly over the gluteus maximus. The subcutaneous tissue is closed in multiple layers and the skin is then closed with either sutures or staples.

Pearls and Pitfalls

- If performed in the prone position, initial internal rotation of the leg during exposure will place the short external rotators in a stretched position and allow easier identification and exposure of the tendinous portions of these muscles.
- Incision of a portion of the gluteus maximus tendinous sling that inserts on the femur may be required if in extremely muscular patients or obese patients in which further posterior retraction of the muscle flap is necessary.
- Placing the patient in a prone position with distal femoral traction pin and peroneal post-traction may facilitate exposure of the hip. Traction can be applied using the table's traction mechanism and the hip joint can be distracted to allow debridement any intra-articular fragments and to assess the femoral head for articular cartilage injuries.

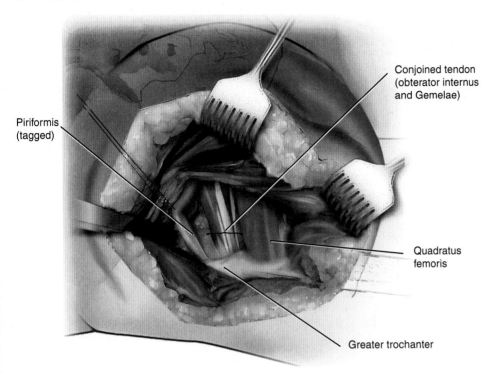

FIGURE 6-23

The piriformis and obturator internus muscles are identified and tagged and incised 1 cm away from their insertion into the femur.

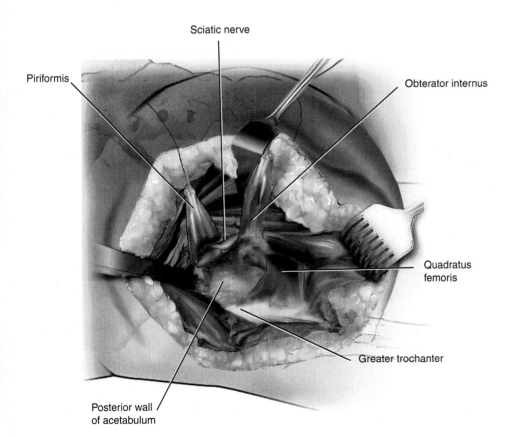

FIGURE 6-24

Dissection underneath the piriformis and obturator internus to the greater and lesser sciatic notches, respectively, with continual traction on the obturator internus to protect the sciatic nerve.

APPROACH TO THE ACETABULUM THROUGH THE EXTENDED ILIOFEMORAL APPROACH

Indications

The extended iliofemoral approach is rarely utilized in the routine treatment of acetabular fractures. The majority of complex fractures can be managed through combined ilioinguinal and Kocher-Langenbeck approaches before an iliofemoral approach would be necessary. However, certain transtectal transverse or T-type acetabular fractures with impaction of the acetabular dome or associated posterior wall fractures are still best treated through the extended iliofemoral approach. This approach may also be useful for treatment of older or malunited fractures.

Position

The extended iliofemoral approach requires the patient to be placed in the lateral position in order to gain access to the entire outer aspect of the ilium.

Landmarks

The iliac crest from the posterior-superior iliac spine to the anterior-superior iliac spine should be identified, as well as the location of the lateral edge of the patella.

Technique

1. Incision: a curvilinear incision from the posterior-superior iliac spine to the anterior-superior iliac spine is the continued in a line towards the lateral border of the patella. The incision will need to be carried to the proximal mid-thigh in order to provide adequate exposure (**Fig. 6-25**).

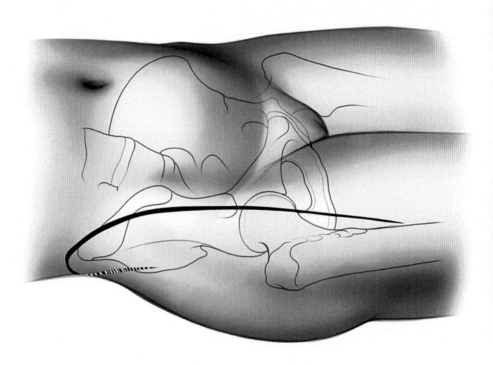

FIGURE 6-25

Patient is placed in the lateral position with the entire iliac crest and thigh prepped into the surgical field. The incision follows the contour of the iliac crest from the posterior superior iliac spine to the anterior superior iliac spine and then down the anterior thigh in a line toward the lateral border of the patella.

2. The tendinous interval between the abdominal and gluteal musculature is identified along the iliac crest and the origins of the gluteal muscles are released and elevated subperiostally to the greater sciatic notch **(Fig. 6-26)**. Continue this elevation anteriorly along the crest to release the tensor fascia lata from its origin on the ilium.

3. Next, identify the fascia of the anterior thigh and incise it longitudinally on the lateral border of the sartorius **(Fig. 6-27)**. Develop the interval between the sartorius and tensor fascia lata with blunt dissection.

4. Ascending branches of the lateral femoral circumflex artery may be encountered in this interval and can safely be ligated to allow further exposure **(Fig. 6-28)**.

5. With the tensor fascia lata retracted laterally and the Sartorius retracted medially, dissection is continued between the rectus femoris medially and gluteus medius laterally. The reflected head of rectus femoris tendon can be released from its origin on the supraacetabular ilium.

6. The gluteus minimus is elevated from the ilium and hip capsule, and its tendon is incised near the insertion on the greater trochanter, leaving a tendinous cuff for later repair. Next, the gluteus medius tendon is incised near its insertion on the greater trochanter, taking care to leave a tendinous cuff on the greater trochanter for later repair **(Fig. 6-29)**.

7. Dissection is now carried posteriorly on the greater trochanter to release the insertion of the piriformis, gemellae, and obturator internus.

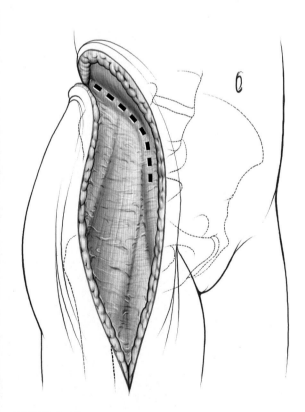

FIGURE 6-26

The gluteal muscles are released at their origin near the aponeurosis of the abdominal musculature and subperiosteal dissection is carried out towards the greater sciatic notch.

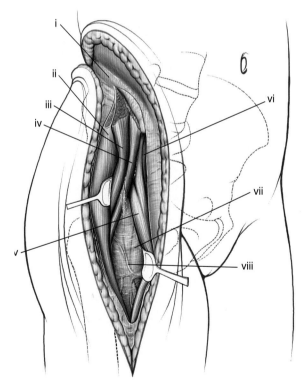

FIGURE 6-27

The fascia over the thigh is split in line with the femur and the interval between the sartorius (medially) and tensor fascia lata (laterally) is developed. (*i*) Avascular white line. (*ii*) Tensor fascia-lata muscle. (*iii*) Gluteus medius muscle. (*iv*) Gluteus minimus muscle. (*v*) Rectus femoris muscle. (*vi*) Sartorius muscle. (*vii*) No-name fascia covering vastus lateralis. (*viii*) Ascending branch of the lateral, femoral, circumflex artery.

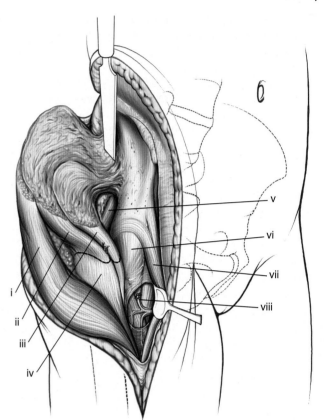

FIGURE 6-28

The ascending branches of the lateral circumflex femoral artery are identified in the interval between the Sartorius and tensor fascia lata and ligated. (*i*) Tensor fascia-lata muscle. (*ii*) Gluteus medius muscle. (*iii*) Gluteus minimus muscle. (*iv*) Greater trochanter. (*v*) Piriformis muscle. (*vi*) Hip joint capsule. (*vii*) Two heads of the rectus muscle. (*vii*) Ligated ascending branch of the lateral, femoral, circumflex artery.

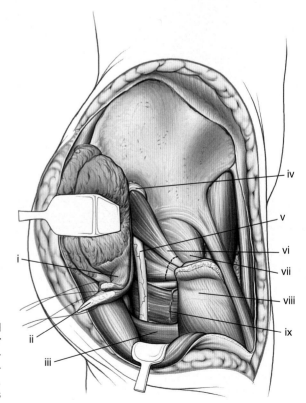

FIGURE 6-29

The tendons of the gluteus minimus and medius are tagged and transected, leaving a cuff of tendon to repair back to the greater trochanter. (*i*) Gluteus minimus tendon. (*ii*) Gluteus medius tendon, (*iii*) Gluteus maximus tendon. (*iv*) Superior-gluteal neurovascular bundle. (*v*) Sciatic nerve. (*vi*) Piriformis and conjoint tendons. (*vii*) Hip-joint capsule. (*viii*) Greater trochanter. (*ix*) Quadratus femoris.

8. These tendons should be released at least 1 cm from their insertions on the femur in order to protect the remaining blood supply to the femoral head. The external rotators can now be elevated off the posterior capsule and retroacetabular surface of the ilium to the greater and lesser sciatic notches **(Fig. 6-30)**.

9. Continuous retraction of the obturator internus posteriorly will provide a protective sling in front of the sciatic nerve and retractors may be placed in the greater or lesser sciatic notches.

10. If further exposure of the anterior column is necessary, the origin of the Sartorius and inguinal ligament may be released from the anterior superior iliac spine. The aponeurotic insertion of the abdominal muscles can be released posteriorly along the iliac crest in a similar fashion to the exposure of the lateral window of the ilioinguinal approach.

11. Superiosteal dissection along the inner table of the ilium will elevate the iliopsoas to the pelvic brim.
    - *Note:* An alternative to complete release of all structures from the anterior-superior iliac spine and iliac crest is to osteotomize the iliac crest while maintaining the inguinal ligament, Sartorius, and abdominal musculature insertions and origins on the ilium. Predrilling the osteotomy will allow easier reduction and fixation during closure.

12. Following fracture reduction and fixation, close attention must be paid to repair of the multiple tendons that have been released from their origins and insertions. Closure begins at the posterior inferior aspect of the greater trochanter. The obturator internus and gemellae common tendon is repaired with a permanent suture, size 0 or larger. The piriformis is repaired next in the same fashion. Working anteriorly on the greater trochanter, the gluteus medius tendon and gluteus minimus tendons are repaired next, respectively. Again, large permanent suture is preferred for this repair, using size 1 suture or larger. Repair of the reflected head of the rectus femoris follows the gluteal tendon repairs.

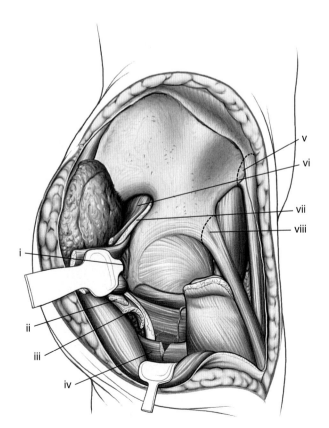

FIGURE 6-30

Retractors can be placed in the greater and lesser sciatic notches to complete the exposure. (*i*) Blunt Homan in lesser sciatic notch. The conjoint tendons have been positioned between the retractor and the sciatic nerve. (*ii*) Gluteus minimus tendon. (*iii*) Gluteus medius tendon. (*iv*) Partial release of gluteus maximus tendon. (*v*) Anterior-superior iliac spine and sartorius muscle origin. (*vi*) Piriformis muscle. (*vii*) Sciatic nerve. (*viii*) Anterior-inferior iliac spine and reflected head of rectus femoris muscle.

13. The hip abductors are repaired back to the abdominal aponeurosis and lumbodorsal fascia using multiple interrupted sutures with the hip held in an abducted position. The fascia over the Sartorius is repaired to complete the deep closure. Layered closure of the subcutaneous tissues and skin follows to complete the procedure.
14. Due to the necessary elevation of the hip abductors from both the ilium and greater trochanter, postoperative protection of the hip is required.
15. After surgery patients should be maintained in a hip abduction pillow in the initial postoperative period and should be restricted from active abduction for 6 weeks or more.
    - *Note:* This exposure has been associated with a high incidence of heterotopic ossification, so consideration of prophylaxis with radiation or indomethacin should be given.

Pearls and Pitfalls

- Multiple tendons need to be released in order to perform this approach appropriately. In order to repair the tendons to the correct place, the tendon cuffs should be tagged as well as the mobile end so the tendons can be put back to the matching location.
- Begin the dissection posteriorly along the ilium and work anteriorly to release the gluteus medius. The interval between the Sartorius and tensor fascia lata can be difficult to determine if the anterior superior iliac spine has not already been identified and exposed. If the interval cannot be determined, follow the Sartorius from the anterior superior iliac spine distally to develop this interval.
- Predrilling the iliac crest osteotomy will allow easier and more accurate reduction and fixation at the end of the case.

RECOMMENDED READING

Cole JD, Bolhofner BR. Acetabular fracture fixation via a modified Stoppa limited intrapelvic approach. Description of operative technique and preliminary treatment results. *Clin Orthop Relat Res* 1994;305:112–123.

Griffin DB, Beaule PE, Matta JM. Safety and efficacy of the extended iliofemoral approach in the treatment of complex fractures of the acetabulum. *J Bone Joint Surg Br* 2005;87(10):1391–1396.

Jimenez ML, Vrahas MS. Surgical approaches to the acetabulum. *Orthop Clin North Am* 1997;28(3):419–434.

Letournel E. The treatment of acetabular fractures through the ilioinguinal approach. *Clin Orthop Relat Res* 1993;292:62–76.

Matta JM. Fractures of the acetabulum: accuracy of reduction and clinical results in patients managed operatively within three weeks after the injury. *J Bone Joint Surg Am* 1996;78(11):1632–1645.

Matta JM. Operative treatment of acetabular fractures through the ilioinguinal approach. A 10-year perspective. *Clin Orthop Relat Res* 1994;305:10–19.

Moed BR, Karges DE. Techniques for reduction and fixation of pelvic ring disruptions through the posterior approach. *Clin Orthop Relat Res* 1996;329:102–114.

Qureshi AA, Archdeacon MT, Jenkins MA, et al. Infrapectineal plating for acetabular fractures: a technical adjunct to internal fixation. *J Orthop Trauma* 2004;18(3):175–178.

7 Hip and Acetabulum

Bernard F. Morrey and Matthew C. Morrey

The basis of the development of this chapter deals principally with the surgical exposures that I and my partners have found useful to manage the majority of the pathology encountered at the hip. Exposures of the acetabulum and pelvis are treated in a separate chapter. Herein we discuss the more functional extensile exposures of the hip generally described as anterolateral, lateral (trochanteric), and posterolateral. Variations exist in each of these which are readily made and modified according to personal preferences once the principals of the exposures are known. In addition to these, three additional limited or minimally invasive exposures are presented. This chapter makes no effort to review every surgical exposure that has been described but those which are useful and relevant for managing the majority of hip problems.

I personally reject the term and even the concept of "minimally invasive" exposures and prefer the term "limited invasive" surgery. The reason is that this conveys to me the reasonable position to limit exposure as able and avoid unnecessary tissue damage but not minimize it at all cost. The three exposures detailed here all have value in that they are effective, have a low complication rate, and are relatively easy to perform. The criteria for the use of any of these exposures are:

1. Abbreviated learning curve
2. No increased complication rate
3. Minimal muscle injury
4. Facilitated rehabilitation

ANTERIOR-LATERAL EXPOSURE (HARDINGE) (1,2)

Indications

Hip joint replacement. Value of anterior exposures: typically more stable than posterior exposures.

Disadvantages

Strength of abduction is regained slower after an anterior compared to a posterior exposure (3).

- *Note:* The Hardinge exposure is an example of the family of anterior lateral approaches and has some similarity to several other anterior lateral exposures including the Mayo limited approach discussed below. In general the anterior lateral exposures vary principally in the manner and effect of releasing the insertion of the gluteus medius while taking care to avoid the superior gluteal nerve which typically runs 3 to 5 cm proximal to the tip of the greater trochanter **(Fig. 7-1)**.

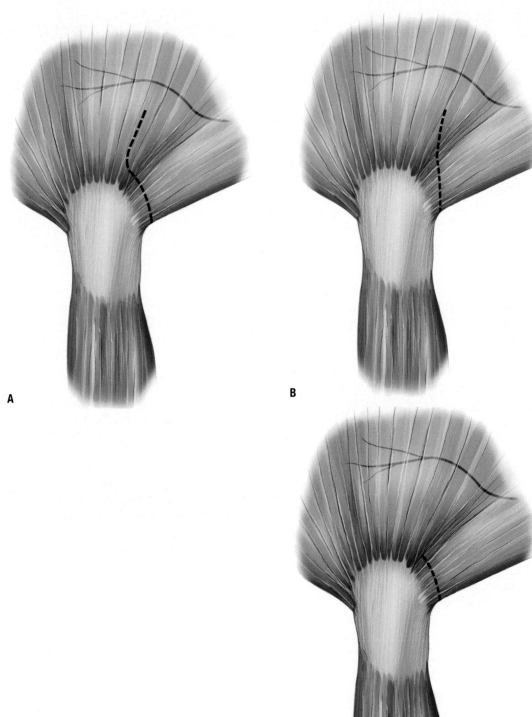

FIGURE 7-1

A

B

C

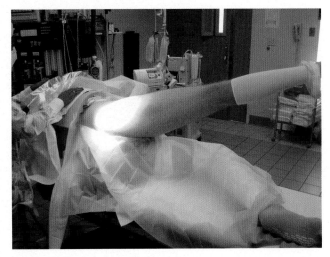

FIGURE 7-2

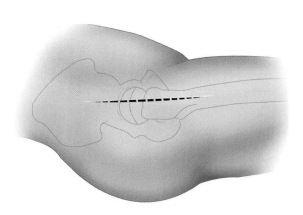

FIGURE 7-3

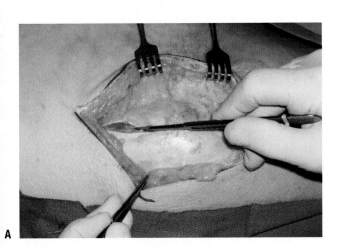

A

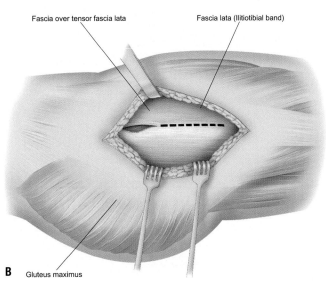

Fascia over tensor fascia lata   Fascia lata (Ilitiotibial band)

B Gluteus maximus

FIGURE 7-4

Position

The patient is placed and supported in the lateral decubitus position; however, the supine position is also acceptable **(Fig. 7-2)**.

Technique

1. Skin incision: the 14 to 16 cm skin incision is centered over the greater trochanter and extends approximately 6 to 8 cm distally along the anterior aspect of the trochanter and down the anterior lateral aspect of the femoral shaft. Proximally, the skin incision extends 6 to 8 cm in line with the fibers of the gluteus maximus muscle **(Fig. 7-3)**.
2. The iliotibial band is entered and split distally and the gluteus maximus muscle is split proximally. The gluteus maximus is retracted posteriorly and the tensor fascia lata retracted anteriorly **(Fig. 7-4)**.

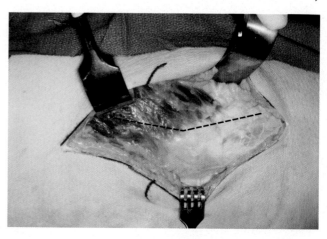

FIGURE 7-5

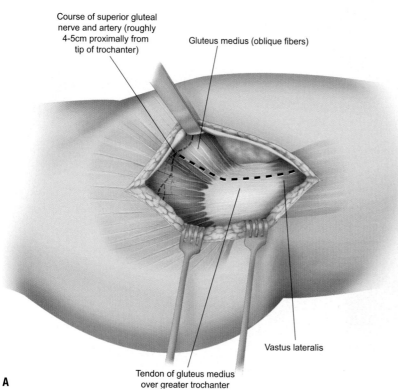

Course of superior gluteal
nerve and artery (roughly
4-5cm proximally from
tip of trochanter)

Gluteus medius (oblique fibers)

Vastus lateralis

Tendon of gluteus medius
over greater trochanter

A

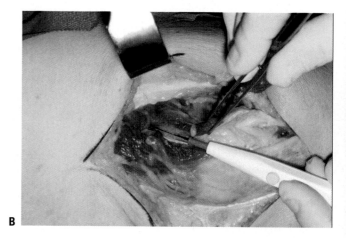

FIGURE 7-6   **B**

- *Note:* If the gluteus is separated from the tensor fascia lata muscle at the site of their interface, the iliotibial band may need to be further released posteriorly to dislocate the hip.

3. The deep exposure begins at the anterior margin of the trochanter and extends distally to include the anterior third of the vastus lateralis muscle (**Fig. 7-5**). Proximally, the incision extends about 4 to 5 cm past the trochanteric tip and splits the gluteus medius musculature in line with its fibers separating its anterior one third from the posterior two thirds.

   - *Note:* Effort is made to maintain continuity of the anterior sleeve of muscle comprising the gluteus medius and anterior portion of the vastus lateralis.

   - *Pitfall:* To avoid injury to the superior gluteal nerve, do not split the gluteus medius more than about 4 to 5 cm proximal to the tip of the trochanter (**Fig. 7-6**)(4).

4. The interval is developed by subperiosteally releasing the antero-oblique fibers of the gluteus medius from the trochanter in line with the remaining anterior fibers of the more proximally fan-shaped portion of the medius musculature.

5. The anterior third of the vastus lateralis muscle is elevated from the trochanter and proximal femur for a distance of about 5 to 7 cm. The sleeve of tissue containing this portion of the abductors and the vastus lateralis is then reflected anteriorly and retracted with a narrow Hohlman retractor (**Fig. 7-7A**). This allows ready access to the anterior capsule (**Fig. 7-7B**).

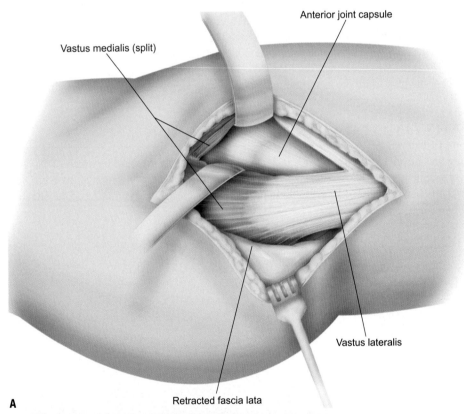

Anterior joint capsule

Vastus medialis (split)

Vastus lateralis

Retracted fascia lata

A

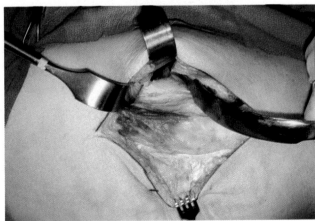

B   FIGURE 7-7

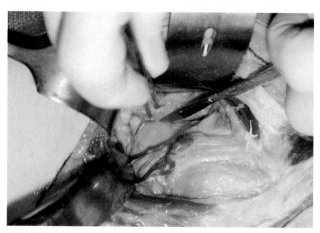

FIGURE 7-8

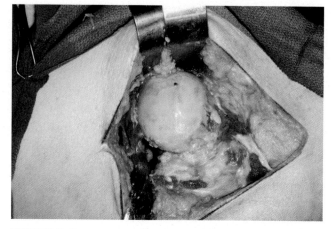

FIGURE 7-9

6. The gluteus minimus muscle is detached from the trochanter beginning anteriorly and separated from the capsule to the extent needed for adequate exposure. A curved Hohlman retractor placed over the femoral neck facilitates retraction of the medius and minimus musculature.
7. The capsule is excised anteriorly, placed over the femoral neck, and further release of the lateral and inferior aspect of the capsule is performed as needed (**Fig. 7-8**).
8. The hip is dislocated by external rotation and flexion. For this exposure the leg may be placed in a sterile pocket anteriorly to prepare the femoral canal (**Fig. 7-9**).
9. Closure: After the procedure the musculature is closed with side-to-side running nonabsorbable sutures.

THE MAYO LIMITED (MINIMAL) ANTERIOR

This exposure was developed by the author in 1995. The goal was to preserve as much of the gluteus medius attachment as possible (**Fig. 7-10**). It is still preferred over the "minimally invasive" approaches currently being popularized as it satisfied the criteria noted at the beginning of the chapter.

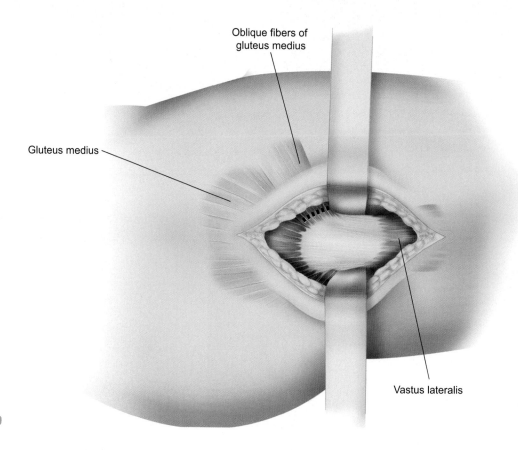

Oblique fibers of
gluteus medius

Gluteus medius

Vastus lateralis

FIGURE 7-10

Indications

Anterior exposure to the hip joint: Incision and drainage; hip joint replacement, typically more stable than posterior exposures.

Position

The patient is placed in the lateral decubitus position. The pelvis is stabilized with method of choice, but should be well fixed vertical to the floor for hip joint replacement (**Fig. 7-11**).

Technique

1. Skin incision: an 8 to 10 cm skin incision is made just anterior to the midline of the trochanter with the distal one-third distal to the tip of the trochanter and the proximal two-thirds over the gluteus medius (**Fig. 7-12**).
2. Through this skin incision the tensor fascia lata is identified (**Fig. 7-13**) and split in the midline from the trochanter distally for a distance of approximately 7 cm. Proximally the muscle of the gluteus maximus is split or alternatively the interval between the gluteus maximus and the tensor fascia lata is identified and split for a distance of approximately an additional 6 cm (**Fig. 7-14**).

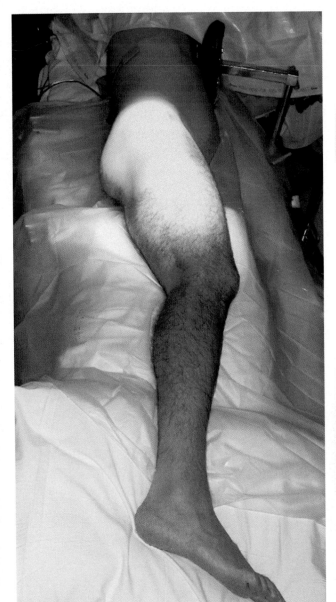

FIGURE 7-11

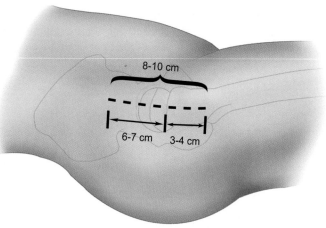

FIGURE 7-12

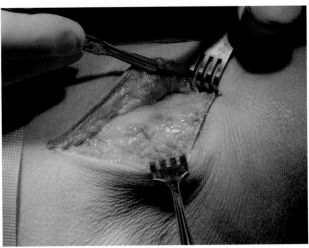

FIGURE 7-13

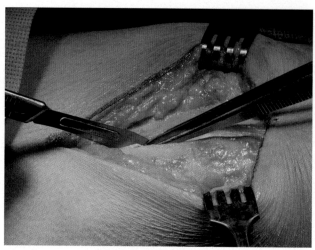
FIGURE 7-14

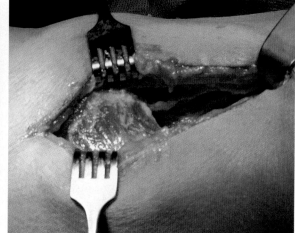
FIGURE 7-15

3. The fascia of the gluteus maximus is reflected posteriorly and the tensor fascia lata is retracted anteriorly.
4. The anterior inferior muscle fibers of the gluteus medius insert almost perpendicular to the long axis of the trochanter **(Fig. 7-15)**. These "anterior-oblique" fibers of the gluteus medius are isolated **(Fig. 7-16)** and released with a cutting cautery leaving a cuff of attachment remaining on the trochanter.

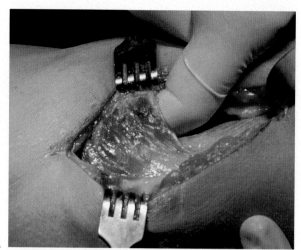
A

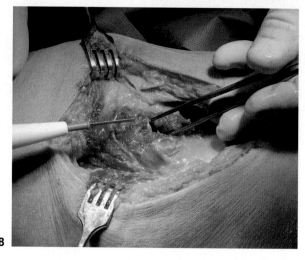
FIGURE 7-16   **B**

5. The release proceeds proximally to the level of the tendinous portion of the gluteus medius and to the leading edge of the gluteus minimis (*arrow*) (**Fig. 7-17**).

   - *Note:* In tight hips a centimeter of the tendinous attachment of the gluteus at the anterior-superior corner of the trochanter may need to be released.

6. The released anterior-oblique fibers of the gluteus medius are reflected proximally and medially. The capsule is identified and is cleaned of soft tissue.

   - *Note:* The key to this exposure resides in the poorly documented or appreciated anatomic feature of the ability to expose the anterior capsule by releasing just those few anterior-oblique fibers.

7. A curved self-retaining retractor is placed between the gluteus minimus and the capsule. A wide self-retaining retractor is placed anteriorly over the rim of the acetabulum allowing ready access to the anterior capsule (**Fig. 7-18**).

8. The hip joint is entered in line with the femoral neck. The anterior portion of the capsule is excised. The inferior capsule is released. The knife is passed blindly over the lateral neck of the femur releasing the lateral capsule. The labrum is incised in several areas radial to its circumference (**Fig. 7-19**).

9. A bone hook is placed around the femoral neck. The hip is externally rotated and the femoral head is delivered into the wound (**Fig. 7-20**). For hip replacement the leg is placed on the table and externally rotated to expose the acetabulum.

   - *Note:* If difficulty of dislocation is encountered, the iliotibial band is released and allowed to slip posterior to the greater trochanter at the time of hip dislocation.

10. Closure: The author prefers to place sutures through the prepared femoral canal and at the margin of the greater trochanter for a transosseous purchase of the nonabsorbable no. 5 suture (**Fig. 7-21**). After reduction of the hip, these sutures are used to repair the antero-oblique fibers of the gluteus medius.

    - *Note:* Of significance is that the majority of the abductors has been left intact with this exposure and generally is not too damaged by femoral canal reaming.

11. Skin closure is routine (**Fig. 7-22**).

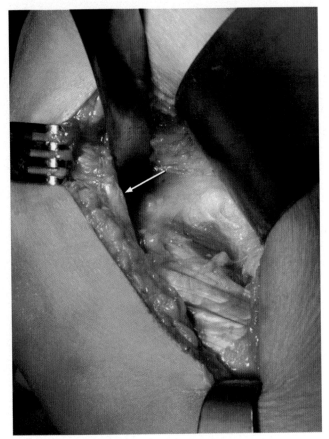

FIGURE 7-17

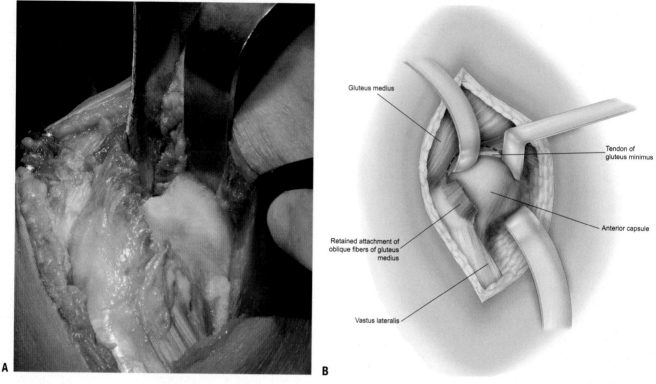

FIGURE 7-18

A

B

Gluteus medius

Tendon of
gluteus minimus

Anterior capsule

Retained attachment of
oblique fibers of gluteus
medius

Vastus lateralis

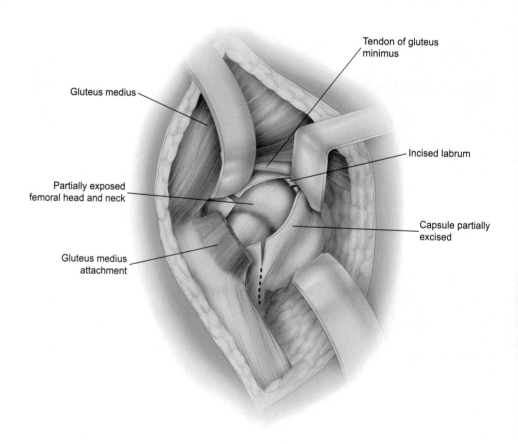

FIGURE 7-19

Tendon of gluteus
minimus

Gluteus medius

Incised labrum

Partially exposed
femoral head and neck

Capsule partially
excised

Gluteus medius
attachment

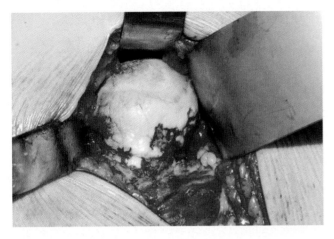

FIGURE 7-20

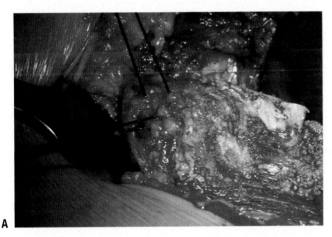

A

FIGURE 7-21

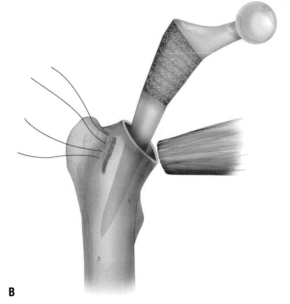

B

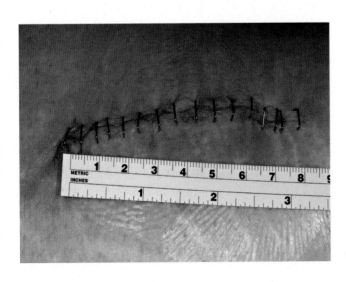

FIGURE 7-22

LIMITED ANTERIOR HIP JOINT EXPOSURE (LIMITED SMITH-PETERSON) (5)

Indications

One of the minimally invasive muscle sparing techniques for hip joint replacement, or for any anterior joint arthrotomy.

Position

The patient is placed supine on the operating table.

Technique

1. The skin incision begins two finger-breadths below the anterior-superior iliac spine (**Fig. 7-23A**) and extends distally for approximately 8 cm in a linear fashion between the tensor fascia lata and the sartorius (**Fig. 7-23B**). This interval can be identified by palpation (**Fig 7-23C**).

   - *Note:* The major disadvantage of this incision is injury to the lateral femoral cutaneous nerve. Although quite variable, this nerve typically exits approximately two finger-breadths below the anterior superior iliac spine and just medial to the sartorius. The lateral branches are variable and can be injured when making the incision in the anterior fascia.

2. The subcutaneous tissue is reflected to the level of the fascia. The sartorius and tensor fascia lata muscles are identified and the fascia investing these two muscles is split longitudinally (**Fig. 7-24**). Splitting the anterior fibers of tensor muscle helps protect against injury to the lateral femoral cutaneous nerve (**Fig. 7-25**) (2).

3. The tensor is separated from the sartorius by sharp and blunt dissection (**Fig. 7-26**). The sartorius is reflected medially, the tensor laterally.

4. Further exposure is straight forward and is usually done by palpating the femoral head and exposing the capsule by blunt dissection.

   - *Note:* The ascending branch of the lateral circumflex artery and vein do cross the field and must be ligated or cauterized (**Fig. 7-27**).

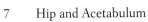

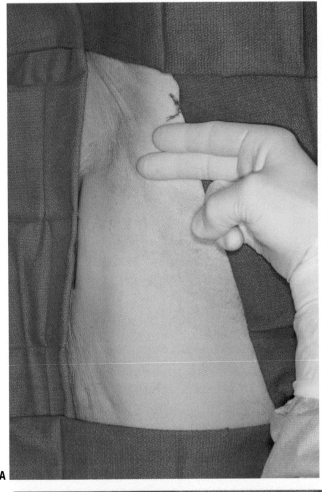

A

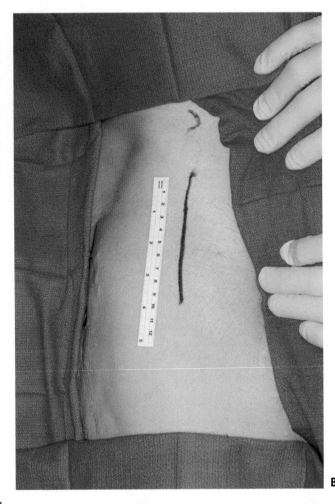

B

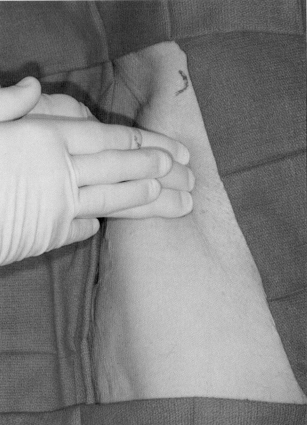

C

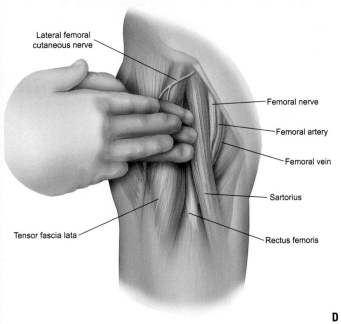

Lateral femoral
cutaneous nerve

Femoral nerve

Femoral artery

Femoral vein

Sartorius

Tensor fascia lata

Rectus femoris

D

FIGURE 7-23

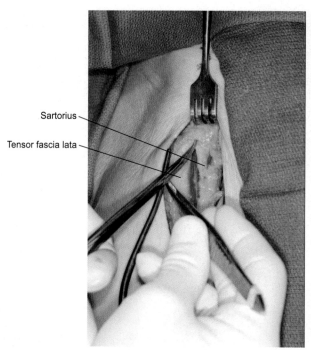

Sartorius

Tensor fascia lata

FIGURE 7-24

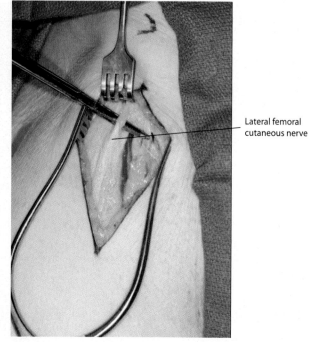

Lateral femoral
cutaneous nerve

FIGURE 7-25

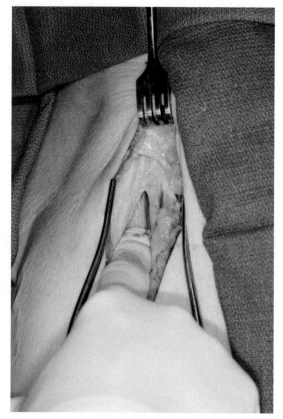

FIGURE 7-26

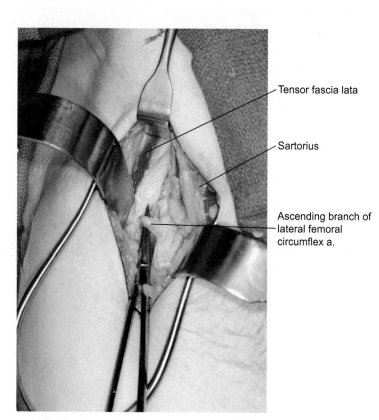

Tensor fascia lata

Sartorius

Ascending branch of
lateral femoral
circumflex a.

FIGURE 7-27

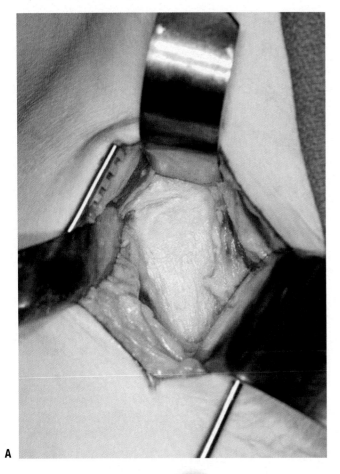

A

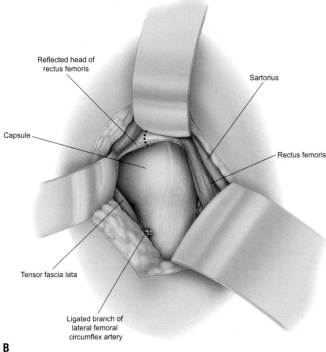

Reflected head of
rectus femoris

Sartorius

Capsule

Rectus femoris

Tensor fascia lata

Ligated branch of
lateral femoral
circumflex artery

FIGURE 7-28

B

5. At the level of the hip joint the gluteus medius and tensor fascia are further reflected laterally. The attachment of the reflected head of the rectus femoris is observed at the superior aspect of the acetabulum and must be incised **(Fig. 7-28)**.

6. The hip joint is then entered by excising the anterior capsule **(Fig. 7-29)**. Dislocation occurs with extension and external rotation **(Fig. 7-30)**.

7. Closure: the closure only requires suture of the skin and subcutaneous tissue.

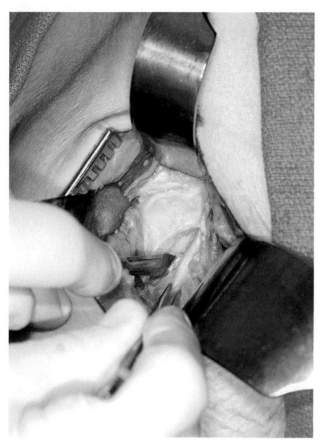

FIGURE 7-29

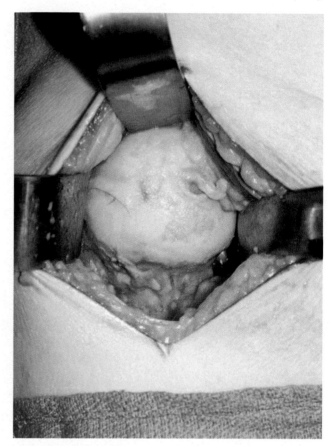

FIGURE 7-30

POSTERIOR APPROACH TO THE HIP (6)

The common feature of posterior exposures is release of the short rotators. Variation is introduced by the manner of developing the exposure dealing with the gluteus maximus muscle and the iliotibial track. The repair of the rotators with capsule is also variably described.

Traditional Exposure

1. Skin incision: variable skin incisions may be used. Typically these are centered over the trochanter just posterior to the midline. The incision is 12 to 14 cm in length and may be straight or follows the fibers of the gluteus maximus and then curves slightly posterior **(Fig. 7-31)**.
2. The dissection exposes the iliotibial band and the proximal gluteus maximus is divided along its fibers posteriorly **(Fig. 7-32)**. The iliotibial band is split and the posterior portion of the gluteus maximus is retracted posteriorly, the anterior fibers of the gluteus maximus and tensor fascia are retracted anteriorly, often with self-retaining retractors.
3. The attachment of the gluteus medius is identified posteriorly and released from the posterior crest of the trochanter with a cutting cautery **(Fig. 7-33)**.
4. The gluteus medius is retracted proximally with a curved retractor placed over the neck of the femur, and the short rotators are exposed. Distally, the quadratus femoris is observed and may or may not be released from the femur. The superior and inferior gemeli; the obturator internus and externus are tagged with two sutures and released more proximally **(Fig. 7-34)**. The piriformis is identified proximally and detached from the styloid process of the greater trochanter.
5. The entire sleeve of short rotator muscles are elevated from the capsule as it is released with a cutting cautery just at its insertion at the posterior margin of the greater trochanter.

   • *Pearl:* To facilitate the all important subsequent reattachment, these muscles and capsule should be tagged before release.

6. The posterior capsule is entered and is excised as needed **(Fig. 7-35)**.

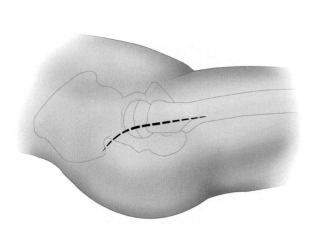

FIGURE 7-31

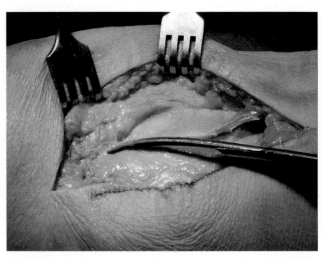

FIGURE 7-32

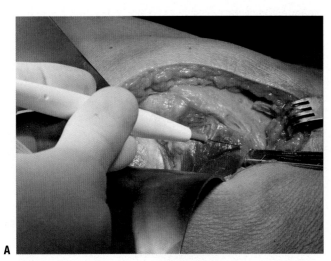

A

B

Gluteus medius

Greater trochanter

Quadratus femoris

Sciatic nerve

Superior gamellus

Obturator internus

Inferior gamellus

Branch from medial femoral circumflex artery

FIGURE 7-33

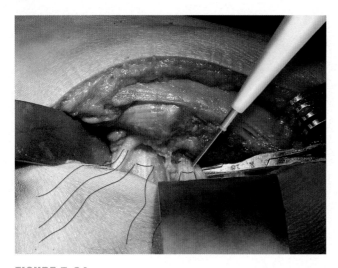

FIGURE 7-34

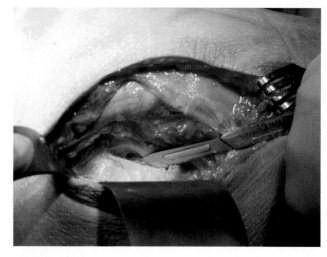

FIGURE 7-35

7. The labrum is incised and with internal rotation of the thigh, the femoral head dislocates posteriorly **(Fig. 7-36)**.

8. Closure: the closure is extremely important with the posterior exposure to lessen the possibility of dislocation. The short rotators are retrieved and are then reattached through bone holes in the posterior margin of the trochanter in the region of their anatomic attachment **(Fig. 7-37)**.

   ● *Note:* The formal and secure reattachment of these muscles with capsular remnants has dramatically decreased the incidence of hip dislocation (7). Several options for reattachment have been described. An alternative to that is illustrated with the minimally invasive exposure (see Fig. 7-48).

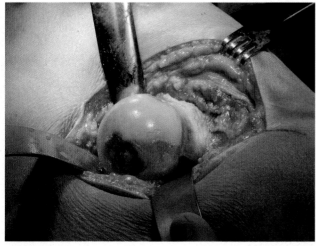

FIGURE 7-36

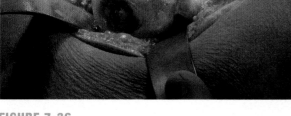

FIGURE 7-37

LIMITED POSTERIOR EXPOSURE (8)

1. As with other limited exposures, special retractors have been developed and modified to facilitate this technique **(Fig. 7-38)**. A limited 7 to 10 cm posterior skin incision is employed.

    - *Pearl:* The key to limited posterior skin incision is the precise placement of the skin incision itself. Typically this parallels the posterior border of the greater trochanter and extends from the tip of the greater trochanter to the tubercle of the vastus lateralis ridge **(Fig. 7-39)**.

2. Deep to the skin, an incision is made through the fibers of the gluteus maximus parallel to the posterior border of the greater trochanter **(Fig. 7-40)**. A retractor is placed anterior to the greater trochanter allowing visualization of the gluteus medius and piriformis tendon posteriorly **(Fig. 7-41)**.

    - *Note:* With this exposure the iliotibial band is not split, the exposure is posterior to this structure through the distal fibers of the gluteus maximus.

3. The gluteus medius is retracted anteriorly exposing the underlying gluteus minimus which is separated from the capsule **(Fig. 7-42)**. The subsequent incision of the hip capsule and external rotators starts from the posterior edge of the gluteus minimus and ends at but does not include the quadratus femoris muscle. Sutures are placed in the short rotators prior to release **(Fig. 7-43)**.

4. The hip capsule and external rotators are incised together from the greater trochanter and these structures are preserved as one layer for later repair **(Fig. 7-44)**.

5. With internal rotation the hip is dislocated posteriorly **(Fig. 7-45)**. The femoral neck cut is carried out in accordance with the preoperative plan regarding neck length.

6. The acetabulum is exposed with a narrow cobra placed at the anterior-inferior iliac spine to retract the femur anteriorly. A specialized sharp-pointed angled retractor is driven into the posterior wall to retract the capsule and external rotators. A broad cobra retractor is placed inferiorly at the level of the transverse ligament to facilitate insertion of acetabular reamers **(Fig. 7-46)**.

7. The femur is exposed with one narrow retractor anteriorly to retract the gluteus maximus and subcutaneous fat. A second narrow angled retractor is placed along the medial neck to retract the preserved

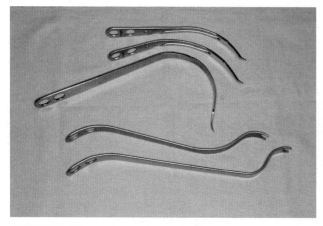

FIGURE 7-38

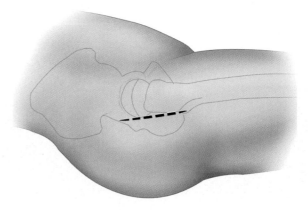

FIGURE 7-39

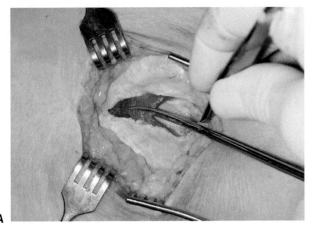
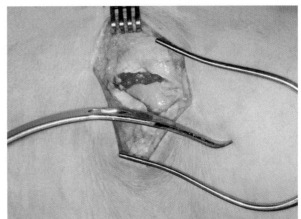

A

B

FIGURE 7-40

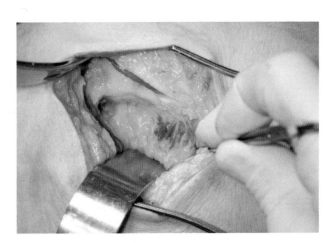

FIGURE 7-41

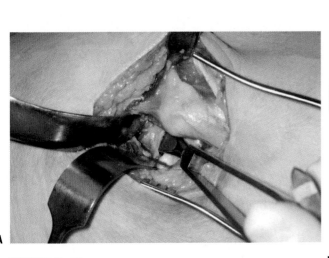

A

FIGURE 7-42

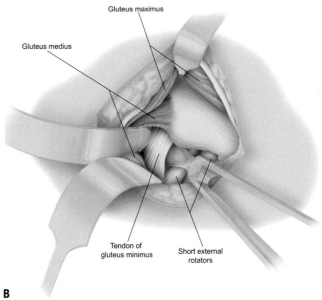

Gluteus maximus

Gluteus medius

Tendon of
gluteus minimus

Short external
rotators

B

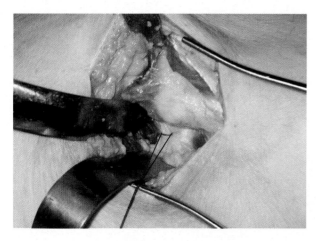

FIGURE 7-43

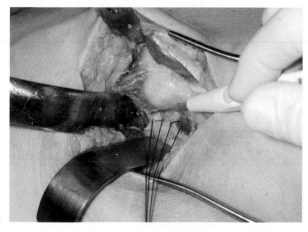

A

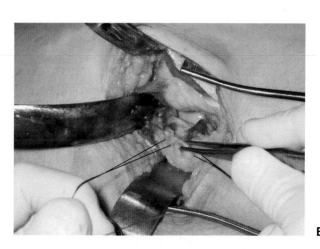

B

FIGURE 7-44

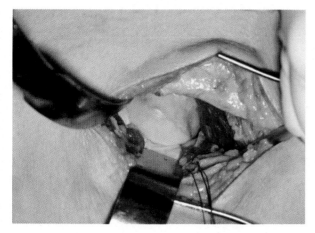

FIGURE 7-45

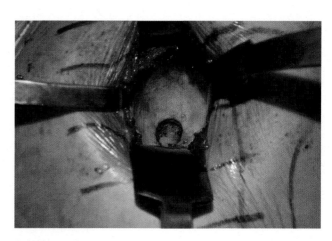

FIGURE 7-46

quadratus femoris muscle. The third retractor is placed beneath the anterior part of the cut femoral neck to retract the skin and posterior edge of gluteus maximus muscle posteriorly (**Fig. 7-47**).

8. Closure: The short rotators are reattached through bone holes as with any posterior hip exposure (**Fig. 7-48A**). Alternatively, the cut edge of gluteus minimus and underlying anterior capsule can be sutured directly to the posterior capsule and overlying external rotators as one layer (**Fig. 7-48B**). This eliminates any dead space between the capsular repair and the prosthetic femoral head.

9. Skin closure is of choice (**Fig. 7-49**).

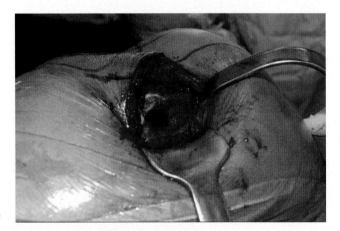

FIGURE 7-47

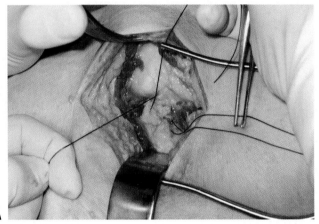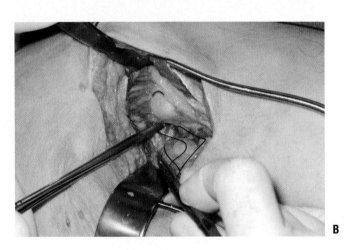

A   B

FIGURE 7-48

FIGURE 7-49

TROCHANTERIC OSTEOTOMY

Today we would recognize three variations of trochanteric osteotomy to have practical utility (**Fig. 7-50**). Two are useful for primary and one for revision hip replacement (9). The first, used by Charnley, simply detaches the trochanter in a way to allow proximal retraction of the gluteus medius and minimus. The second is an osteotomy in continuity leaving the attachment of the gluteus medius proximally and of the vastus lateralis distally. The extended osteotomy is the third version and is reserved for revision procedures and includes the trochanter with the gluteus attachments but also extends distally to maintain the attachment of the vastus lateralis. The osteotomy is initiated posteriorly just anterior to the intermuscular septum and is hinged anteriorly. This exposure has realized great popularity in recent years to facilitate removal of well-fixed femoral components.

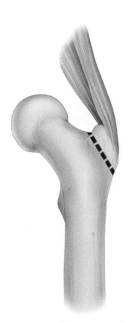
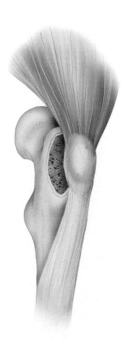
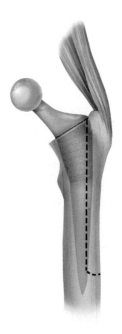

FIGURE 7-50

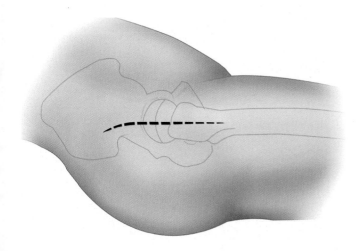

FIGURE 7-51

"Simple" Trochanteric Osteotomy (Charnley)

Proximal reflection: this osteotomy was used and popularized by Sir John Charnley during the development of the total hip (low friction arthroplasty) era (10).

Position   Typically the patient is in the lateral decubitus position although the osteotomy can be performed in a supine position as well.

Technique

1. Incision: the incision is of choice. A straight or slightly posterior curved skin incision measuring 14 to 16 cm is usually adequate since the trochanter is to be reflected proximally so the incision will be centered somewhat more proximally referable to the trochanter (**Fig. 7-51**).
2. The fascia is split distally for approximately 4 to 6 cm and proximally the gluteus maximus is either split from the tensor fascia lata or simply split the gluteus maximus muscle in line with its fibers (**Fig. 7-52**).
3. The iliotibial band is separated with a self-retaining retractor. The trochanteric bursa is resected to allow clear identity of the origin of the vastus lateralis at the crest of the greater trochanter (**Fig. 7-53**). The vastus lateralis is then released distally from its attachment at the crest of the greater trochanter (**Fig. 7-54**).
4. Posteriorly the styloid to which the periformis attaches is identified. A wide 40 to 50 mm osteotome is driven under the trochanter originating at the trochanteric crest and proceeds to and through the styloid process. The depth of the osteotomy can be accurately facilitated by placing a periosteal retractor under the styloid process (**Fig. 7-55**).

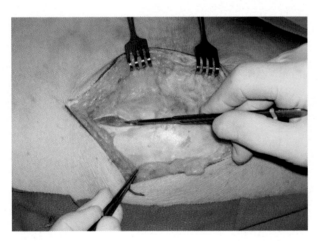

FIGURE 7-52

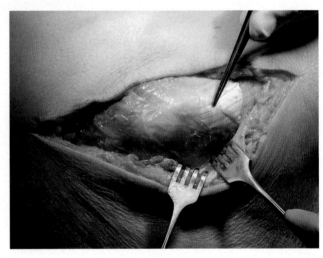

FIGURE 7-53

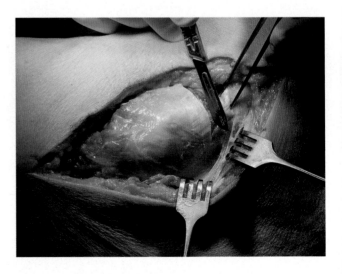

FIGURE 7-54

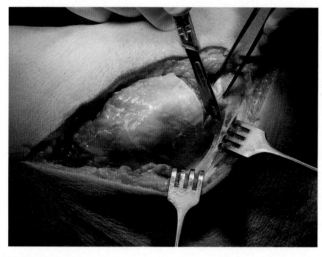
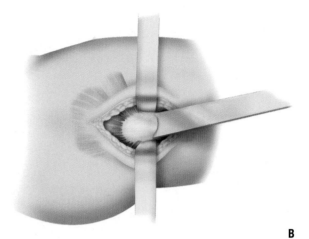

A   B

FIGURE 7-55

- ● *Pearl:* Care should be taken not to make this osteotomy too thick since, with an implant in place, the osteomized bed may be compromised exposing the implant and nonhealing may ensue.

5. The trochanter is retracted proximally and the anterior fibers of the gluteus medius are released both anteriorly (**Fig. 7-56A**) and posteriorly (**Fig. 7-56B,C**).
6. On further retraction of the trochanter proximally, the gluteus minimus is separated from the capsule with scissors (**Fig. 7-57**).

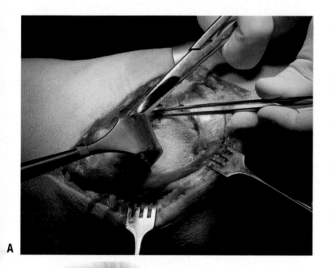
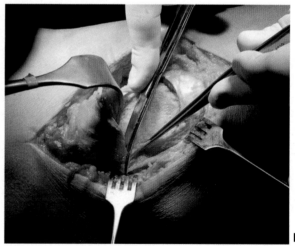

A   B

FIGURE 7-56

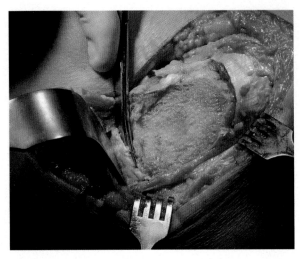

FIGURE 7-57

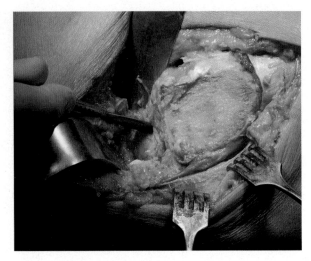

FIGURE 7-58

7. The capsule is excised **(Fig. 7-58)** and the femoral head is dislocated anteriorly by external rotation of the thigh.
8. Reattachment: Several options have been successfully used. Monofilament no. 14 wire is effective if placed through bone and distributed both vertically and transversely **(Fig. 7-59)** (11,12). Alternatively, specially designed "claws" have been designed just for this purpose **(Fig. 7-60)**.

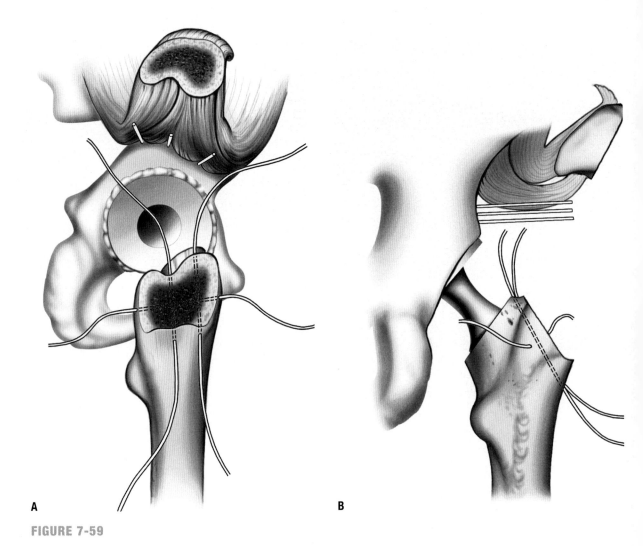

A   B

FIGURE 7-59

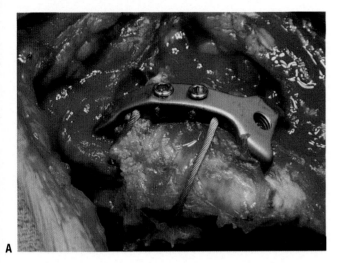

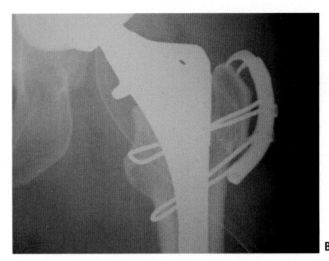

A   B

FIGURE 7-60

- *Pearl:* I prefer the monofilament wire rather than cables or special constraints as it is effective, less expensive, and less likely to cause trochanteric bursitis than is the "claw" or braided wire.

The Trochanteric Osteotomy in Continuity (8,13,14)

Rationale   The attachment of the vastus lateralis helps compress the osteotomy and assure healing of the osteotomy.

Technique

1. Incision: an exposure is used similar to that which was used for simple osteotomy with proximal retraction (**see Fig. 7-51**).

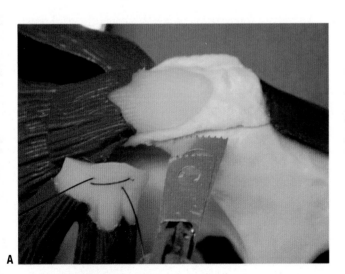

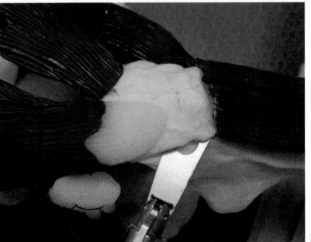

A   B

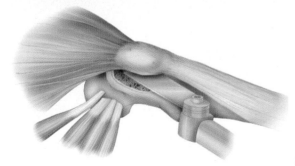

C   **FIGURE 7-61**

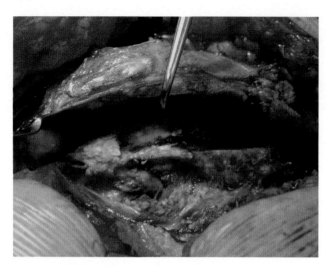

FIGURE 7-62

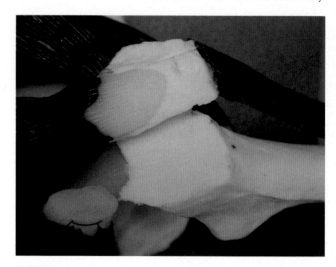

FIGURE 7-63

2. The trochanter is freed of its soft tissue posteriorly and the short rotators are released. An oscillating saw separates the trochanter with the attachments of the gluteus medius and minimus proximally and the vastus lateralis distally (**Fig. 7-61**). The fragment is mobilized from posterior to anterior.

   ● *Note:* The depth of the trochanteric osteotomy can be variable but detaching the short rotators is required in all instances (**Fig. 7-62**).

3. The capsule is exposed and excised posteriorly and laterally (**Fig. 7-63**).
4. The hip dislocates posteriorly with internal rotation of the thigh.
5. Reattachment. For this osteotomy two circumferential monofilament wires are effective and easy to apply (**Fig. 7-64**).

   ● *Note:* The osteotomy in continuity does allow compression of the osteotomy site with proximal and distal muscle contracture which is the reason that this osteotomy is preferred by some.

Extended Trochanteric Osteotomy

This osteotomy involves the posterior-lateral one third of the circumference of the femur (9,15–17) (see Fig. 7-51). This osteotomy is used for revision of the femoral component and involves the posterior-lateral one third.

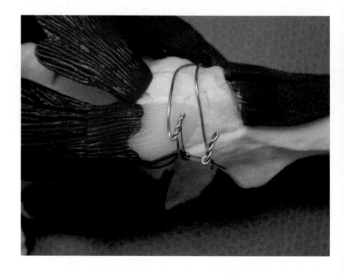

FIGURE 7-64

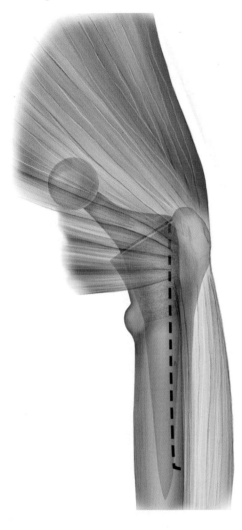

FIGURE 7-65

Technique

1. The exposure is similar as described above. Posteriorly the gluteus musculature is identified and the trochanter is osteotomized from its posterior border distally along the linea aspira to a length necessary for adequate exposure of the proximal or fixed portion of the femoral stem **(Fig. 7-65)**.
2. Anteriorly, a series of drill holes are used to allow the osteotomy to hinge anteriorly **(Fig. 7-66)**.
3. An osteotomy is performed with an oscillating saw, and usually a drill hole is placed in the posterior distal corner to avoid a stress riser effect **(Fig. 7-67)**.

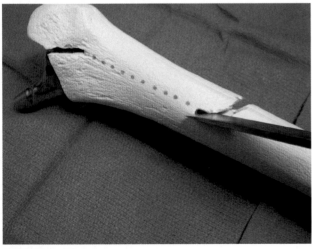

FIGURE 7-66

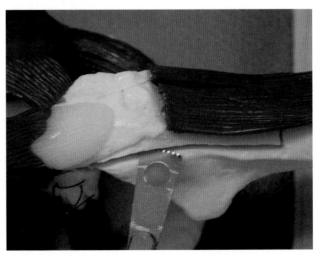

FIGURE 7-67

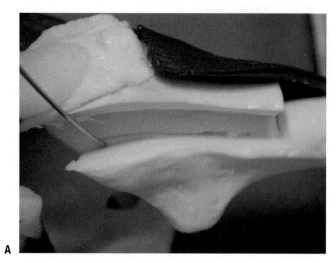
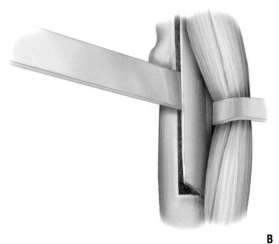

FIGURE 7-68

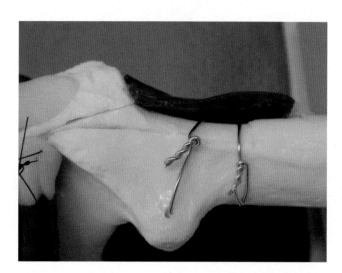

FIGURE 7-69

4. The transverse cut is then made distally to the level of the anterior drill holes.
5. The osteotomized segment is elevated anteriorly with one or several osteotomes and the retraction of this extended trochanteric osteotomy is from posterior to anterior **(Fig. 7-68)**. The vastus lateralis muscle remains attached to the fragment.
6. The hip is dislocated posteriorly with internal rotation.
7. At completion, the trochanter is "reduced" to its original bed and secured with at least three circumferential monofilament wires **(Fig. 7-69)**.

   ● *Note:* While healing rates are high in excess of 90%, care should be taken to attain as accurate a reduction as is possible. This may be difficult if the revised implant has different dimensions than the one removed.

REFERENCES

1. Glassman AH, Engh CA, Bobyn JD. A technique of extensile exposure for total hip arthroplasty. *J Arthroplasty* 1987;2:11–21.
2. Jensen NF, Harris WH. A system for trochanteric osteotomy and reattachment for total hip arthroplasty with a ninety-nine percent union rate. *Clin Orthop* 1986;(208):174–181.
3. Lindgren U, Svenson O. A new transtrochanteric approach to the hip. *Int'l Orthopaedics* 1988;12(1):37–41.
4. Hardinge K. The direct lateral approach to the hip. *J Bone Joint Surg* 1982;64B:17–19.
5. Pellici PM, Bostrom M, Poss R. Posterior approach to total hip replacement using enhanced posterior soft tissue repair. *Clin Orthop* 1998;355:224–228.
6. Fulkerson JP, Crelin ES, Keggi KJ. Anatomy and osteotomy of the greater trochanter. *Archives of Surg* 1979;114(1):19–21.
7. Chiu FY, Chen CM, Chung TY, et al. The effect of posterior capsulorrhaphy in primary total hip arthroplasty: A prospective randomized study. *J Arthroplasty* 2000;15:194–199.
8. Dorr LD. *Hip Arthroplasty: Minimally Invasive Techniques and Computer Navigation.* Philadelphia: Elsevier Health Sciences, 2006.
9. McGrory BJ, Morrey BF, Cahalan TD, et al. Effect of femoral offset on range of motion and abductor muscle strength after total hip arthroplasty. *J Bone Joint Surg* 1995;77B(6):865–869.
10. Charnley J, Ferreira A, De SD. Transplantation of the greater trochanter in arthroplasty of the hip. *J Bone Joint Surg* 1964;46B:191.
11. Jacobs LG, Buxton RA. The course of the superior gluteal nerve in the lateral approach to the hip. *J Bone Joint Surg* 1989;71A:1239–1243.
12. Smith-Peterson MN. Approach to and exposure of the hip joint for mold arthroplasty. *J Bone Joint Surg* 1949;31A:40.
13. English TA. The trochanteric approach to the hip for prosthetic replacement. *J Bone Joint Surg* 1975;57A:1128–1133.
14. Light TR, Keggi KJ. Anterior approach to hip arthroplasty. *Clin Orthop* 1980;152:255–260.
15. Chen WM, McAuley JP, Engh CA Jr, et al. Extended slide trochanteric osteotomy for revision total hip arthroplasty. *J Bone Joint Surg* 2000;82A:1215–1219.
16. Gibson A. Posterior exposure of the hip joint. *J Bone Joint Surg* 1950;32B:183.
17. Wroblewski BM, Shelley P. Reattachment of the greater trochanter after hip replacement. *J Bone Joint Surg* 1985;67B(5):736–740.
15. McGrory J, Bal BS, Harris WH: Trochanteric osteotomy for total hip arthroplasty: Variations and indications for their use. *JAAOS* 1996;4:258–267.
19. Younger TI, Bradford MS, Magnus RE, et al: Extended proximal femoral osteotomy: A new technique for femoral revision arthroplasty. *J Arthroplasty* 1995;10:329–338.

8 Femur

Joseph R. Cass

ANTEROMEDIAL APPROACH TO THE FEMUR

Indications

Situations in which combined exposure of the knee and femoral shaft is necessary, such as for the placement of large revision knee arthroplasty components.

Extension

The exposure can be extended distally to complete a medial parapatellar approach to the knee. Proximal extension is limited by the femoral artery crossing the wound.

Anatomy

The anteromedial approach is distant from any important neurovascular structures and it involves a transmuscular plane to the femur. This approach to the femur is performed between the vastus medialis and rectus femoris in the superficial layer and involves splitting the vastus intermedius in the deep layer to access the femur.

Technique

1. Incision: if it is possible to determine the location of the medial border of the vastus medialis the incision should follow this contour, extending proximally from a point just proximal and medial to the superomedial pole of the patella. If the vastus medialis contour is unable to be determined, the incision should be carried in a longitudinal fashion from a point medial and proximal to the superomedial pole of the patella (**Fig. 8-1**).

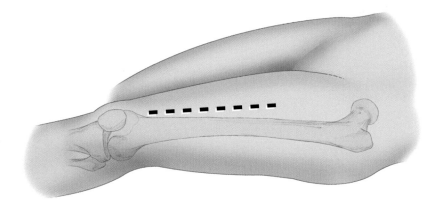

FIGURE 8-1

The skin incision typically extends proximally as needed from a point just medial and superior to the superomedial aspect of the patella.

2. The deep fascia of the thigh is incised in line with the skin incision and flaps are elevated medially and laterally **(Fig. 8-2)**. The interval between the vastus medialis and rectus femoris is identified and is developed with blunt dissection proximally.
3. As this interval is continued distally, the quadriceps tendon is incised close to its medial border, leaving adequate amount of tendon medially and laterally for later closure **(Fig. 8-3)**.
4. Deep to the vastus medialis and rectus femoris, the vastus intermedius is split in line with its fibers **(Fig. 8-4)**.
5. Subperiosteal dissection along the femoral shaft elevates the vastus intermedius off the femur **(Fig. 8-5)**. Retraction of the vastus medialis in the lateral and medial direction allows complete exposure of the anterior aspect of the distal femur.

Closure

Muscle reapproximation of the vastus intermedius is not possible. Closure consists of first repairing the incision in the quadriceps tendon, followed by reapproximating the deep fascia.

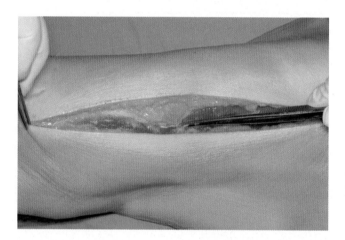

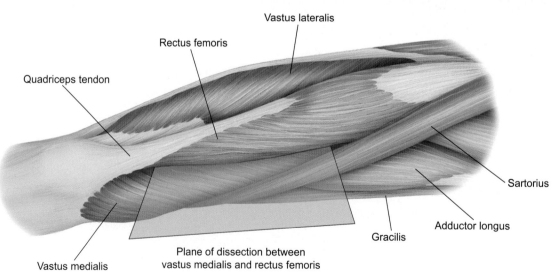

FIGURE 8-2

The deep fascia of the thigh is split to expose the interval between the vastus medialis and rectus femoris. Distally, the muscles join to form the quadriceps tendon.

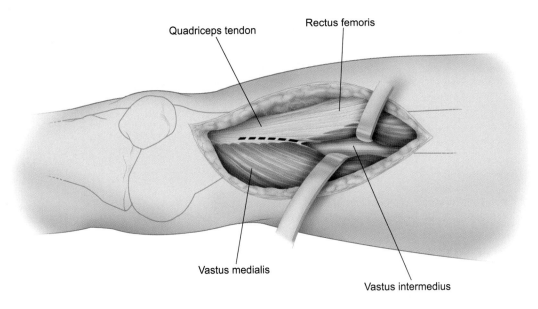

Quadriceps tendon   Rectus femoris

Vastus medialis

Vastus intermedius

FIGURE 8-3

The interval between the vastus medialis and rectus femoris is developed with blunt dissection. Distally, the quadriceps tendon may need to be split in order to access the distal femur and articular surface.

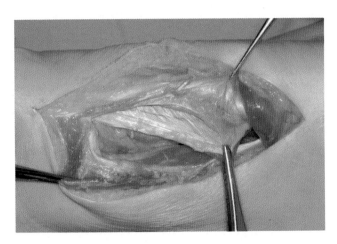

FIGURE 8-4

The vastus intermedius is deep to the interval developed.

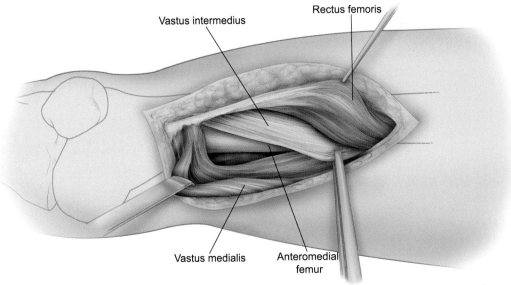

Vastus intermedius   Rectus femoris

Vastus medialis   Anteromedial femur

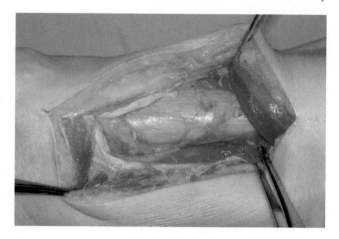

FIGURE 8-5
Subperiosteal dissection of the vastus intermedius medially and laterally allows exposure of the anterior femur.

ANTEROLATERAL APPROACH TO THE FEMUR

Indications

Fractures, bone grafting, total femoral replacement, and extensor mechanism repair.

Extension

The exposure can be extended proximally to expose the hip joint and distally to expose the knee joint through a lateral parapatellar approach.

Anatomy

The interval between the rectus femoris and vastus lateralis is developed in order to expose the vastus intermedius. The approach involves splitting the fibers of the vastus intermedius to access the femoral shaft. The descending branch of the lateral femoral circumflex artery crosses the plane between the rectus femoris and the vastus lateralis in the proximal thigh. The artery enters the vastus lateralis along with the motor branch of the nerve to the vastus lateralis and should be preserved as it enters the vastus lateralis. A branch of the vessel continues along the medial side of the vastus lateralis to join the arterial anastomosis around the knee.

Technique

1. Incision: the incision is made along a line from the anterior-superior iliac spine to the lateral aspect of the patella. The length of the incision is determined by the pathology being addressed. The skin and subcutaneous tissue are incised in the line described **(Fig. 8-6)** to expose the deep fascia of the thigh.
2. The fascia is split in line with the skin incision and the interval between the rectus femoris and vastus lateralis is identified **(Fig. 8-7)**.

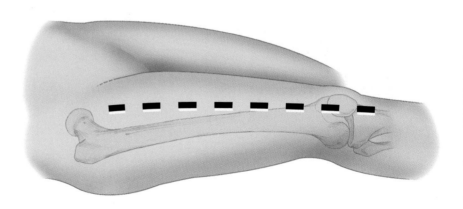

FIGURE 8-6

The skin incision is made along a line connecting the anterior-superior iliac spine and the lateral edge of the patella. The location of the incision along this line depends on the region of the femur that needs to be exposed.

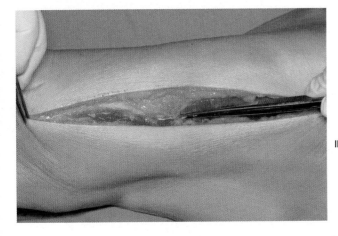

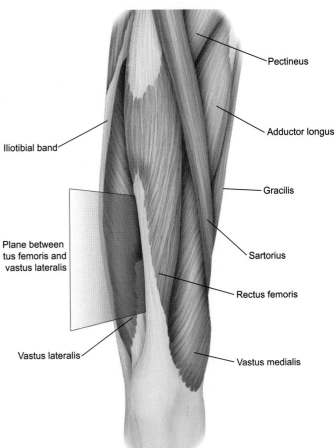

Pectineus

Adductor longus

Iliotibial band

Gracilis

Plane between
tus femoris and
vastus lateralis

Sartorius

Rectus femoris

Vastus lateralis

Vastus medialis

FIGURE 8-7

The deep fascia of the thigh is split in line with the skin incision and the rectus femoris and vastus lateralis muscles
are identified.

3. This interval is easily developed in the middle of the thigh. In the distal thigh, the muscles are adherent, connected by an aponeurotic sheet of tissue. This connection will need to be split in order
   to access the vastus intermedius in the distal thigh **(Fig. 8-8)**. Proximally, care should be taken in
   order to prevent injury to the descending branch of the lateral femoral circumflex artery and motor nerve to the vastus lateralis as they cross from the rectus femoris to the vastus lateralis together.
4. The vastus intermedius muscle belly is split in line with its fibers to expose the anterior femoral
   shaft. Subperiosteal dissection medially and laterally to elevate the vastus intermedius will further expose the anterior aspect of the femur **(Fig. 8-9)**.

Closure

Muscle reapproximation of the vastus intermedius is not possible. Closure consists of reapproximating the deep fascia followed by routine subcutaneous tissue and skin closures.

POSTEROLATERAL APPROACH TO THE FEMUR

Indications

Reduction and internal fixation of femoral shaft fractures, subtrochanteric and intertrochanteric fractures, and biopsy and treatment of bone tumors.

Extension

The posterolateral approach to the femur can be extended proximally and combined with multiple
hip exposures to expose the proximal femur. Distally, the exposure is easily extended to a lateral
parapatellar approach to the knee joint.

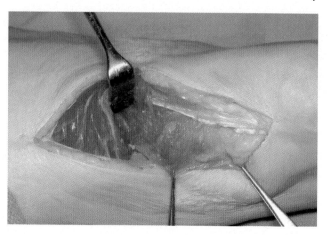

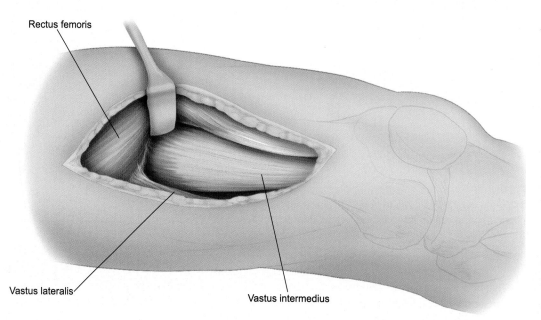

Rectus femoris

Vastus lateralis

Vastus intermedius

FIGURE 8-8

In the proximal thigh, the plane between the rectus femoris and vastus lateralis is easily developed. It is recommended to begin developing the interval proximally and then working in a distal direction. Distally, the muscles are adherent and separation requires sharp dissection. Once divided, the vastus intermedius is visible.

FIGURE 8-9

The vastus intermedius has been split along the anterior aspect of the femur in line with its fibers. Subperiosteal dissection medially and laterally allows elevation of the vastus intermedius and exposure of the anterior femur.

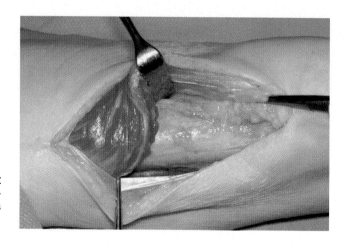

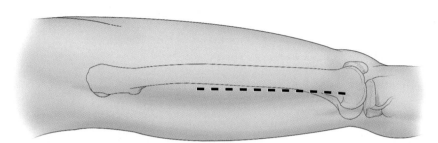

FIGURE 8-10

The skin incision is located along a line from the posterior edge of the greater trochanter to the posterior aspect of the lateral femoral condyle, parallel to the femoral shaft.

Anatomy

The posterolateral approach to the femur utilizes the plane between the vastus lateralis and the posterior intermuscular septum. There are no important nerves at risk in this exposure. Perforating vessels which pierce the lateral intermuscular septum are at risk during this approach and need to be ligated in order to access the femoral shaft.

Positioning

The patient is placed in the supine position with a sandbag under the ipsilateral hip.

Technique

1. Incision: the incision is parallel to the femoral shaft on a line from the posterior aspect of the greater trochanter to the posterior edge of the lateral femoral condyle (**Fig. 8-10**). Depending on the part of the femur that needs exposure, the location of the incision can be adjusted proximally and distally along this line. The subcutaneous tissue and fat are dissected in line with the skin incision towards the fascia lata and posterolateral aspect of the femoral shaft.
2. The fascia lata is split in line with its fibers along the posterolateral aspect of the femur. This will allow for exposure of the posterior margin of the vastus lateralis (**Fig. 8-11**).
3. The femoral shaft should be palpated through the fascia lata prior to splitting the fascia lata.

   - *Note:* Opening the fascia lata too anteriorly will cause difficulty in dissection of the vastus lateralis posteriorly to the linea aspera. Separating the fascia lata proximally will require splitting the tensor fascia lata in line with its muscle fibers.

4. The fascia over the vastus lateralis is exposed beneath the fascia lata and incised in line with the fibers close to the lateral intermuscular septum. Blunt dissection using elevators allows separation of the vastus lateralis muscle from the fascia and lateral intermuscular septum towards the linea aspera (**Fig. 8-12**). Elevation of the muscle fibers is accomplished with distal to proximal elevation to elevate the fibers as they originate from the femur and intermuscular septum.
5. As the linea aspera is approached, the perforating vessels are encountered. Careful blunt dissection along the interval between the muscle and lateral intermuscular septum will expose the vessels as they perforate the lateral intermuscular septum, allowing them to be carefully ligated (**Fig. 8-13**).

   - *Pearl:* Proper control of the perforators cannot be overstated. Inadvertent transaction may result in retraction of the vessels, making hemostasis problematic.

6. Subperiosteal elevation anteriorly along the femur will allow retractor placement over the anterior aspect of the femur for exposure and anterior retraction of the entire vastus lateralis (**Fig. 8-14**).

Closure

The muscle belly of the vastus lateralis is allowed to fall posteriorly against the lateral intermuscular septum. Repair of the fascia of the vastus literalist is performed next, followed by the closure of the fascia lata. Separation of the fascia lata in a line more anteriorly than the vastus lateralis fascia will allow the vastus lateralis fascia and fascia lata closure to be in separate, overlapping layers.

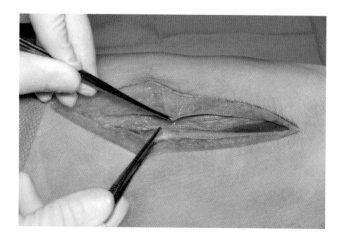

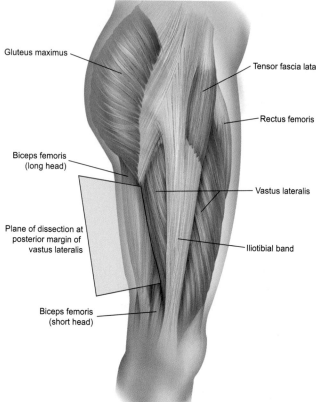

FIGURE 8-11

The fascia lata has been split in line with its fibers along the posterolateral border of the femur, exposing the fascia over the vastus lateralis deep in the wound. The interval formed by the posterior margin can then be elevated to gain access to the posterolateral femur.

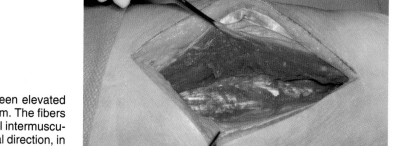

FIGURE 8-12

The posterior margin of the vastus lateralis has been elevated from its insertion on the lateral intermuscular septum. The fibers of the vastus lateralis are separated from the lateral intermuscular septum using an elevator in the distal to proximal direction, in order to elevate all the fibers as a unit and not separate the muscle fibers.

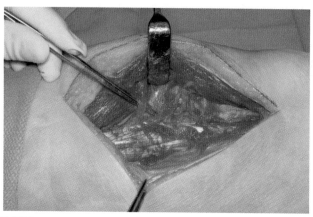

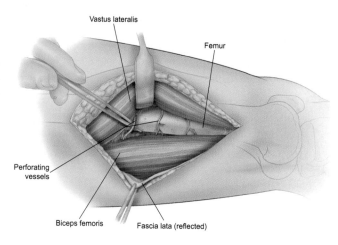

FIGURE 8-13

Perforating and crossing vessels should be identified as they emerge between the bone and intermuscular septum. These vessels are ligated to allow subperiosteal dissection toward the linea aspera for exposure of the lateral femur.

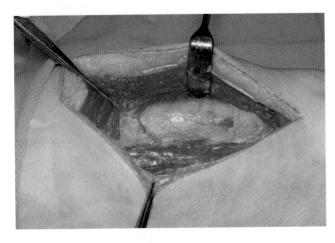

FIGURE 8-14
Retractors placed over the femur will retract the vastus lateralis anteriorly in order to expose the femur.

POSTERIOR APPROACH TO THE FEMUR

Indications

The direct posterior approach to the femur is rarely used. It can be used to access the femoral shaft for posterior bone grafting of nonunions.

Anatomy

Understanding the position of the sciatic nerve as is passes through the posterior thigh is paramount in performing the posterior approach successfully. In the proximal thigh, the posterior approach requires dissection lateral to the long and short heads of the biceps femoris, with the sciatic nerve retracted medially and protected by the two heads of the biceps femoris. When the exposure is performed in the distal aspect of the thigh, the dissection is carried medial to the long and short heads of the biceps femoris and the sciatic nerve is retracted laterally and again protected by the two heads of the biceps femoris.

Technique

1. Incision: the skin incision is centered over the posterior aspect of the femur and is directed longitudinally, beginning at the gluteal fold and extending to the popliteal crease **(Fig. 8-15)**. The subcutaneous tissue beneath the skin is dissected in line with the skin incision to the deep fascia of the thigh.
2. The deep fascia of the thigh is split longitudinally to expose the long head of the biceps femoris. The posterior femoral cutaneous nerve of the thigh lies in the groove between the long head of the biceps and the semitendinosus **(Fig. 8-16)**. Care must be taken when opening the deep fascia as the posterior femoral cutaneous nerve lies just beneath the fascia.
3. In the proximal thigh, the dissection is carried into the interval between the long head of the biceps femoris and the vastus lateralis **(Fig. 8-17)**. The long head of the biceps femoris is retracted medially to expose the short head.
4. At this deeper level, the interval between the short head of the biceps femoris and the vastus lateralis is developed to access the linea aspera of the femoral shaft. Perforating and crossing vessels near the linea aspera should be identified and ligated as the short head of the biceps femoris is retracted medially **(Fig. 8-18)**. The sciatic nerve will be protected by the medial retraction of the long and short heads of the biceps femoris. Subperiosteal dissection of the short head of the biceps off the posterior femur will allow placement of retractors medially and laterally along the femoral shaft.
5. If access to the posterior aspect of the distal femoral shaft is necessary, the deep fascia is again split in the longitudinal direction and the long head of the biceps femoris is again identified **(Fig. 8-19)**. The dissection is then carried in the interval between the two heads of the biceps femoris

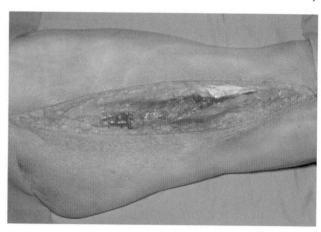

FIGURE 8-15

The skin incision is centered over the posterior aspect of the femur and may be extended from the gluteal fold to the popliteal crease.

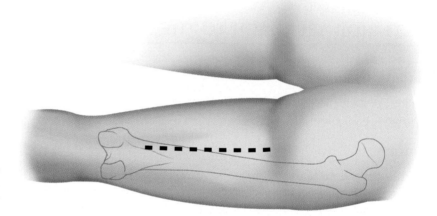

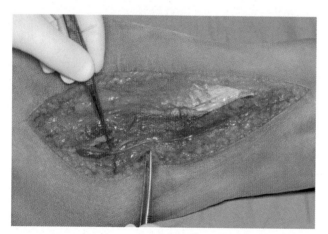

FIGURE 8-16

The deep fascia of the thigh is split to expose the long head of the biceps femoris. The posterior femoral cutaneous nerve of the thigh lies just deep to the deep fascia and should be preserved.

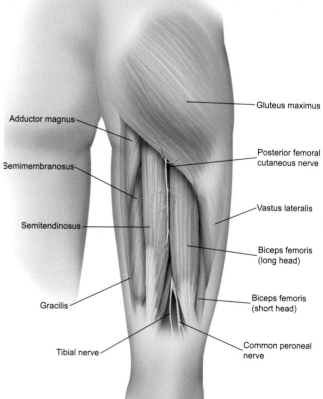

Gluteus maximus

Adductor magnus

Posterior femoral cutaneous nerve

Semimembranosus

Vastus lateralis

Semitendinosus

Biceps femoris (long head)

Biceps femoris (short head)

Gracilis

Common peroneal nerve

Tibial nerve

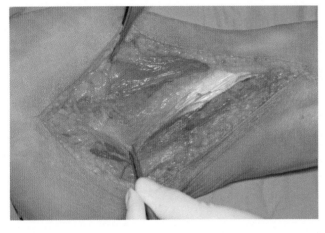

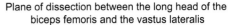
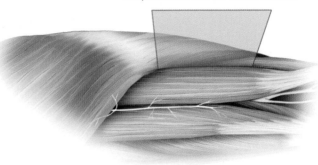

Plane of dissection between the long head of the
biceps femoris and the vastus lateralis

FIGURE 8-17

In the proximal thigh, the plane between the long head of the biceps femoris and the vastus lateralis is developed, exposing the short head of the biceps femoris. Dissection should be carried out lateral to the short head of the biceps femoris.

laterally and the semitendinosus and semimembranosus medially. The sciatic nerve is lateral to the plane of dissection, surrounded by fatty tissue.

6. Lateral retraction of the biceps femoris and sciatic nerve allows exposure of the linea aspera (**Fig. 8-20**).

7. Subperiosteal dissection along the linea aspera medially results in the elevation of the adductor magnus, while lateral subperiosteal elevation lifts the short head of the biceps off the femur to expose the femoral shaft (**Fig. 8-21**).

Closure

Closure of this approach requires only reapproximation of the deep fascia of the thigh followed by routine closure of the subcutaneous tissue and skin.

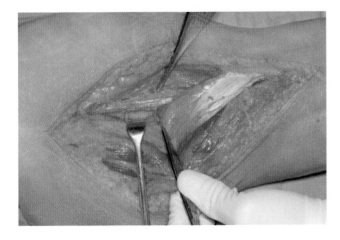

FIGURE 8-18

Perforating and crossing vessels should be ligated to allow subperiosteal dissection along the linea aspera for exposure of the posterior femur.

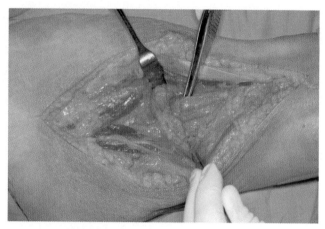

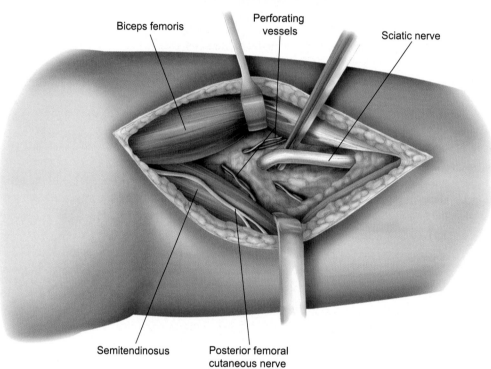

Biceps femoris

Perforating
vessels

Sciatic nerve

Semitendinosus

Posterior femoral
cutaneous nerve

FIGURE 8-19

In the distal thigh, the plane of dissection is between the biceps femoris laterally and the semitendinosus and semimembranosus medially. Care should be taken to identify the sciatic nerve which is encountered between the biceps and semitendinosus.

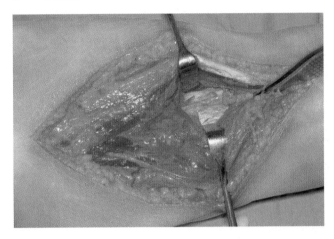

FIGURE 8-20

The plane between the long head of the biceps and hamstrings is developed and the long head is retracted laterally to expose the short head of the biceps femoris.

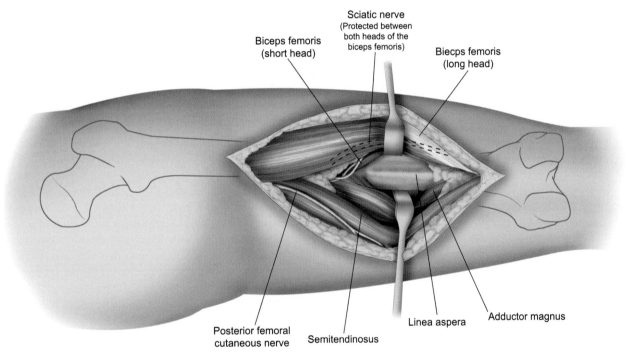

Sciatic nerve
(Protected between both heads of the biceps femoris)

Biceps femoris (short head)

Biecps femoris (long head)

Posterior femoral cutaneous nerve

Semitendinosus

Linea aspera

Adductor magnus

FIGURE 8-21

The short head of the biceps femoris is retracted laterally and the semimembranosus and semitendinosus are retracted medially to expose the femur. Subperiosteal dissection along the posterior shaft of the femur allows retraction of these muscle groups as well as the adductor magnus. The sciatic nerve is retracted laterally, protected by the two heads of the biceps femoris.

MEDIAL APPROACH TO THE FEMUR

Indications

For internal fixation of distal femoral fractures requiring medial buttress plating, supracondylar osteotomies, and resection of benign tumors of the femur.

Extension

Proximally, extension of this approach is limited by the femoral artery crossing from anterior to posterior. Distally, the exposure can be extended to combine with a medial subvastus approach to the knee.

Anatomy

The interval utilized is between the vastus medialis and the medial intermuscular septum. The saphenous nerve crosses from anterior to posterior, entering and exiting the sartorius as it passes distally in the leg. The femoral vessels cross from anterior to posterior through the hiatus in the adductor magnus tendon. The medial superior genicular artery and the articular branch of the descending genicular artery cross deep in the wound on the surface of the medial femur.

Technique

1. Incision: the skin incision is parallel to the femoral shaft, located midway between the posterior border of the medial femoral condyle and the medial aspect of the patella, near the adductor tubercle. It can be extended proximally 10 to 13 cm from the knee joint, limited by the location of the femoral artery crossing the wound (**Fig. 8-22**).
2. The deep fascia of the thigh is split in line with the skin incision. The adductor magnus tendon and the vastus medialis muscle belly are identified, as the dissection will continue in the plane between these two structures. The saphenous nerve should be identified and retracted posteriorly in the wound (**Fig. 8-23**).
3. The muscle fibers of the vastus medialis are elevated off the medial intermuscular septum from distal to proximal. Blunt elevation of these fibers will allow identification of the perforating arteries so ligation can be completed (**Fig. 8-24**).
4. As the femur is approached, the muscular branch of the descending genicular artery is encountered and ligation can be performed (**Fig. 8-25**).
5. Subperiosteal dissection along the medial and anterior femur allows retraction of the vastus medialis anteriorly, exposing the distal femoral shaft.

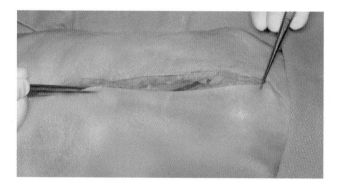
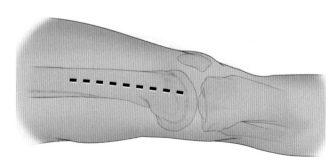

FIGURE 8-22

The skin incision is made over the adductor tubercle, at a point halfway between the medial border of the patella and the posterior aspect of the medial femoral condyle. The incision is made parallel to the femur and may extend 10 to 13 cm proximally from the knee joint.

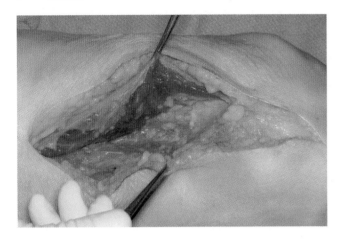

FIGURE 8-23

The deep fascia of the thigh is split in line with the skin incision and the interval between the vastus medialis and adductor magnus is identified. The saphenous nerve is identified crossing from anterior to posterior in the wound and retracted posteriorly.

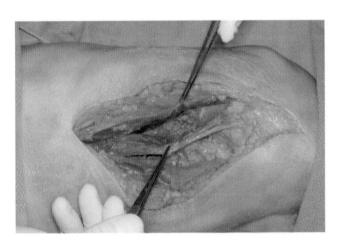

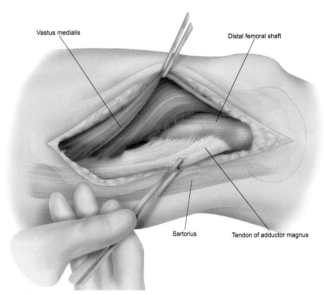

FIGURE 8-24

The muscle fibers of the vastus medialis are elevated off the medial intermuscular septum. Using an elevator, the muscle can be teased off the septum with distal to proximal strokes of the elevator to minimize damage to the muscle.

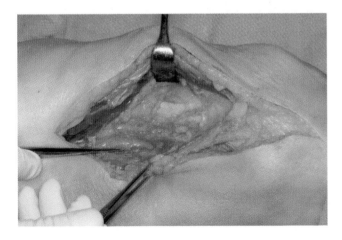

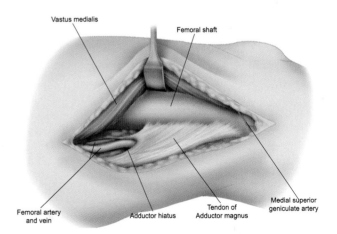

FIGURE 8-25

Subperiosteal dissection along the femur allows anterior retraction of the vastus medialis to expose the femur. Note femoral vessels as it enters adductor hiatus.

RECOMMENDED READING

Chapman MW, Finkemeier CG. Treatment of supracondylar nonunions of the femur with plate fixation and bone graft. *J Bone Joint Surg Am* 1999;81(9):1217–1228.

Checroun AJ, Mekhail AO, Ebraheim NA, et al. Extensile medial approach to the femur. *J Orthop Trauma* 1996;10(7):481–486.

Della Valle CJ, Berger RA, Rosenberg AG. Surgical exposures in revision total knee arthroplasty. *Clin Orthop Relat Res* 2006;446:59–68.

Kregor PJ. Distal femur fractures with complex articular involvement: management by articular exposure and submuscular fixation. *Orthop Clin North Am* 2002;33(1):153–175, ix.

O'Beirne J, O'Connell RJ, White JM, et al. Fractures of the femur treated by femoral plating using the antero-lateral approach. *Injury* 1986;17(6):387–390.

Wang JW, Weng LH. Treatment of distal femoral nonunion with internal fixation, cortical allograft struts, and autogenous bone-grafting. *J Bone Joint Surg Am* 2003;85A(3):436–440.

9 Knee

Mark W. Pagnano

GENERAL OBSERVATIONS REGARDING SKIN INCISION

Whenever possible an anterior midline incision should be used for extensive operations that involve the knee joint itself. By extending the skin incision proximally or distally and developing full thickness skin flaps it is possible to reach anterior, medial, and lateral sided structures around the knee. Many patients who require an open operation on the knee as young adults ultimately come to require total knee arthroplasty and the utility of the anterior midline incision should be remembered. If an incision is made medially or laterally it should be far from the midline such that a substantial skin bridge ($\geq$7 cm) is present to accommodate a subsequent anterior midline incision. Rarely today should a surgeon choose to make an oblique or sharply angled incision around the knee as such incisions are difficult to accommodate should future surgery, such as total knee arthroplasty, be required.

STANDARD MEDIAL PARAPATELLAR ARTHROTOMY

Indications

The medial parapatellar arthrotomy has long been the standard arthrotomy for total knee arthroplasty. Modifications of this approach are useful for a variety of procedures including intramedullary nailing of the tibia and articular cartilage transplant.

Position

Supine.

Technique

1. Incision: the extensor mechanism is exposed through an anterior midline incision.
2. The extensor mechanism is exposed both proximally and distally by developing moderate skin flaps. The arthrotomy parallels the medial border of the patellar tendon beginning at the insertion of the pes anserine tendons (**Fig. 9-1**).
3. The arthrotomy is continued along the medial border of the patella where most surgeons leave a 1 cm sleeve of soft tissue attached to the patella in order to facilitate later closure.
   - *Note:* Some surgeons prefer the technique popularized by Insall where the arthrotomy is carried over the medial edge of the patella itself as that approach improves visualization of the medial border of the patella for patellar resurfacing.

The quadriceps tendon is divided for a distance of 8 cm above the superior pole of the patella (**Fig. 9-2**).

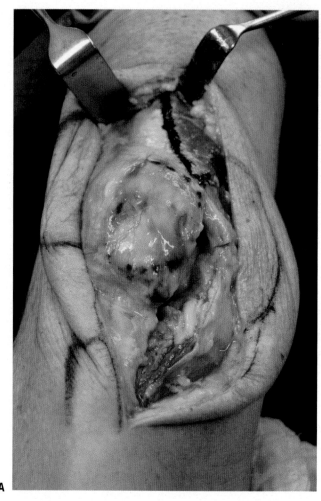

FIGURE 9-1

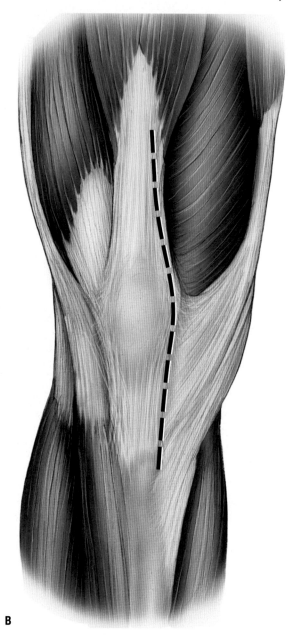

B

4. Most surgeons leave a small cuff of tendon medially (1 to 2 cm) with the vastus medialis and the great preponderance of the tendon in continuity laterally with the rectus femoris and the vastus lateralis. The retropatellar fat pad is split, the patella is everted, and the knee can be flexed **(Fig. 9-3)**.

 ● *Note:* An everted patella puts the patellar tendon at risk for avulsion as the tendon is apt to peel from its attachment to the tubercle. If excessive tension is noted in the tendon, the patella should just be subluxed and not everted or the exposure converted to a quadriceps snip.

5. During total knee arthroplasty, a subperiosteal release of the deep portion of the medial collateral ligament can be carried out. As the knee is progressively flexed the tibia can be rotated externally, the anterior cruciate ligament can be excised, and the posteromedial corner of the tibia can be sub-luxed anterior to the femur **(Fig. 9-4)**.

6. A retractor positioned around the tibial attachment of the posterior cruciate ligament can lever the tibia forward and improve visualization during resection of the proximal tibia **(Fig. 9-5)**.

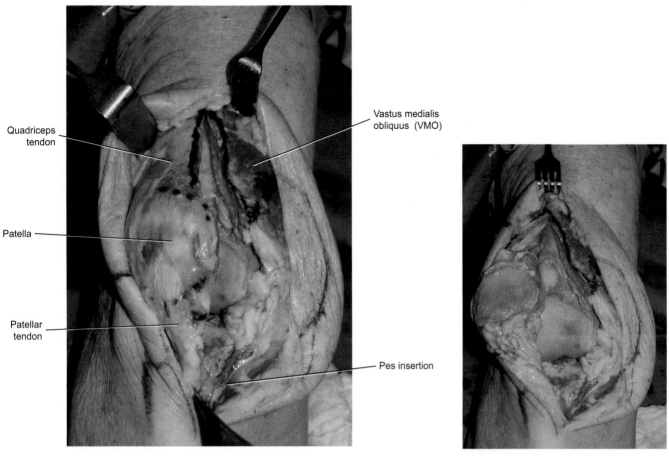

Quadriceps tendon

Vastus medialis obliquus (VMO)

Patella

Patellar tendon

Pes insertion

FIGURE 9-2

FIGURE 9-3

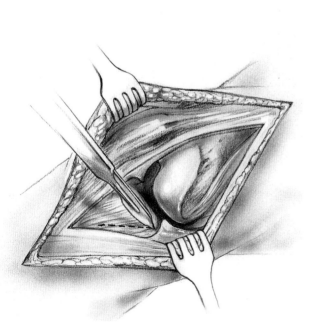

FIGURE 9-4

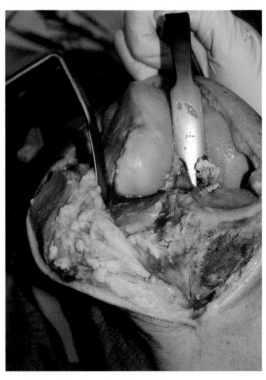

FIGURE 9-5

The Quadriceps Snip

In cases where there is excessive tension on the patellar tendon when subluxing or everting the patella, it is useful to perform a proximal quadriceps snip. This approach was introduced by Insall and is particularly useful in knees that are stiff from prior surgery.

1. A standard medial parapatellar arthrotomy is done.
2. At the proximal portion of the split in the quadriceps the arthrotomy is then extended proximally and laterally across the remaining extensor mechanism and up into the muscle fibers of the vastus lateralis (**Fig. 9-6**).
3. The angle of the cut is the same as the angle of insertion of the vastus lateralis fibers (60 degrees) such that the quadriceps snip can extend itself further into the vastus lateralis if needed (**Fig. 9-7**).

   - *Note:* The quadriceps snip is quite versatile. The vast majority of difficult total knees and revision total knees can be done with a quadriceps snip coupled with adequate debridement of scar tissue from the lateral gutter and around the patella.

4. The arthrotomy can be closed with multiple interrupted sutures and there is no need to alter the patient's weight-bearing status after using the quadriceps snip exposure.

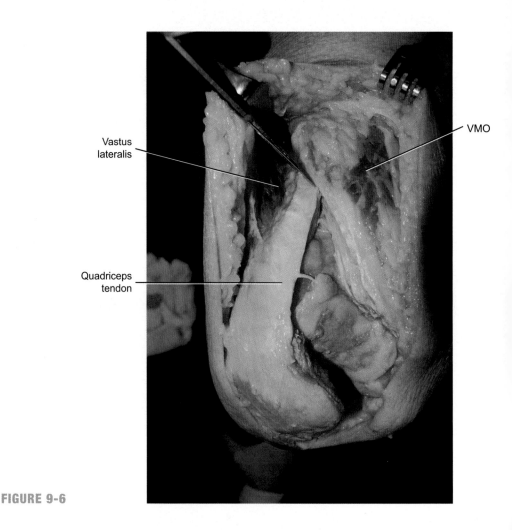

Vastus
lateralis

VMO

Quadriceps
tendon

FIGURE 9-6

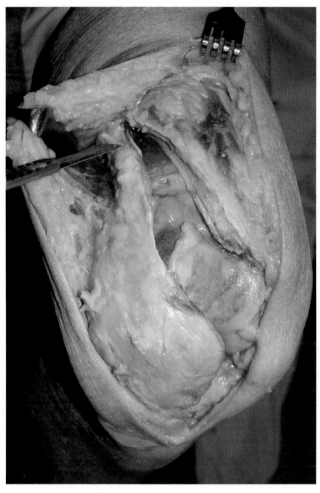 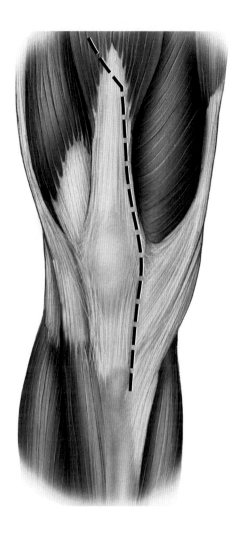

FIGURE 9-7

SUBVASTUS APPROACH

Indications

This approach can be used for routine total knee arthroplasty and medial unicompartmental knee arthroplasty.

Because it preserves the entire extensor mechanism's attachment on the patella, the subvastus approach has an anatomic edge on other arthrotomies of the knee joint. Recent anatomic studies at the Mayo Clinic have confirmed that the tendon of the vastus medialis extends all the way to the midpole of the patella. Thus any arthrotomy that extends proximal to the midpole disrupts part of the extensor mechanism.

Technique

1. Incision: the standard subvastus approach is done through a midline incision.
2. Care is taken to develop a medial skin flap to truly define the inferior border of the vastus medialis obliquus (VMO) **(Fig. 9-8)**.

   - *Note:* The VMO attaches to the patella at a 50 degree angle and always extends more distally and more medially than the surgeon is inclined to think. The subvastus arthrotomy is made by incising the retinaculum and joint capsule at the VMO muscle edge from proximal to distal at the same 50 degree angle as the VMO itself. Care should be taken to extend the arthrotomy to the midpole of the patella and not to cheat the arthrotomy up toward the superior pole of the patella.

3. At the midpole of the patella the arthrotomy is turned distally and parallels the medial border of the patellar tendon **(Fig. 9-9)**.

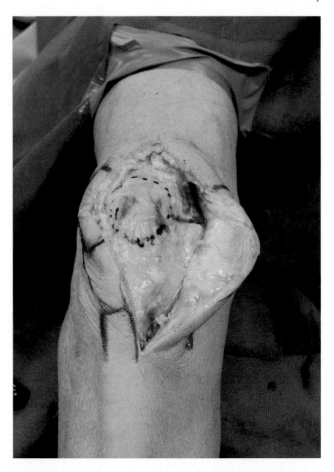

FIGURE 9-8

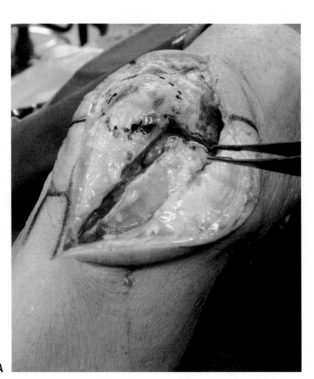

A

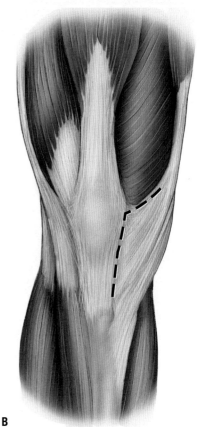

B

FIGURE 9-9

4. The fat pad is split and the patella can be subluxed into the lateral gutter of the knee. In cases where the patella is difficult to sublux laterally, the surgeon will usually find a tight band of tissue proximal-medially (the medial patellofemoral ligament) that must be released. Once the medial patellofemoral ligament is released the patella will sublux laterally with relatively little force **(Fig. 9-10)**.

5. If desired the patella can be everted at this stage and the knee flexed **(Fig. 9-11)**.

   - *Note:* Everting the patella is difficult in heavily muscled patients and markedly obese patients. In those patients the patella should just be subluxed into the lateral gutter. In patients with substantial patella baja the subvastus approach is not recommended.

6. When closing the subvastus arthrotomy it is useful to tension and tie the capsular sutures with the knee in 90 degrees of flexion to avoid overtightening the medial capsule.

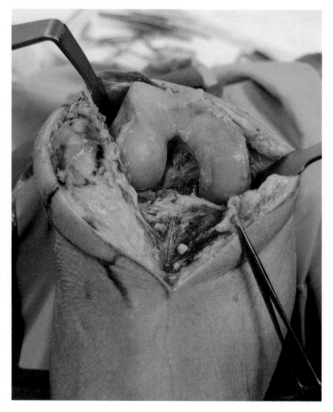

FIGURE 9-10

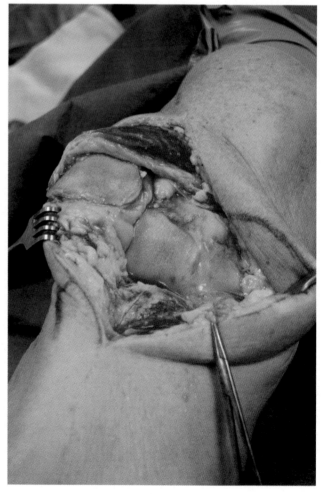

FIGURE 9-11

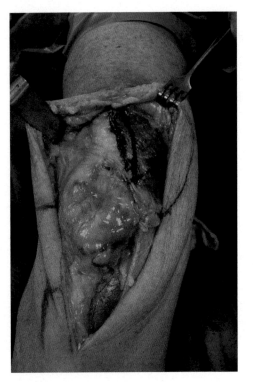

FIGURE 9-12

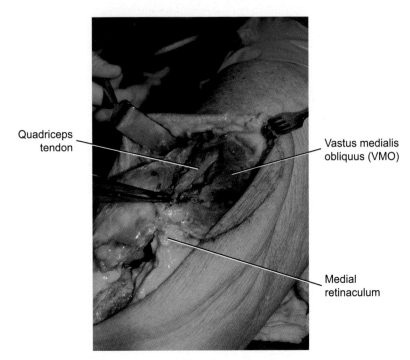

FIGURE 9-13

TRIVECTOR RETAINING APPROACH

The trivector approach can be used for total knee and medial unicompartmental knee arthroplasty.

Technique

1. Incision: an anterior midline incision is made and the vastus medialis muscle and tendon are identified.
2. The knee is flexed to 90 degrees and, beginning three finger-breadths proximal to the patella, the arthrotomy is made from proximal to distal 2 cm medial to the quadriceps tendon **(Fig. 9-12)**.
3. This means the arthrotomy involves transection vastus medialis muscle fibers proximal and medial to the patella **(Fig. 9-13)**.
4. The arthrotomy is extended distally along the medial border of the patella and the medial edge of the patellar tendon. The fat pad is split, the patella is everted with the knee in extension, and then the knee can again be flexed.
5. At the time of closure the surgeon will see that the edge of the quadriceps tendon actually extends medially under the cut muscle fibers of the vastus medialis. Thus there is reasonable tissue through which to place sutures and close the joint itself.

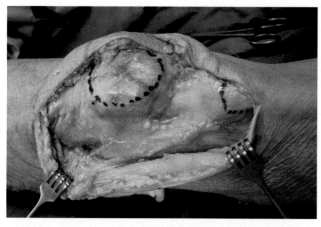

FIGURE 9-14

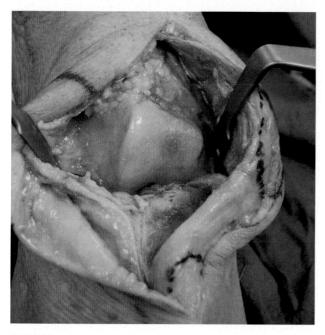

FIGURE 9-15

FIGURE 9-16

LATERAL APPROACH FOR TOTAL KNEE ARTHROPLASTY IN THE VALGUS KNEE

Indications

For patients with substantial valgus deformity who require total knee arthroplasty some surgeons use an anterolateral approach.

Technique

1. Incision: an anterior midline incision is made and a skin flap is developed on the lateral side (**Fig. 9-14**).
2. The quadriceps tendon is divided beginning 6 to 8 cm above the superior pole of the patella. Most surgeons leave a small cuff of quadriceps tendon laterally (1 to 2 cm) with the vastus lateralis and the great preponderance of the tendon in continuity medially with the rectus femoris and the vastus medialis.
3. The arthrotomy is continued along the lateral border of the patella leaving a 1 cm sleeve of soft tissue attached to the patella in order to facilitate later closure (**Fig. 9-15**).
4. Distally the arthrotomy parallels the patellar tendon. The patella can be subluxed medially or everted medially and the knee flexed, but each of those maneuvers is more difficult than with a standard medial parapatellar arthrotomy (**Fig. 9-16**).

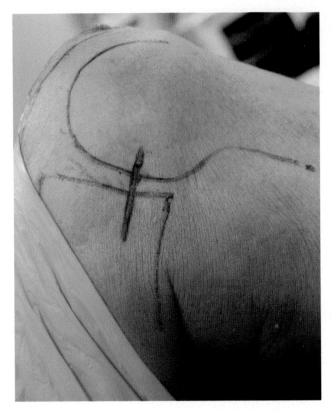

FIGURE 9-17

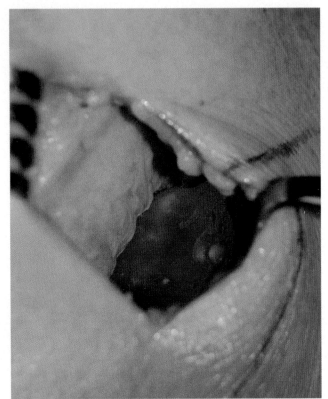

FIGURE 9-18

LIMITED MEDIAL APPROACH TO THE KNEE FOR ARTHROSCOPIC MENISCAL REPAIR

Indications

Exposure of the posteromedial corner of the knee is needed for arthroscopic inside-out suture repair of medial meniscal tears.

Technique

1. Insertion: the knee is flexed 90 degrees and the arthroscope can be advanced to light the posteromedial corner of the knee just posterior to the medial collateral ligament. If the operating room lights are dimmed, it is possible to transilluminate the skin at the level where the incision should be made.
2. A short (3 to 4 cm) vertical incision is made (**Fig. 9-17**). Care is taken to avoid damage to the saphenous nerve and vein.
3. The fascia along the superior border of the sartorius is divided and blunt finger dissection is carried out to expose the posteromedial joint capsule itself.
4. A simple retractor made from a tablespoon with its handle bent 120 degrees can be placed against the posteromedial corner of the knee to catch and deflect the flexible needles used to carry out the inside-out meniscal repair (**Fig. 9-18**).

LIMITED LATERAL APPROACH TO THE KNEE FOR ARTHROSCOPIC MENISCAL REPAIR

Indications

Exposure of the posterolateral corner of the knee is needed for arthroscopic inside-out suture repair of lateral meniscal tears.

Technique

1. Insertion: the knee is flexed 90 degrees and the arthroscope can be advanced to light the posterolateral corner of the knee just posterior to the lateral collateral ligament and anterior to the popliteus tendon.
2. If the operating room lights are dimmed it is possible to transilluminate the skin at the level where the incision should be made.
3. A short (3 to 4 cm) vertical incision is made **(Fig. 9-19)**. The fibular collateral ligament is identified and the posterolateral capsule and arcuate ligament complex lie just posterior.
4. A simple retractor made from a tablespoon with its handle bent 120 degrees can be placed against the posterolateral corner of the knee to catch and deflect the flexible needles used to carry out the inside-out meniscal repair **(Fig. 9-20)**.

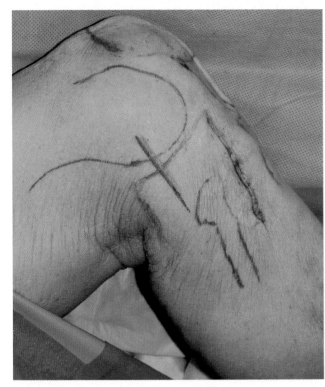

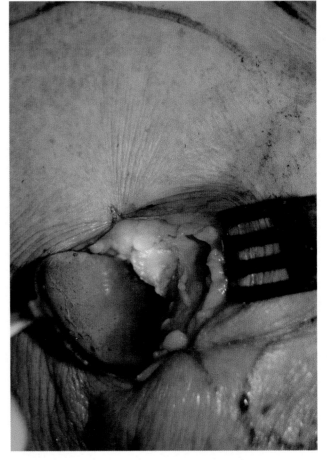

FIGURE 9-19   **FIGURE 9-20**

MINIMALLY INVASIVE APPROACHES FOR TOTAL KNEE ARTHROPLASTY

There has been considerable interest among patients and surgeons alike in minimally invasive approaches for total knee arthroplasty. The exact definition of minimally invasive total knee arthroplasty continues to be debated but most would agree that it involves a short skin incision, avoiding eversion of the patella, and limiting the amount of surgical dissection in the suprapatellar pouch. Alteration of the surgical approach alone however is not enough for intraoperative success and, thus, manufacturers have introduced modified or new instruments for minimally invasive total knee arthroplasty. Patients who have had prior open knee surgery, who have patella baja, who have a very stiff knee, or who have poor skin quality are not good candidates for a minimally invasive total knee arthroplasty approach. Most surgeons would be well served to pursue specialized cadaver training before using minimally invasive total knee arthroplasty approaches in clinical practice.

Mini Subvastus Approach

Indications   The minimally invasive subvastus approach provides good exposure of both condyles, preserves the entire extensor insertion on the patella, is made easier by avoiding patellar eversion, and allows rapid and reliable knee joint closure.

- *Comment:* As in all minimally invasive techniques, retractor placement and leg position are important in facilitating visualization throughout the procedure. Surgeons can learn this technique in a step-wise fashion by making a standard incision using the subvastus exposure without everting the patella and then gradually decreasing incision size over time.

Technique

1. Incision: an anterior midline incision is made from the superior pole of the patella to the top of the tibial tubercle (**Fig. 9-21**).

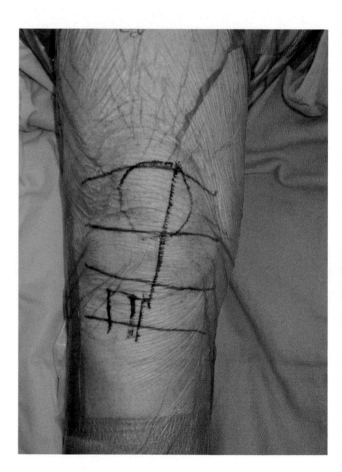

FIGURE 9-21

2. A medial skin flap is raised and the inferior border of the vastus medialis muscle is identified **(Fig. 9-22)**.
3. Beginning 5 to 8 cm medial to the patella border, the fascia is incised at the inferior border of the vastus medialis and the arthrotomy is continued over to the midpole of the patella at a 50 degree angle paralleling the angle of insertion of the vastus medialis muscle fibers **(Fig. 9-23)**.
4. Care must be taken to preserve the triangle of tendon that inserts down to the midpole of the patella as this is where the retractor will rest. If the tendon is not preserved, the retractor will slide proximally and macerate the vastus medialis obliquus muscle itself. The distal portion of the arthrotomy parallels the patellar tendon.
5. A 90 degree bent Homan retractor is placed into the lateral gutter of the knee and the patella and distal portion of the extensor mechanism are retracted with relatively little tension on the vastus muscle itself **(Fig. 9-24)**.
6. The patella is not everted. Another bent Homan retractor is placed medially and the knee can be flexed to expose both femoral condyles simultaneously and the distal femur is cut.
7. The proximal tibia is exposed with subperiosteal elevation of the deep medial collateral ligament and then bent Homans are placed medially and laterally against the tibia and a pickle-fork retractor is placed posteriorly around the posterior cruciate ligament (PCL) attachment levering the tibia forward **(Fig. 9-25)**.
8. The tibia is cut and that then provides more working room for sizing and rotating the femur (typically the most difficult part of any minimally invasive total knee procedure) **(Fig. 9-26)**.
9. After the femoral cuts are made, a laminar spreader is placed in the flexion space and the notch osteophytes, cruciate ligament(s), medial and lateral menisci, and posterior osteophytes can be excised under direct vision. The trial components can be assembled and the knee reduced.
10. The patella is then turned up 90 degrees but not everted and cut from medial to lateral for patellar resurfacing **(Fig. 9-27)**.
11. Cementing is done first on the tibial tray, then femur, insertion of the tibial polyethylene, and finally the patella. The tourniquet is let down and the subvastus space is specifically examined to ensure there are no bleeders.

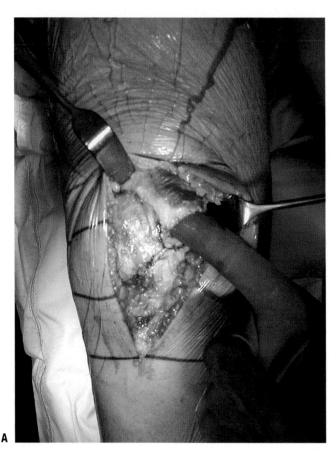
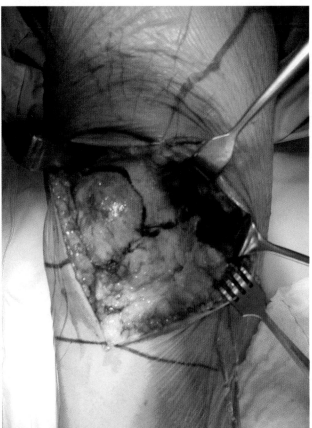

A   B

FIGURE 9-22

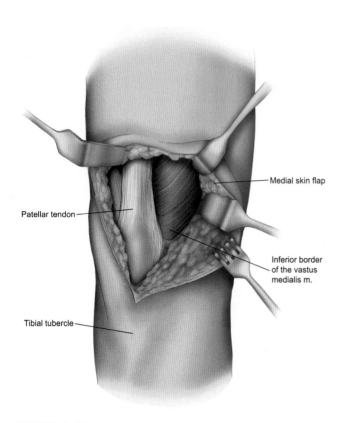

Medial skin flap

Patellar tendon

Inferior border
of the vastus
medialis m.

Tibial tubercle

FIGURE 9-23

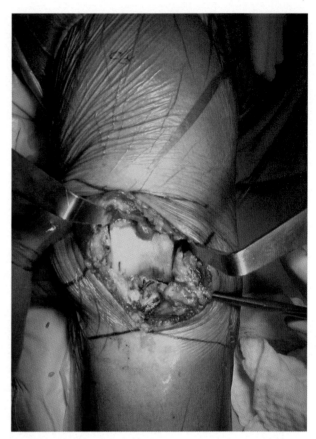

FIGURE 9-24

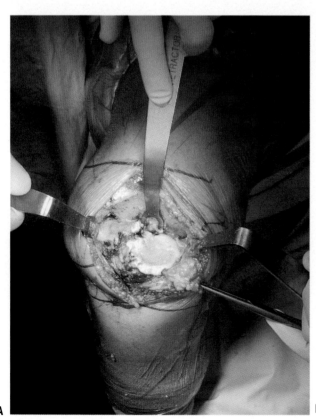

A

FIGURE 9-25

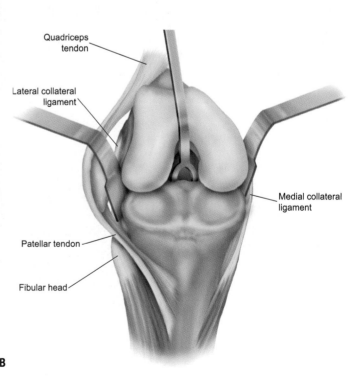

Quadriceps
tendon

Lateral collateral
ligament

Medial collateral
ligament

Patellar tendon

Fibular head

B

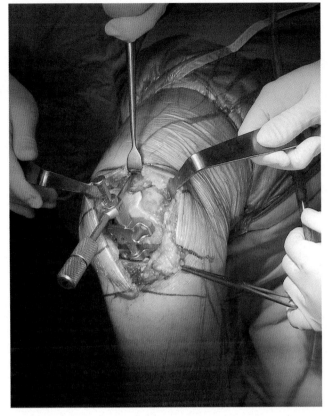

FIGURE 9-26

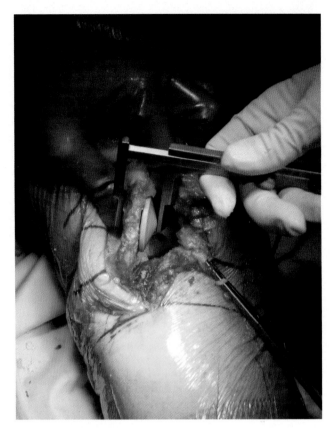

FIGURE 9-27

12. The arthrotomy is closed with multiple interrupted sutures and it is useful to tension and tie these sutures with the knee in 90 degrees of flexion to avoid overtightening the medial capsule **(Fig. 9-28)**. The wound is closed in layers **(Fig. 9-29)**.

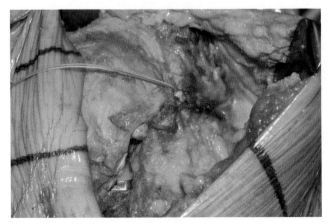

FIGURE 9-28

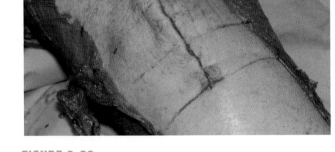

FIGURE 9-29

Mini Midvastus Approach

Technique

1. Incision: a midline incision is made from the superior pole of the patella to the midpoint of the tibial tubercle distally.
2. A medial arthrotomy is begun distally 5 mm medial to the tibial tubercle and extended proximally just medial to the patellar border (**Fig. 9-30**).
3. At the superomedial corner of the patella the arthrotomy is turned proximal-medially and a 2 cm split is made between the muscle fibers of the vastus medialis (**Fig. 9-31**).
4. The patella is retracted laterally with a bent Homan but not everted, the fat pad is excised, and the anterior horns of the medial and lateral menisci are incised (**Fig. 9-32**).
5. The distal femur is prepared with the leg in 70 to 90 degrees of flexion. The anteroposterior axis of the knee as described by Whitesides is used to assess femoral rotation.
6. The distal cutting guide is placed and the cut made. The femur is then sized, with variations in knee flexion angle needed to accommodate the guide, and the finishing cuts are made.
7. The tibia is exposed with bent Homan retractors placed medially and laterally at the tibial margins and a posterior retractor is used to lever anteriorly.
8. A tibial cutting guide specifically modified for small incision surgery is of great assistance here. The lateral portion of the tibia is the most difficult to cut safely and a narrow saw blade is useful in maneuvering around the patellar tendon.

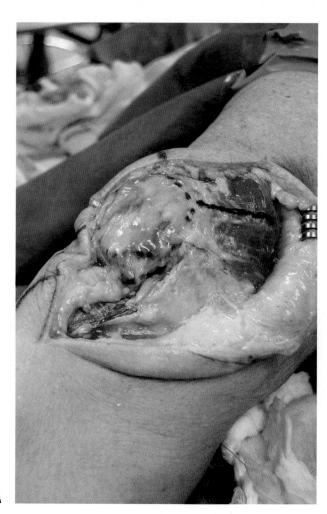

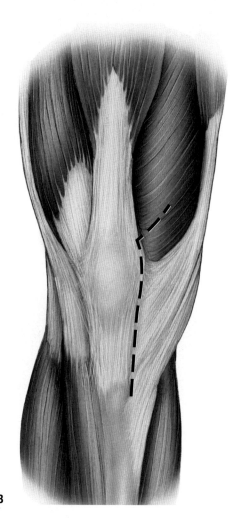

A   B

FIGURE 9-30

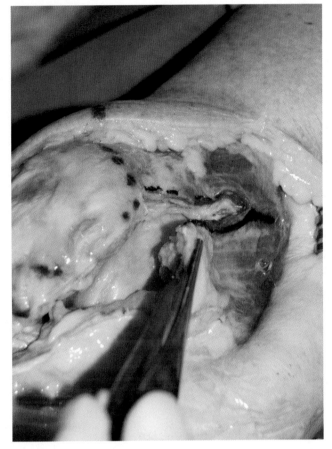

FIGURE 9-31

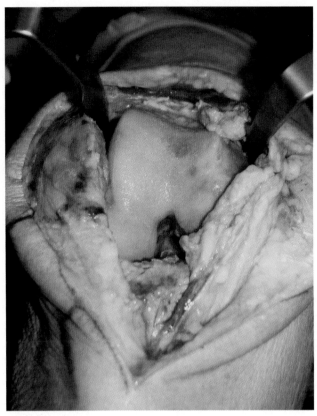

FIGURE 9-32

9. After removing the proximal tibial fragment a laminar spreader can be placed in the flexion space and the osteophytes, cruciate ligaments, and posterior menisci removed under direct vision.

10. The trial components are assembled and the knee reduced.

11. The patella is prepared last. Cementing is done first on the tibia followed by the femur and then the patella.

Mini Medial Parapatellar Approach

Indications   The mini medial parapatellar approach has the advantage that it can be quickly converted to a standard medial parapateller approach at any time. The indications are similar to the other mini-incision approaches for total knee arthroplasty.

Technique

1. Incision: a midline or slightly medially biased incision is made from the just above the superior pole of the patella to the top of the tibial tubercle.
2. The medial parapatellar arthrotomy is done similar to the standard parapatellar approach except that the proximal extent of the quadriceps tendon incision is only 2 to 4 cm (versus the 8 to 10 cm in the standard approach) (**Fig. 9-33**).
   - *Note:* If there is difficulty subluxing the patella laterally then the arthrotomy is extended more proximally.
3. Modified instruments are used to make the bone cuts according to the surgeon's normal sequence. Some prefer to cut the tibia first and that can be done with this approach.
4. There is adequate exposure to safely cut the tibia with bent Homan retractors placed medially and laterally to protect the collateral ligaments and a pickle-fork retractor placed posteriorly.
5. Cutting the tibia first provides more working room in both flexion and extension for the remainder of the procedure.

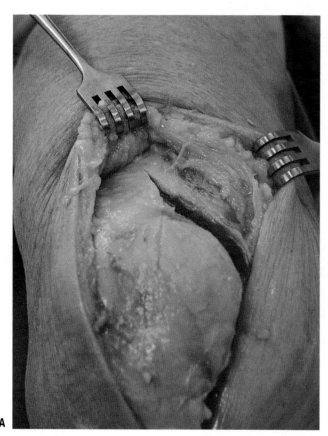
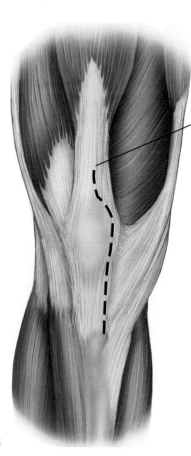

2-4 cm proximal extent of arthrotomy

FIGURE 9-33

6. The exposure exists to reference the anteroposterior axis and the posterior condyles for rotational positioning of the femur **(Fig. 9-34)**.
7. The epicondylar axis can be identified after appropriate retractor placement. Appropriate soft tissue balancing is done and the trial components are assembled.
8. The patella can be prepared by turning the patella up 90 degrees and cutting from medial to lateral or by everting the patella with the knee in full extension after the trial components have been removed.
9. Typically the tibia is cemented first followed by the femur and patella.

- *Note:* In all of the mini total knee approaches the surgeon should specifically look for retained cement laterally around both the femoral and tibial components before closing. That area often is obscured when the patella is subluxed and not everted.

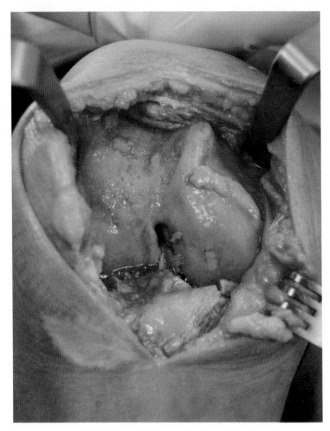

FIGURE 9-34

Alternative

1. An even more limited medial parapatellar exposure has been used by some surgeons with the arthrotomy stopping at the superior pole of the patella (**Fig. 9-35**). That approach has been given the trademarked term quad-sparing because it does involve the detachment of the vastus medialis obliquus tendon which inserts along the medial patella from the superior pole to the midpole.
2. That approach affords the poorest visualization of any of the minimally invasive approaches for total knee arthroplasty (**Fig. 9-36**).
   - *Note:* Because of that limited visualization the procedure must be carried out with instruments that cut from medial to lateral and demands partial cuts through resection guides followed by free-hand finishing cuts. In addition, the patella must be cut first with this approach raising the possibility of inadvertent damage to the cut patellar surface from poorly placed retractors.

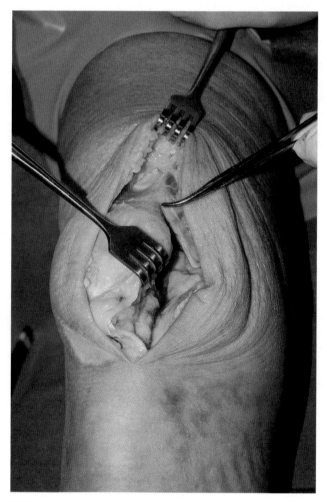

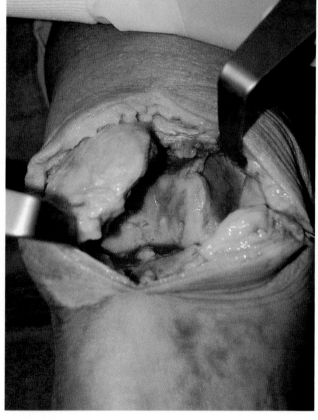

FIGURE 9-35   **FIGURE 9-36**

Mini Lateral Approach

Technique

1. Incision: an 8 to 10 cm incision is made from just below Gerdy's tubercle and extends proximally to the lateral epicondyle.
2. The iliotibial band is split in line with the skin incision and then elevated from Gerdy's tubercle to allow exposure of the proximal tibia. The fat pad and the anterior horn of the lateral meniscus are excised.
3. A retractor is placed across the knee joint to retract the patellar tendon anteromedially and allow the anterior horn of the medial meniscus to be excised.
4. The synovium overlying the distal anterior femur is removed and the patella is mobilized medially. Specialized cutting guides are required to allow cutting in a lateral to medial direction.
5. The distal femur is resected first.
6. The tibia is cut next and that is done with a partial cut through the resection guide followed by a free-hand finishing cut. The femur is then sized and the femoral finishing guide is rotated relative to the anteroposterior axis. The notch osteophytes, anterior cruciate ligament, meniscal remnants, and posterior osteophytes are excised and the trial components inserted.
7. The patella is turned up 90 degrees and cut from lateral to medial.
8. Cementing of the tibia is done first followed by the femur and patella. Care is taken to look for excess cement medially after this approach.

EXTENSILE LATERAL APPROACH TO THE KNEE FOR POSTEROLATERAL CORNER RECONSTRUCTION

Indications

Wider exposure of the posterolateral corner of the knee is required for repair or reconstruction of the stabilizing ligamentous and capsular structures of the posterolateral corner.

Technique

1. Incision: the skin incision follows the posterior 10% of the iliotibial band proximally and extends between the fibular head and Gerdy's tubercle distally (**Fig. 9-37**).
2. The iliotibial band is split longitudinally to allow access to the lateral collateral and popliteus insertion sites at the lateral epicondyle (**Fig. 9-38**).
3. The biceps tendon is identified as is the peroneal nerve which runs just posterior to that tendon. The posterior corner of the knee is readily assessed.

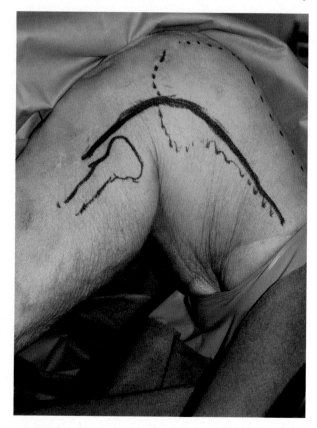

FIGURE 9-37

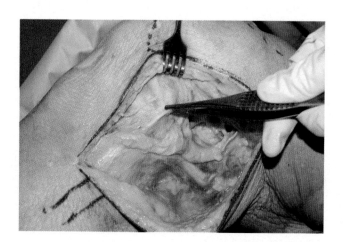

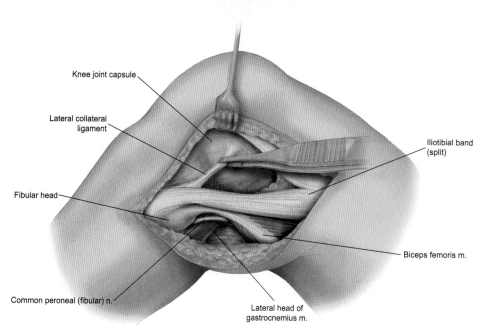

Knee joint capsule

Lateral collateral
ligament

Fibular head

Iliotibial band
(split)

Biceps femoris m.

Common peroneal (fibular) n.

Lateral head of
gastrocnemius m.

FIGURE 9-38

POSTERIOR APPROACH TO THE POPLITEAL FOSSA AND POSTERIOR CRUCIATE LIGAMENT ORIGIN

Indications

The posterior approach allows access to the neurovascular structures of the popliteal fossa and direct visualization of the posterior cruciate ligament's tibial attachment site.

Technique

1. Incision: an S-shaped incision is used to cross the flexion crease (**Fig. 9-39**).
2. The fascia overlying the popliteal fossa is incised, exposing the neurovascular bundle (**Fig. 9-40**).
3. In the midline is the small saphenous vein which is often found in association with the medial sural cutaneous nerve which can be followed back to the tibial nerve. The popliteal artery and vein will lie deep to the tibial nerve. The scissors mark the medial head of the gracilis medius (**Fig. 9-41**).
4. The neurovascular structures can be retracted laterally to allow direct access to the posterior aspect of the knee (**Fig. 9-42**).
5. Alternatively, when approaching the tibial attachment of the posterior cruciate ligament, the dissection can begin medial to the medial head of the gastrocnemius muscle.
6. The medial gastrocnemius is then retracted laterally past the midline allowing exposure of the tibial attachment of the posterior cruciate while also protecting the neurovascular structures.

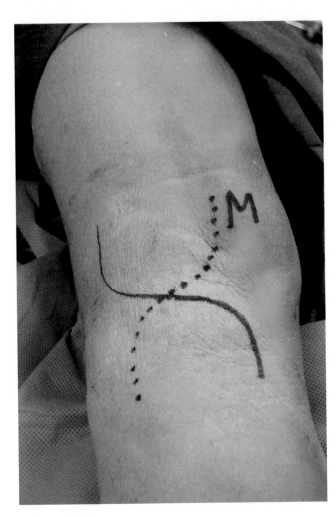

FIGURE 9-39

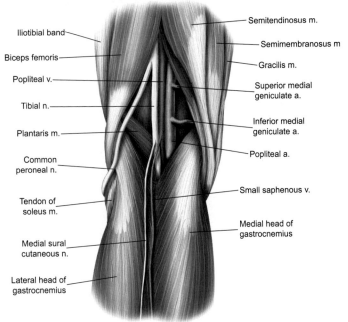

FIGURE 9-40

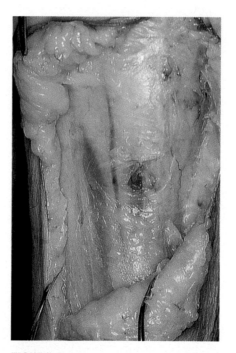

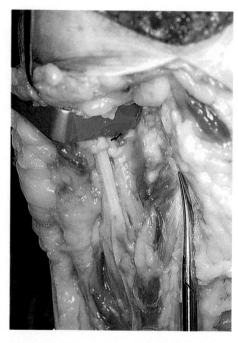

FIGURE 9-41   **FIGURE 9-42**

RECOMMENDED READING

Bezwada HP, Mont MA, Bonutti PM, et al. Minimally invasive lateral approach to total knee arthroplasty. In: Berger RA, Scuderi GR, Tria AJ, eds. *MIS Techniques in Orthopedics*. New York: Springer, 2006.

Boerger TO, Aglietti P, Mondanelli N, et al. Mini-subvastus versus medial parapatellar approach in total knee arthroplasty. *Clin Orthop Relat Res* 2005;440:82–87.

Buechel FF. Lateral approach. In: Lotke PA, ed. *Master Techniques in Orthopedic Surgery: Knee Arthroplasty*. New York: Raven Press, 1995.

Hoffman AA, Plaster RI, Murdock LE. Subvastus approach for primary total knee arthroplasty. *Clin Orthop* 1991;269:70.

Fisher DA, Trimble SM, Breedlove K. The medial trivector approach in total knee arthroplasty. *Orthopedics* 1998;21(1):53–56.

Garvin KL, Scuderi GR, Insall JN. Evolution of the quadriceps snip. *Clin Orthop Relat Res* 1995;321:131–137.

Insall JN. A midline approach to the knee. *J Bone Joint Surg* 1971;53-A;1584–1586.

Jacob RP. The arthroscopic meniscal repair: Techniques and clinical experience. *Am J Sports Med* 1991;16:137–141.

Laskin RS, Beksac B, Phongjunakorn A, et al. Minimally invasive total knee replacement through a mini-midvastus incision: an outcome study. *Clin Orthop* 2004;428:74–81.

Roysam GS, Oakley MJ. Subvastus approach for total knee arthroplasty: a prospective randomized and observer blinded trial. *J Arthroplasty* 2001;16:454–457.

Scuderi GR, Tenholder M, Capeci C. Surgical approaches in mini-incision total knee arthroplasty. *Clin Orthop Relat Res* 2004;428:61–67.

10 Tibia and Fibula

Joseph R. Cass, Luke Wolff, and Michael Torchia

O ptimal exposure for any surgical technique requires both a grasp of the pertinent anatomy and knowledge of possible approaches. Whether the operative procedure is done for a congenital abnormality, an acute fracture or nonunion, or for a complex joint reconstruction, the surgeon desires the best view with the least trauma to the tissues.

RELEVANT ANATOMY

Before attempting any surgical exposure in the lower extremity one must have an absolute knowledge of the relevant anatomy of the entire lower extremity. The direction of approach will be dictated by location and pathology. The soft tissue and bony architecture are reasonably predictable from one patient to the next with little variability except in pathologic processes. A thorough understanding of normal anatomy is required to recognize abnormal anatomy.

Vascular Supply

The popliteal artery trifurcates posterior to the knee as it branches to enter the anterior and posterior aspects of the leg. The posterior tibial artery enters the deep posterior compartment of the leg, traveling just posterior to the tibialis posterior muscle. The deep peroneal artery also runs in the deep compartment, lateral to the tibial nerve. The anterior tibial artery crosses superior to the interosseous membrane and travels just anterior to it. In the distal third of the leg it begins to proceed anteriorly.

Innervation

The saphenous nerve is the large sensory continuation of the femoral nerve, which innervates the medial aspect of the distal thigh around the level of Hunter's canal and continues distally in a curvilinear pattern to provide sensation along the medial leg and proximal ankle. One of its larger branches, the infrapatellar branch of the saphenous nerve, crosses medially to laterally across the anterior aspect of the leg near the level of the inferior pole of the patella. This is frequently transected during anterior approaches of the knee. The saphenous nerve travels primarily down the medial aspect of the leg on the medial head of the gastrocnemius, along with the greater saphenous vein.

The tibial nerve runs in the deep posterior compartment, just lateral to the posterior tibial artery. The sural cutaneous nerve is a branch of the tibial nerve, which is located in the midline of the posterior aspect of the leg and is usually lateral to the small saphenous vein, supplying cutaneous branches through the fascia to the posterior aspect of the calf.

The superficial peroneal nerve is one of two branches of the common peroneal nerve at the level of the proximal fibula. Along with innervating the muscles of the lateral compartment of the leg, the nerve continues to the dorsum of the foot after piercing the anterior fascial compartment approximately 10 to 12 cm proximal to the tip of the lateral malleolus. Its cutaneous innervation is to the dorsum of the foot, excluding the first webspace. The deep peroneal nerve runs in the anterior compartment with the anterior tibial artery and becomes superficial only after it passes through the anterior compartment and to the extensor retinaculum where it supplies cutaneous sensation to the first webspace.

The sural nerve continues its course down the posterior aspect of the leg with the lesser saphenous vein. At approximately the level of the junction of the proximal two-thirds and distal one-third of the leg, the nerve begins to take a lateral course with the vein curving posterior and then distal to the lateral malleolus, supplying sensation to the lateral ankle as well as the lateral aspect of the hindfoot. Transection of this nerve during exposure of the ankle or calcaneus may result in painful neuroma and/or numbness along the lateral aspect of the foot, which may have irritating consequences.

Musculature of the Leg

The lower extremity from the knee to the ankle may also be compartmentalized to simplify the anatomy, as well as the surgical approaches. The leg may be divided into four anatomical compartments.

The anterior compartment is made up of the tibialis anterior, extensor hallucis longus, and extensor digitorum. Its nerve supply is a branch of the common peroneal nerve, the deep peroneal, and its vascular supply is from the anterior tibial artery.

The lateral compartment is comprised of the peroneus longus and the peroneus brevis, which are supplied by the second branch of the common peroneal nerve, the superficial peroneal nerve.

The posterior aspect of the leg is divided into superficial and deep compartments with the superficial compartment being comprised to the two heads of the gastrocnemius muscle, as well as the soleus and plantaris. The deep posterior compartment is occupied by the tibialis posterior, the flexor digitorum longus, and the flexor hallucis longus muscles. The posterior compartment has its vascular supply from the posterior tibial artery and the nerve supply is from the tibial nerve. The medial and lateral intermuscular septae are more defined in the leg than in the hip. The lateral intermuscular septum is pierced by the superficial peroneal nerve, approximately 12 cm proximal from the tip of the lateral malleolus as it crosses from the lateral to the anterior compartment of the distal leg.

POSTEROMEDIAL APPROACH TO THE PROXIMAL TIBIA

Indications

Fractures of the proximal tibia occasionally require two incisions for reduction and fixation, one anterolaterally, described below, and another posteromedially.

Position

For the posteromedial approach a sandbag or bump is placed under the contralateral buttock of the supine patient (**Fig. 10-1A–C**).

Technique

1. Incision: the incision is made in line with the posterior aspect of the tibial shaft. As it is parallel to the pes tendons, the saphenous nerve is encountered and retracted anterosuperiorly (**Fig. 10-1D**).
2. The pes tendons are mobilized anteriorly; the medial gastrocnemius fascia is released from the proximal tibia.
3. With posterior retraction of the gastrocnemius, the posteromedial proximal tibia is thus exposed (**Fig. 10-1E**). Parts of the semimembranosus insertion may have to be elevated as well (**Fig. 10-1F,G**).

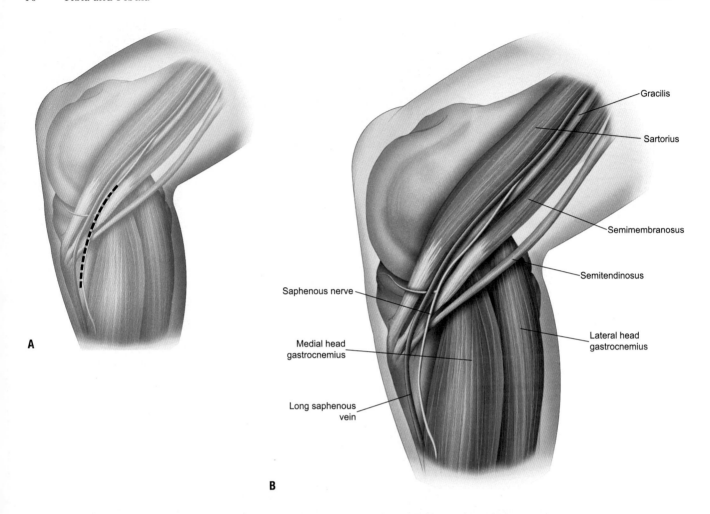

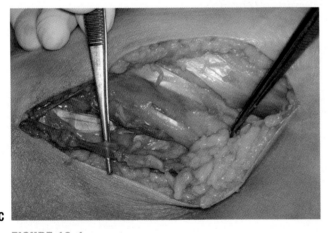

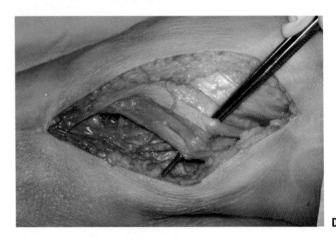

FIGURE 10-1

A–C: Patient in supine position with the leg flexed and externally rotated. Proximal is to the viewer's right, posterior to the bottom of the photograph. Forceps to the right is on the pes tendons, forceps to the left is on the saphenous nerve. **D:** Forceps is elevating the pes tendons.

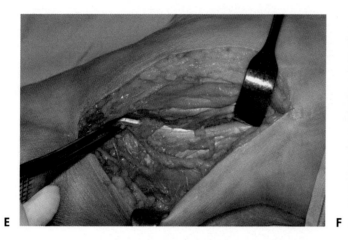

E

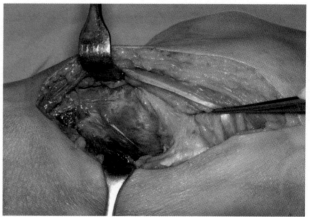

F

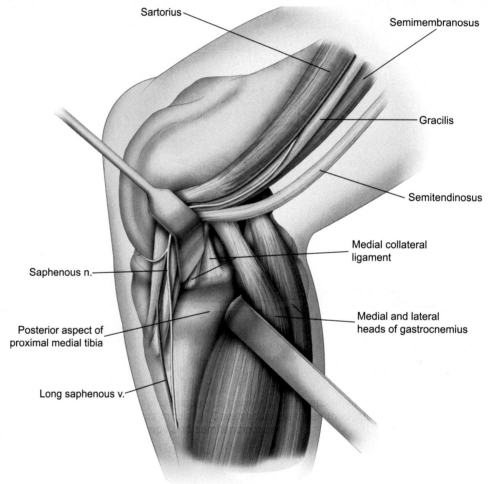

Sartorius

Semimembranosus

Gracilis

Semitendinosus

Medial collateral
ligament

Saphenous n.

Medial and lateral
heads of gastrocnemius

Posterior aspect of
proximal medial tibia

Long saphenous v.

G

FIGURE 10-1

(Continued) **E:** Retractor to the right is holding the pes tendons. Forceps to the left is pointing out the medial gastrocnemius fascia. **F,G:** Gastrocnemius retracted posteriorly demonstrating exposure of proximal medial tibia on posterior aspect. The oblique portion of the medial collateral ligament is just distal to the forceps.

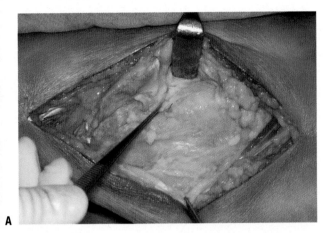
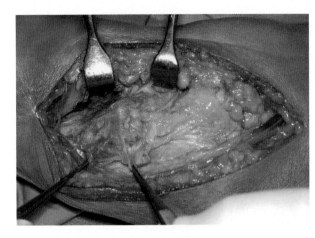

A   B

FIGURE 10-2
A: Patient is prone; proximal is to the viewer's right, the medial is the the bottom of the photo. The medial head of the gastrocnemius fascia is held by the forceps, the medial collateral ligament is beneath the pes tendons which are being held by the forceps at the bottom of the photograph. **B:** Medial head of the gastrocnemius retracted to the superior side of the photograph, forceps at the knee joint line.

- *Note:* Variations of this exposure have also been described. Placing the patient in the prone position makes the exposure easier but also requires a second positioning if one desires to expose the anterolateral tibia as well (**Fig. 10-2**).

ANTEROLATERAL APPROACH TO PROXIMAL TIBIA

Indications

Fractures of the lateral tibial plateau are typically exposed via this route.

Technique

1. Incision: a straight or lazy S-shaped incision is usually centered over the lateral epicondyle and extended distally in line with the iliotibial band toward Gerdy's tubercle (**Fig. 10-3A,B**). Extension of the incision distally is dictated by the amount of metadiaphyseal exposure needed.
2. Full thickness soft tissue flaps are elevated to expose the iliotibial band. This is then split in line with its fibers (**Fig. 10-3C,D**). If an arthrotomy is desired, a submeniscal entry is preferred.
3. The coronary ligament is incised and the meniscus is retracted superiorly to visualize the joint surface (**Fig. 10-3E**).
4. The origins of the anterior compartment muscles are elevated and retracted posterolaterally as needed to visualize the proximal tibia (**Fig. 10-3F**).

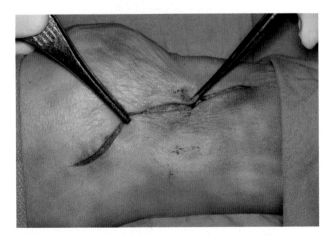

FIGURE 10-3
A: Incision for anterolateral proximal tibia exposure.   **A**

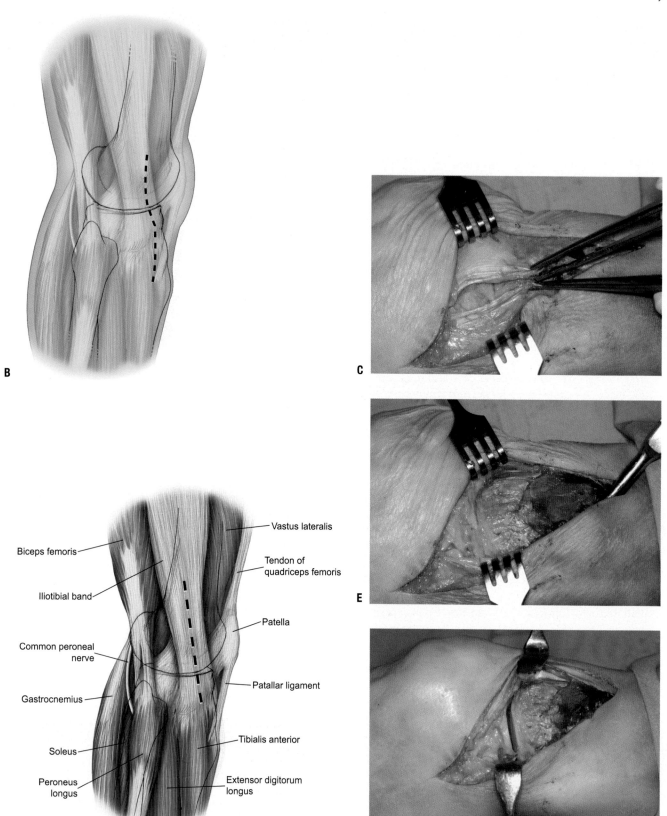

B

C

D

E

F

Biceps femoris

Iliotibial band

Common peroneal
nerve

Gastrocnemius

Soleus

Peroneus
longus

Vastus lateralis

Tendon of
quadriceps femoris

Patella

Patallar ligament

Tibialis anterior

Extensor digitorum
longus

FIGURE 10-3

(Continued) **B:** Incision for anterolateral proximal tibia exposure. **C,D:** Iliotibial band split in line with its fibers. **E:** Iliotibial band freed from Gerdy's tubercle, the extensor muscle attachment seen to the viewer's right can be elevated as needed for exposure of the proximal tibia. **F:** A sub-meniscal arthrotomy has been performed as well. The lateral tibial plateau articular surface is visible. This opening can be increased by application of a varus force to the knee.

POSTEROLATERAL APPROACH TO THE PROXIMAL TIBIA

Position

For approaches to the posterolateral proximal tibia and proximal tibio-fibular joint, the patient can be positioned prone.

Technique

1. Incision: a curvilinear incision is made proximally over the biceps tendon, and then curving slightly medially over the proximal fibula (**Fig. 10-4A,B**).
2. The peroneal nerve is identified (**Fig. 10-4A,B**).
3. The lateral head of the gastrocnemius is retracted medially (it may have to be released) and the soleus freed from its origin (**Fig. 10-4C**). The popliteus tendon can be retracted proximally and medially or released (to be repaired at the time of closure). The posterior-lateral tibial articular surface can then be exposed by a submeniscal arthrotomy, releasing the coronary ligament inferior to the meniscus and medial to the popliteal tendon hiatus. The breadth of exposure of the posterolateral tibia is relatively small.

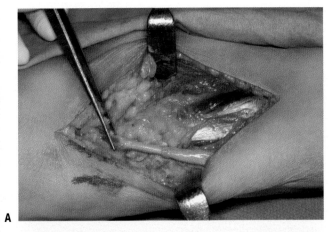

A

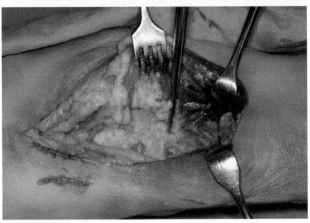

C

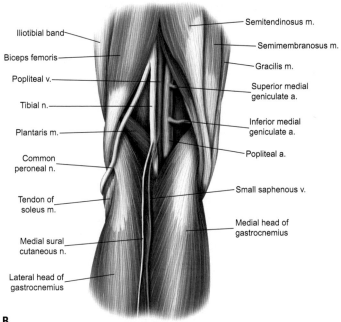

B

FIGURE 10-4

A,B: Proximal is to the viewer's left. The common peroneal nerve is held by the forceps. The fascia of the lateral head of the gastrocnemius is visible. **C:** The lateral head of the gastrocnemius had been retracted to the superior side of the photograph. The forceps is on the knee joint line but the distal (to the viewer's right) extent of the tibial exposure is limited. One can release the lateral head of the gastrocnemius, but the popliteal artery is medial and anterior tibial artery branches off, proceeding anteriorly and laterally relative to the retractor.

SURGICAL EXPOSURES OF THE TIBIAL AND FIBULAR DIAPHYSIS

Anteromedial Approach

The anterior approach to the leg is relatively simple due to the superficial location of the anterior border of the triangular-shaped tibia. The anteromedial border can easily be palpated from the proximal medial aspect of the tibia at the pes anserine insertion all the way distal to the medial malleolus. The skin incision is typically made in a longitudinal fashion just medial to the bony prominence to help facilitate soft tissue closure. The entire anterior two-thirds may then be easily exposed by performing a subperiosteal dissection off the medial side of the tibia. Except for the pes anserine insertion proximally, the anteromedial surface is free of any soft tissue attachments. The saphenous nerve and vein are the only neurovascular structures at risk with this exposure. Skin and bone vascularity are an issue with this approach so although the tibia is easily exposed via this route, it is less frequently used.

Anterolateral Approach

If one desires better soft tissue coverage of an implant, the anterolateral approach allows for placement of the device between the tibialis anterior muscle and the bone. The incision is made just lateral to the tibial crest. The anterolateral aspect of the tibialis anterior is elevated off the surface of the bone. The main neurovascular structures at risk during this approach are the deep peroneal nerve and anterior tibial artery, which will remain unharmed if dissection is carried out subperiosteally in the anterior compartment.

Posteromedial Approach

Orientation   Proximal is to the viewer's left.

Technique

1. Incision: for release of the posterior compartments of the leg, or for exposure of the posterior part of the diaphysis of the tibia, one can make an incision just posterior to the tibia. If one is releasing both compartments, the incision is made about 2 cm posterior to the posterior tibial border. If one is approaching the posterior tibia, the incision is at or just posterior to the tibial border.
2. Care should be taken to identify the greater saphenous vein which courses along the medial aspect of the tibia. After skin retraction, the posterior aspect of the tibia is identified and the fascia incised (**Fig. 10-5A–C**). Both the superficial compartment and the deep compartment can be released through this incision.
3. If access to the tibia is desired, the deep muscles are retracted posteriorly. The neurovascular bundle of the deep posterior compartment is located lateral and slightly posterior to the first muscle belly encountered—that of the flexor digitorum longus (**Fig. 10-5D**).

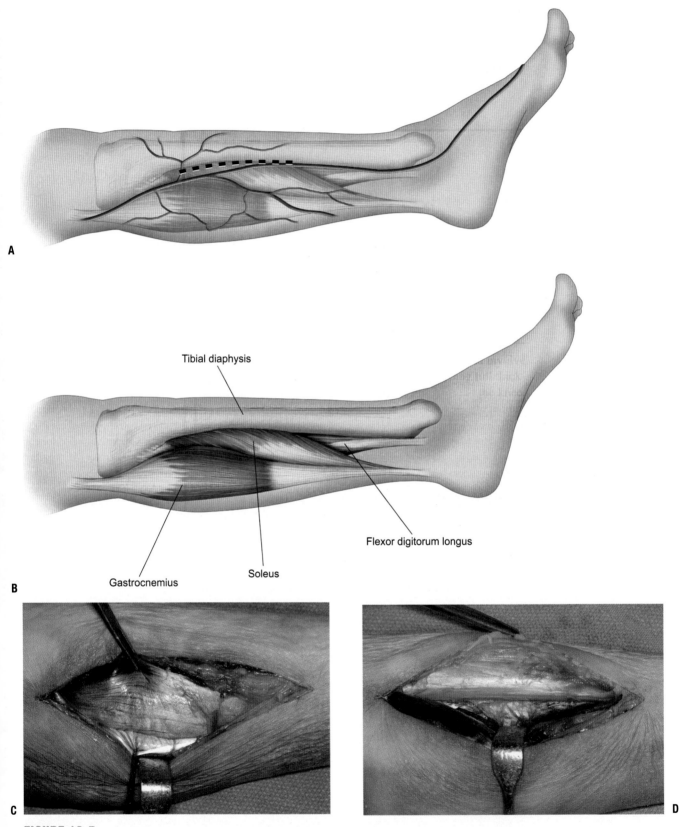

FIGURE 10-5

A–C: Posteromedial approach to the tibia diaphysis. The soleus muscle is held by the upper forceps, the gastrocnemius fascia by the lower forceps. **D:** The deep compartment muscles are retracted toward the bottom of the photograph. The posterior and posteromedial aspect of the tibial shaft are visible.

LATERAL APPROACH TO THE TIBIA

Indications

The posterolateral approach to the tibia is most frequently used in the posttraumatic setting where bone grafting of the tibia is performed in a patient with compromised anteromedial soft tissues.

Orientation

Proximal is to the viewer's left.

Position

The patient is positioned prone or in the lateral decubitus position.

Technique

1. Incision: the incision is longitudinal, centered just posterior to the fibula.
2. Dissection is carried down through the overlying fascia, which is split in line with the skin incision. The plane between the soleus and the peronei is entered. The soleus is dissected free from the fibula and the deep posterior compartment is entered. The flexor hallucis muscle is released from the fibula (**Fig. 10-6A**).
3. The peroneal artery and vein are deep to this great toe flexor muscle. The remaining deep flexor musculature is dissected off of the interosseous membrane and the tibia approached (**Fig. 10-6B**).

   - *Pearls/Pitfalls:* Often, because of the scarring, it is easier to approach the involved site from proximally, where the anatomical planes are more distinct. Although a similar approach can be carried out anterior to the interosseous membrane, as well through a more anterior lateral incision, the neurovascular bundle is at much more risk via this route.

RELEASE OF ANTERIOR AND LATERAL COMPARTMENT FASCIA

For double incision fasciotomy, the anterior and lateral compartments are released via a longitudinal incision centered midway between the tibia and fibula. The anterior intermuscular septum is identified and the fascia released both anterior and posterior to the septum.

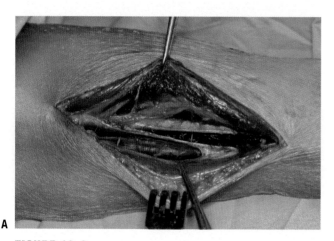
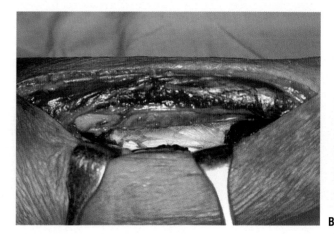

A   B

FIGURE 10-6

A: Posterolateral approach to the tibia. The peronei are retracted anteriorly (upper aspect of photograph). The soleus is retracted posteriorly and the fibula is visible in the middle of the wound. **B:** By staying directly on the fibula as its posteromedial surface angles anteriorly, one will come to the interosseous membrane. The posterior musculature is elevated from the membrane until the tibia is visible. Here the tibial diaphysis is visible in the base of the wound.

SURGICAL APPROACH TO THE FIBULA

Surgical exposure of the fibula for fracture reduction and internal fixation, osteotomy for nonunion of the tibia, or for vascularized bone grafting is made through a direct lateral approach. The typical skin incision is made approximately just posterior to the fibula and may be extended from the tip of the lateral malleolus proximally to the head of the fibula. There is very little subcutaneous dissection distally. Care must be taken proximally to avoid injury to the common peroneal nerve, as it is located in a subcutaneous location while it crosses the fibular neck. The muscular interval used to gain access to the fibula is between the soleus posteriorly and the peroneal muscles anteriorly. The majority of the soft tissue attachments will be found on the proximal two-thirds of the fibula. The distal one-third exposure is easily made after incising the deep fascia of the leg. At this level the peroneal musculature is retracted posteriorly to access the bone. Again, the amount of soft tissue elevation and dissection from the fibula should be dictated by the least amount of exposure needed. In the distal portion of the incision, at a variable length above the mortise, the superficial peroneal nerve will be encountered.

ANTEROMEDIAL APPROACH TO THE DISTAL TIBIA

Indications

The standard anterior approach to the ankle joint involves entering via the plane between the tibialis anterior medially and the neurovascular bundle and toe extensors laterally. This works well for intra-articular ankle procedures but not as well for distal tibial fracture reduction and fixation. The anteromedial approach works well for medial plating and fractures of the distal tibia in which the medial side has failed in compression and requires plating and bone grafting.

Position

The patient is supine.

Technique

1. Incision: the 8 to 10 cm incision is made medial, rather than lateral, to the tibialis anterior tendon (**Fig. 10-7A–C**).
2. That tendon is retracted laterally along with the other structures lateral to it (**Fig. 10-7D**).
3. One must identify and preserve the saphenous nerve; otherwise, the medial malleolus and medial distal tibia are well presented via this approach. The tubercle of the Chaput is not as well visualized via this approach, however.

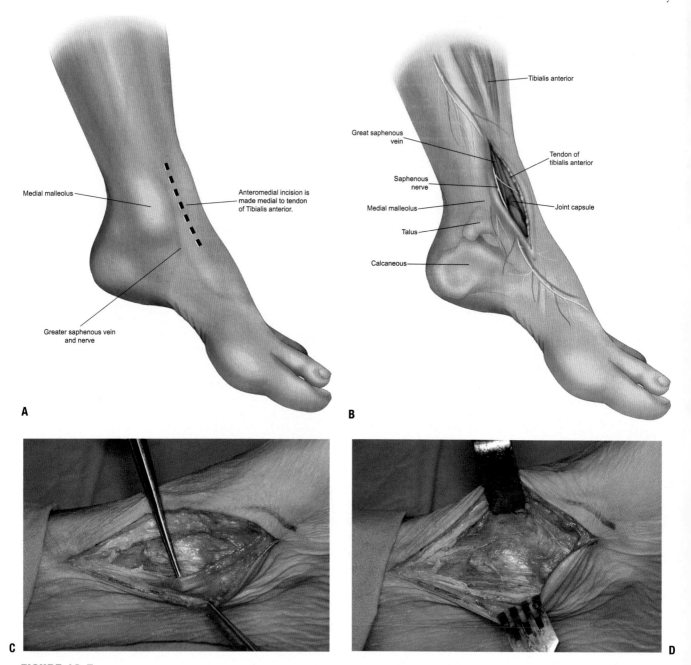

A

Medial malleolus

Anteromedial incision is made medial to tendon of Tibialis anterior.

Greater saphenous vein and nerve

B

Tibialis anterior

Great saphenous vein

Tendon of tibialis anterior

Saphenous nerve

Joint capsule

Medial malleolus

Talus

Calcaneous

C

D

FIGURE 10-7

A–C: Anteromedial approach to the distal tibia. Proximal is to the viewer's left. The forceps is elevating the saphenous nerve and vein. **D:** The knee retractor is holding the anterior tibial tendon and ankle capsule is directly below it in this photograph.

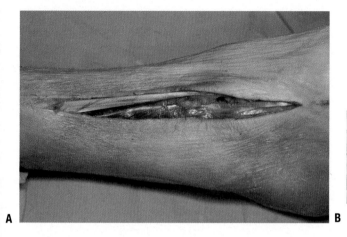
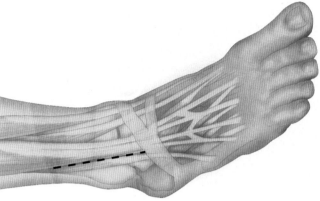

A   **B**

FIGURE 10-8
A,B: Incision for anterolateral approach to the distal tibia.

ANTEROLATERAL APPROACH TO THE DISTAL TIBIA

Indications

Pilon fractures with compression failure laterally can be easily exposed anterolaterally. The window is opened by retracting the extensors of the ankle and toes medially along the neurovascular bundle.

● *Pearls/Pitfalls:* One has to watch out for the superficial peroneal nerve as it crosses the fibula and proceeds distally and medially. The peroneus tertius is retracted laterally.

This is an excellent exposure for application of anterolateral periarticular plates.

Orientation

Proximal is to the viewer's left.

Technique

1. Incision: the incision is made in line with the fourth metatarsal distally. It is a straight incision, crossing the ankle joint (**Fig. 10-8A,B**).
2. It can be extended proximally as necessary, freeing up the anterior compartment muscles as necessary. It can be extended distally and allows access to the dorsal lateral aspect of the talar neck as well, if necessary.
3. After incising the skin, the retinaculum is encountered and incised as well. The tendons and neurovascular structures are retracted as noted (**Fig. 10-8E,F**).

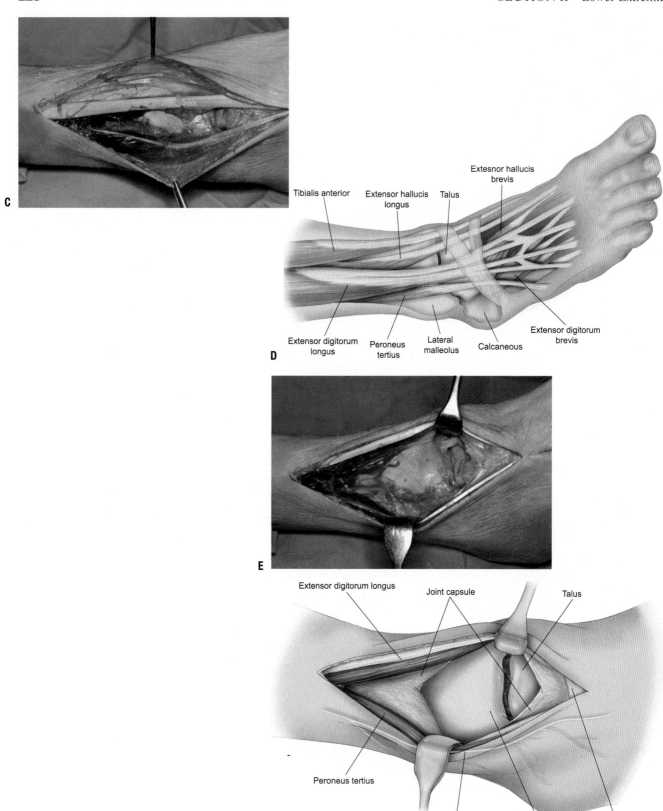

C

Tibialis anterior

Extensor hallucis
longus

Talus

Extesnor hallucis
brevis

Extensor digitorum
longus

Peroneus
tertius

Lateral
malleolus

Calcaneous

Extensor digitorum
brevis

D

E

Extensor digitorum longus

Joint capsule

Talus

Peroneus tertius

Superficial peroneal
nerve

Tibia

Extensor
retinaculum

F

FIGURE 10-8

(Continued) **C,D:** Extensor muscles to the top of the photograph, peroneus
tertius to the bottom, anterolateral tibia and talus are easily visible. **E,F:** With
retraction, the whole anterior tibia is exposed. The superficial peroneal nerve
is behind the lower retractor, with the peroneus tertius tendon.

POSTERIOR MEDIAL APPROACH TO THE DISTAL TIBIA

Indications

Occasionally it is necessary to approach the tibia or the talus via a posterior medial approach. This can be accomplished with the patient prone or supine.

Position

If the patient is positioned supine, a bump can be placed under the opposite hip. The ipsilateral leg is then flexed and externally rotated.

Orientation

Proximal is to the viewer's right.

Technique

1. Incision: the incision is made at approximately the midpoint between the Achilles tendon and the medial malleolus, with care taken to avoid the saphenous vein (**Fig. 10-9A–C**).
2. The plane past the neurovascular bundle can either be via the flexor digitorum longus medially and the neurovascular bundle laterally, between the neurovascular bundle and the flexor hallucis longus, or by retracting the flexor hallucis medially and protecting the nerve and artery (**Fig. 10-9D**).

   - *Note:* One cannot directly visualize the intracuticular aspect of the distal tibia directly via this approach but it works well for indirect reduction techniques and also for posteromedial fractures of the talus.

3. It is also possible by making the incision more anteriorly over the posterior aspect of the medial malleolus, to access the posterior distal tibia and the medial malleolus both, by releasing the cephalad attachments of the posterior tibial sheath, and retracting the tendon distally and posteriorly (**Fig. 10-9E**). One can, by retracting the malleolar fragment distally, directly assess the reduction of the articular surface at the posterior aspect.

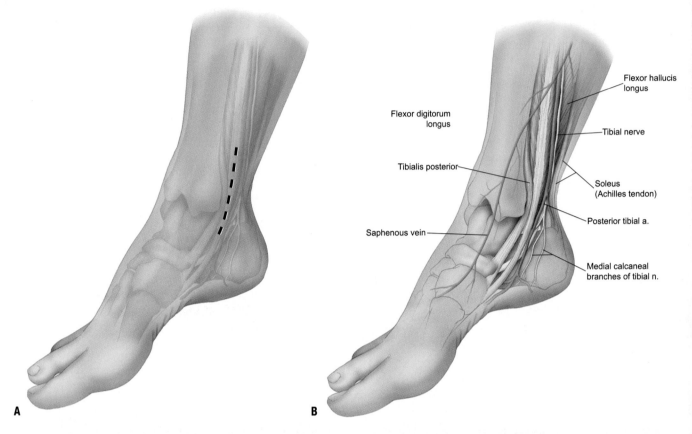

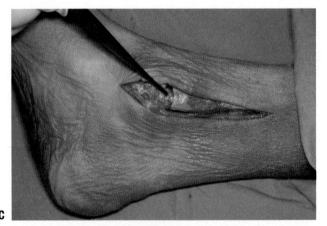

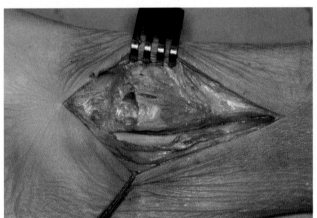

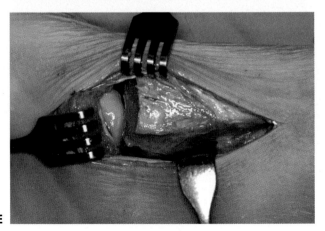

FIGURE 10-9

A–C: Posteromedial approach to the distal tibia, this exposure allows access to both the posterior tibia and the articular surface if there is a medial malleolar fracture present, or an osteotomy performed. **D:** Posterior tibial tendon visible along the posterior aspect of the tibia. **E:** Both the tibial and talar articular surfaces are visible, along with the posterior tibia, through this approach. This approach works well for the supination-adduction type ankle fracture pattern where there is medial plafond depression that has to be elevated.

POSTEROLATERAL APPROACH TO THE DISTAL TIBIA

Indications

One can access pilon fractures and fibular fractures through the posterolateral corner of the ankle as well.

Position

Typically the patient is positioned prone, although supine positioning can be utilized with a bump under the ipsilateral hip. The patient can also be placed in a sloppy lateral position. Positioning may depend on the patient's other injuries.

Technique

1. Incision: an incision is made between the fibula and the Achilles tendon (**Fig. 10-10A,B**).
2. The dissection is carried medial to the peroneal musculature. The sural nerve must be identified and protected (**Fig. 10-10C,D**).
3. The flexor hallucis longus muscle is elevated as needed and retracted medially (**Fig. 10-10E**). Both the posterior-lateral tibia and the posterior aspect of the fibula can be approached from this direction.

   - *Note:* Like with the posteromedial approach, the articular surface of the distal tibia won't be directly seen with this exposure. Both of these approaches work well if one is applying a buttress plate, however. Reduction and plating of fibula can be accomplished as well and one can maintain a very wide skin bridge between anterior and posterior incisions.

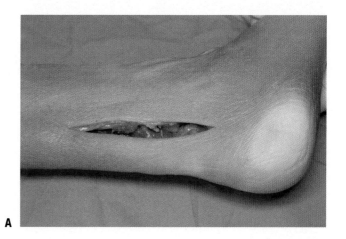

A

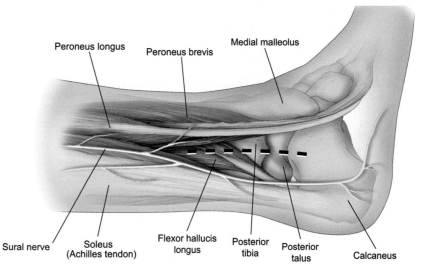

FIGURE 10-10

A,B: Incision for approach to postero-lateral distal tibia.　**B**

Labels: Peroneus longus — Peroneus brevis — Medial malleolus — Sural nerve — Soleus (Achilles tendon) — Flexor hallucis longus — Posterior tibia — Posterior talus — Calcaneus

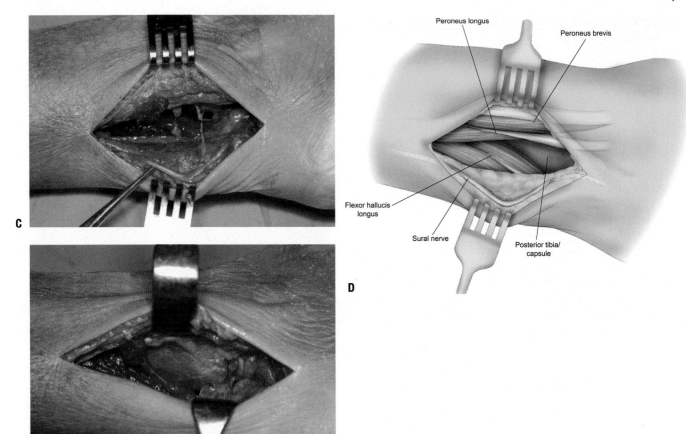

FIGURE 10-10

(Continued) **C,D:** Sural nerve shown next to forceps. Peroneal tendons superiorly in the photograph. **E:** The peroneal tendons retracted anteriorly, the flexor hallucis muscle belly is elevated and retracted posteromedially. The posterior distal tibia is visible along with the posterior aspect of the talus.

RECOMMENDED READING

Barei DM, Nork SE, Mills WJ, et al. Complications associated with internal fixation of high-energy bicondy-lar tibial plateau fractures utilizing a two-incision technique. *J Ortho Traumaa* 2004;18: 649–657.

Carlson DA. Bicondylar fracture of the posterior aspect of the tibial plateau: A case report and a modified op-erative approach. *J Bone Joint Surg* 1998;80A:1049–1052.

Fakler JK, Ryzewicz M, Hartshorn C, et al, Optimizing the management of Moore type I postero-medial split fracture dislocations of the tibial head: Description of the Lobenhoffer approach. *J Ortho Trauma* 2007;21:330–335.

Hollinshead WH. Knee, leg, ankle and foot. In: *The Back and Limbs: Anatomy for Surgeons*, Vol. 3. New York: Harper and Rowe, 1969:796–831.

Nelson G, Kelly P. Blood supply of the human tibia. *J Bone Joint Surg* 1960;42A:625–635.

Wiss DA, ed. *Master Techniques in Orthopaedic Surgery: Fractures*. Philadlephia: Lippincott Williams & Wilkins, 2006.

11 Foot and Ankle

Julie E. Adams, Joseph R. Cass, and Harold Kitaoka

ANATOMIC CONSIDERATIONS

The ankle is stabilized by anatomic congruence of the talus in the mortise as well as the strong ligaments and capsular attachments. The medial ligaments coalesce into a strong single ligament known as the deltoid ligament (1,2). It has superficial and deep fibers (1,2). The lateral collateral ligament is comprised of three discrete components; the anterior talofibular ligament, the calcaneofibular ligament, and the posterior talofibular ligament (1,3). The thin anterior talofibular ligament is most commonly disrupted with ankle sprains. Other stabilizers of the ankle joint include the syndesmosis and interosseous membrane.

Soft Tissue Anatomy

The muscles of the foot may be divided into the intrinsic muscles, whose origins and insertions lie in the foot, and extrinsic muscles, whose bellies lie proximal and tendons extend into the foot to exert their influences. Plantarly, the musculature of the foot is arranged in four layers, from plantar to dorsal: (a) abductor hallucis, flexor digitorum brevis, abductor digit minimi; (b) flexor digitorum longus, flexor hallucis longus, quadratus plantae, and the lumbricals; (c) flexor digiti minimi brevis, adductor hallucis, flexor hallucis brevis; and (d) the four dorsal and three plantar interossei muscles. Dorsally, the extensor digitorum brevis and extensor hallucis brevis lie in a relatively superficial plane (**Fig. 11-1**).

Overlying the tendons of the ankle are the retinacula, which prevent bowstringing of the tendons. The superior extensor retinaculum lies anteriorly and is split by the tibialis anterior tendon. The inferior extensor retinaculum lies over the dorsum of the foot and is Y shaped. It stretches from the lateral os calcis to the medial malleolus and to the plantar aponeurosis (**Fig. 11-2**). The flexor retinacula are lateral and consist of the superior peroneal retinaculum, which is a thickening of deep fascia stretching from the tip of the lateral malleolus to the calcaneus, and the inferior peroneal retinaculum, which crosses from the peroneal tubercle to lateral calcaneus.

The potential internervous planes include *medially*, between the tibial nerve innervated flexors (tibialis posterior) and the deep peroneal nerve innervated extensors (tibialis anterior); *posterolaterally* between the flexors (flexor hallucis longus) and the superficial peroneal nerve innervated everters (peroneus brevis); and *laterally*, between the extensors (peroneus tertius) and the everters (peroneus brevis) (4).

Neurovascular Anatomy

Anteriorly, the anterior tibial artery and the deep branch of the peroneal nerve course toward the foot, crossing the ankle joint midway between the malleoli (see Fig. 11-1) (4–6). The anterior tibial artery lies between the tibialis anterior tendon and the extensor hallucis longus proximal to joint and then between the extensor hallicus longus (EHL) and the extensor digitorum longus (EDL) distal to the

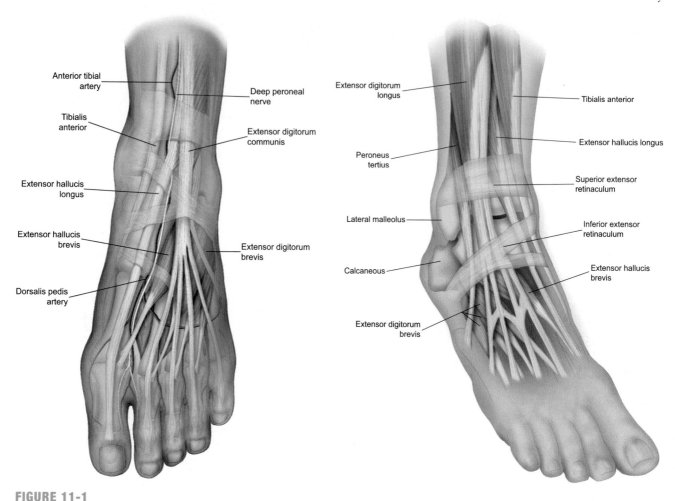

FIGURE 11-1

FIGURE 11-2

joint. It becomes the dorsalis pedis artery distally as it enters the foot. The deep peroneal nerve supplies the extensor digitorum brevis (EDB) and extensor hallucis brevis and provides cutaneous sensation to the first web space.

Posteromedially, the neurovascular bundle includes the posterior tibial artery and the tibial nerve and courses posterior to medial malleolus, lying between the tendons of the flexor digitorum longus (FDL) and flexor hallucis longus (FHL) **(Fig. 11-3)**. The posterior tibial artery passes behind the tendon of the flexor digitorum longus before entering the sole of the foot and dividing into medial and lateral plantar arteries. Analogous to the hand, the lateral plantar nerve supplies sensation to 1.5 digits, while the medial plantar nerve supplies 3.5 digits (1,3).

Several superficial structures are important to identify and preserve. The saphenous nerve, the terminal branch of femoral nerve, runs with the long saphenous vein anterior to medial malleolus. Proximally, it pierces the deep fascia between the sartorius and gracilis tendons. The branches of the nerve are closely associated with those of the long saphenous vein throughout their courses. The saphenous nerve passes anterior to the medial malleolus to provide cutaneous sensation to the medial first ray and base of the big toe. The nerve divides into two branches at the level of the medial malleolus and thus supplies sensation to the medial midfoot as well **(Fig. 11-4)**.

The superficial peroneal nerve is a terminal branch of the common peroneal nerve. It pierces the deep fascia of the anterior compartment at the distal one-third of the leg and distally crosses the ankle anteriorly at the mid-malleolar line. It is superficial and lateral to the anterior tibial neurovascular bundle. It divides into the medial and intermediate dorsal cutaneous nerves, which provide sensation to the dorsum of the foot (see Fig. 11-4).

The sural nerve is the terminal branch of tibial nerve and runs over the lateral aspect of the leg and foot, posterior to the lateral malleolus. It pierces the deep fascia in the posterior calf then travels distally, lateral to the Achilles tendon. The sural nerve travels with the short saphenous vein, with which its branches are closely bound. Its path curves anteriorly distal to the lateral malleolus along the fifth

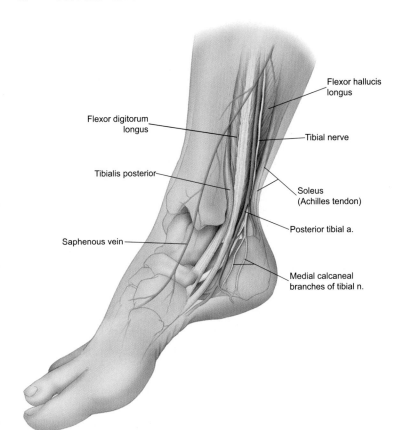

Flexor hallucis
longus

Flexor digitorum
longus

Tibial nerve

Tibialis posterior

Soleus
(Achilles tendon)

Posterior tibial a.

Saphenous vein

Medial calcaneal
branches of tibial n.

FIGURE 11-3

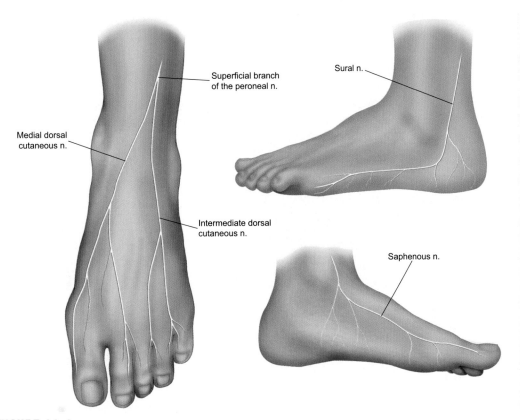

Superficial branch
of the peroneal n.

Sural n.

Medial dorsal
cutaneous n.

Intermediate dorsal
cutaneous n.

Saphenous n.

FIGURE 11-4

ray to finally become the lateral dorsal cutaneous nerve of the foot and provides sensation to the lateral aspect of the foot (see Fig. 11-4) (1,2,4,5).

APPROACHES TO THE DISTAL TIBIA/ANKLE JOINT (5,7–10)

Anteromedial Approach to the Distal Tibia/Ankle Joint

Indications   The standard anterior approach to the ankle joint involves entering via the plane between the tibialis anterior medially and the neurovascular bundle and toe extensors laterally. This works well for intraarticular ankle procedures but not as well for distal tibial fracture reduction and fixation. This anteromedial approach works well for medial plating and fractures of the distal tibia in which the medial side has failed in compression and requires plating and bone grafting.

Technique

1. The incision is made medial, rather than lateral, to the tibialis anterior tendon (**Fig. 11-5A**).
2. That tendon is retracted laterally along with the other structures lateral to it. One must identify and preserve the saphenous nerve; otherwise the medial malleolus and medial distal tibia are well presented via this approach (**Fig. 11-5B**). The tubercle of Chaput is not as well visualized via this approach, however.
3. The knee retractor may be utilized to retract the anterior tibial tendon laterally and the ankle capsule is readily visible (**Fig. 11-5C**).

Anterolateral Approach to the Distal Tibia/Ankle Joint

Indications   Pilon fractures with compression failure laterally can be easily exposed anterolaterally. This is an excellent exposure for application of anterolateral periarticular plates. The interval is defined by retracting the extensors of the ankle and toes medially along with the neurovascular bundle.

- *Note:* One has to watch out for the superficial peroneal nerve as it crosses the fibula and proceeds distally and medially. The peroneus tertius is a part of the extensor digitorum communis.
- *Note:* This anterolateral exposure has been described both as between the tertius and communis tendons, or lateral to those tendons.

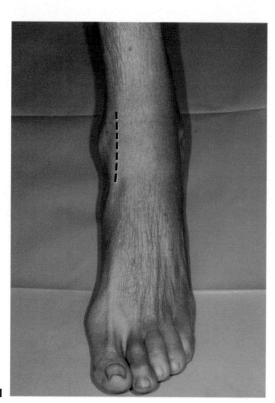
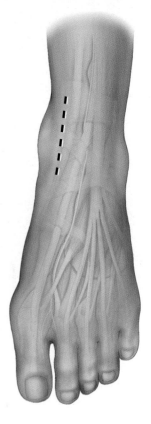

FIGURE 11-5 A1   **A2**

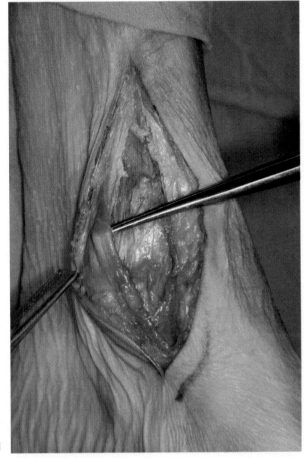

B1

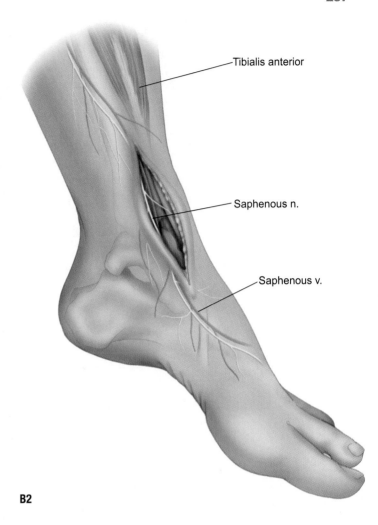

Tibialis anterior

Saphenous n.

Saphenous v.

B2

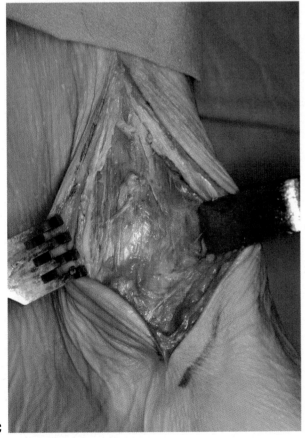

C

FIGURE 11-5 *(Continued)*

Technique

1. The incision is made in line with the fourth metatarsal distally (**Fig. 11-6A**). It is a straight incision, crossing the ankle joint.
   - *Note:* It can be extended proximally as necessary, freeing up the anterior compartment muscles as necessary. It can be extended distally and allows access to the dorsal lateral aspect of the talar neck as well, if necessary.
2. After incising the skin, the retinaculum is encountered and incised as well (**Fig. 11-6B**). The tendons and neurovascular structures are identified (**Fig. 11-6C**).
3. The extensor muscles are retracted laterally and the peroneus tertius medially.
4. With retraction, the joint and anterior distal tibia are easily observed. The superficial peroneal nerve is behind the lateral retractor along with the peroneus tertius tendon (**Fig. 11-6D**).

Posteromedial Approach to the Distal Tibia/Ankle Joint

Indications   Occasionally it is necessary to approach the tibia or the talus via a posterior medial approach, usually for medial malleolar fractures or possibly to expose the talus with a medial malleolar osteotomy.

Position   This can be accomplished with the patient prone or supine. If the patient is positioned supine, a bump can be placed under the opposite hip. The ipsilateral leg is then flexed and externally rotated.

Technique

1. The incision is made at approximately the midpoint between the Achilles tendon and the medial malleolus (**Fig. 11-7A**).
   - *Note:* The plane past the neurovascular bundle can either be via the flexor digitorum longus medially and the neurovascular bundle laterally, between the neurovascular bundle and the flexor hallucis longus, or by retracting the flexor hallucis medially and protecting the nerve and artery (**Fig. 11-7B**).
2. The malleolus is readily exposed by a periosteal elevator (**Fig. 11-7C**). One cannot directly visualize the intraarticular aspect of the distal tibia directly via this approach but it works well for indirect reduction techniques and also for posteromedial fractures of the talus.
   - *Note:* It is also possible, by making the incision more anteriorly over the posterior aspect of the medial malleolus, to access both the posterior distal tibia and the medial malleolus.
3. Release the cephalad attachments of the posterior tibial sheath (**Fig. 11-7D**) and retract the tendon distally and posteriorly.
4. The malleolus is osteotomized, and by retracting the malleolar fragment distally, the posterior reduction of the articular surface may be assessed (**Fig. 11-7E**).
   - *Note:* Both the tibial and talar articular surfaces are visible, along with the posterior tibia, through this approach. This approach works well for the supination-adduction type ankle fracture pattern where there is medial plafond depression that has to be elevated.

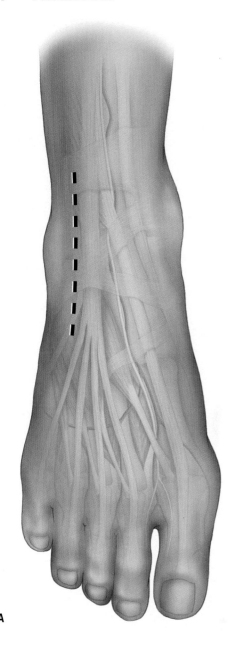

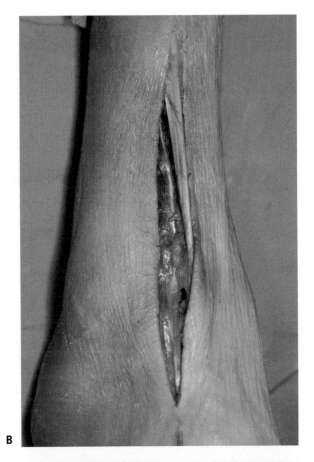

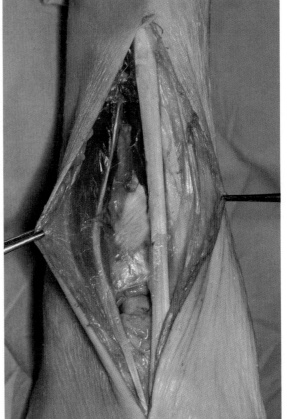

A

B

C

FIGURE 11-6

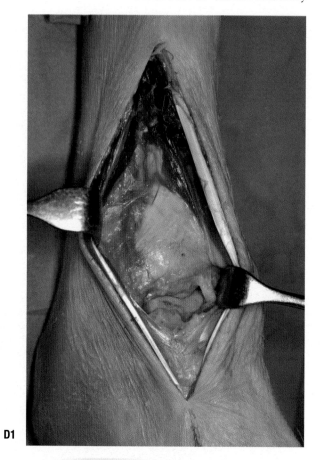

D1

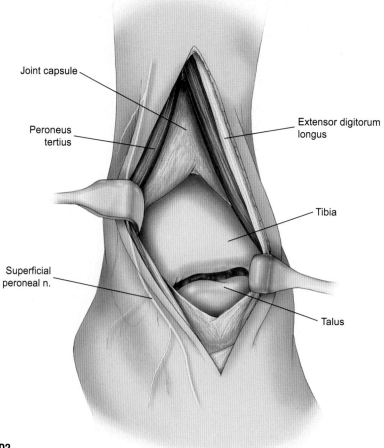

Joint capsule

Peroneus
tertius

Extensor digitorum
longus

Tibia

Superficial
peroneal n.

Talus

FIGURE 11-6 *(Continued)*   **D2**

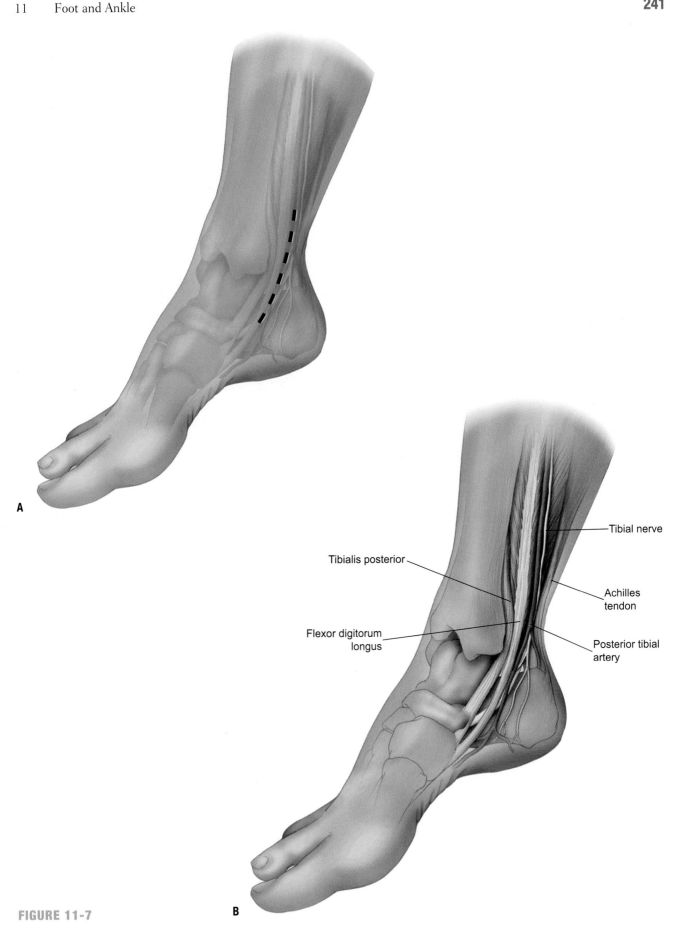

Tibial nerve

Tibialis posterior

Achilles tendon

Flexor digitorum longus

Posterior tibial artery

A

B

FIGURE 11-7

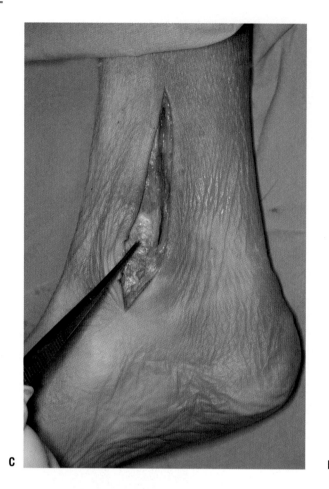

C

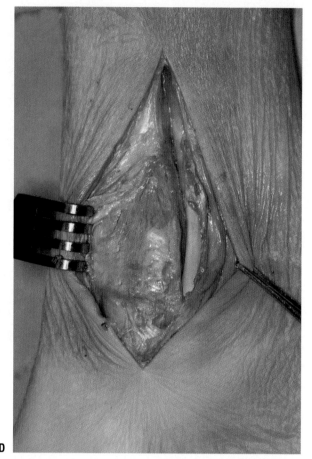

D

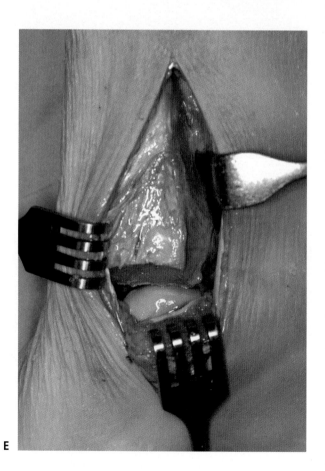

E

FIGURE 11-7 *(Continued)*

Posterolateral Approach to the Distal Tibia/Ankle Joint (4,11)

Indications   One can access pilon fractures and fibular fractures through the posterolateral corner of the ankle as well.

Positioning   Typically the patient is positioned prone, although supine positioning can be utilized with a bump under the ipsilateral hip. The patient can also be placed in a sloppy lateral position. Positioning may depend on the patient's other injuries.

Technique

1. An incision is made between the fibula and the Achilles tendon **(Fig. 11-8A)**. The dissection is carried medial to the peroneal musculature **(Fig. 11-8B)**.
2. The sural nerve must be identified and protected **(Fig. 11-8C)**.
3. The flexor hallucis longus muscle is elevated as needed and retracted medially **(Fig. 11-8D)**.
   - *Note:* Both the posterior-lateral tibia and the posterior aspect of the fibula can be approached from this direction. Like with the posteromedial approach, the articular surface of the distal tibia won't be directly seen with this exposure. Both of these approaches work well if one is applying a buttress plate, however. Reduction and plating of fibula can be accomplished as well and one can maintain a very wide skin bridge between anterior and posterior incisions.

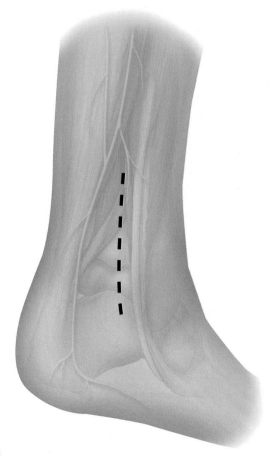

A

FIGURE 11-8

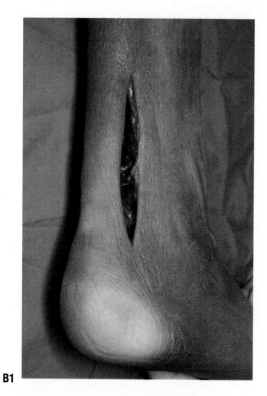

B1

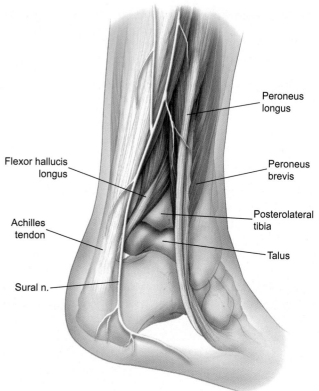

Peroneus
longus

Flexor hallucis
longus

Peroneus
brevis

Achilles
tendon

Posterolateral
tibia

Talus

Sural n.

B2

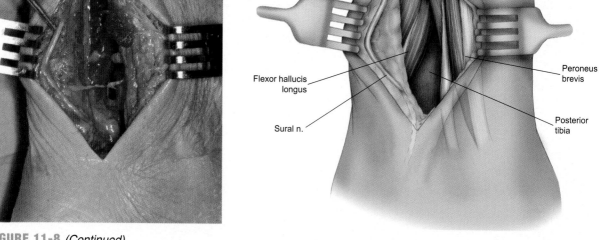

C1

Peroneus
longus

Flexor hallucis
longus

Sural n.

Peroneus
brevis

Posterior
tibia

C2

FIGURE 11-8 *(Continued)*

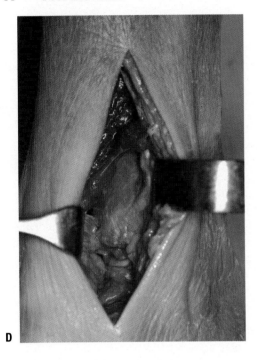

D   **FIGURE 11-8** *(Continued)*

Anterior Approach to the Distal Tibia/Ankle Joint

This approach has been described utilizing two intermuscular planes: between the tibialis anterior tendon and extensor hallucis longus tendon, or between the extensor hallucis longus and extensor digitorum communis tendons. The structure at risk is the anterior neurovascular bundle, consisting of the anterior tibial artery (dorsalis pedis) and the deep peroneal nerve.

Indications

- Ankle arthrodesis
- Ankle arthroplasty (2,12)
- Address intraarticular pathology (loose body excision, synovectomy, septic arthritis decompression/debridement)
- Open reduction and internal fixation of pilon or talar body fractures

Position   The patient is positioned supine, with bony prominences well padded. A soft bolster under the ipsilateral hip is helpful.

Landmarks   The medial and lateral malleoli are palpable. A transverse line is drawn connecting the malleoli. The center of this bimalleolar line corresponds to the position of the neurovascular bundle. The plane of dissection for this approach is between either the tibialis anterior and EHL, or the EHL and the extensor digitorum communis (**Fig. 11-9A**).

Technique

1. An incision of appropriate length is made anteriorly through skin only, bisecting the distance between malleoli. An incision is made through the extensor retinaculum to expose the appropriate intermuscular plane. The superficial peroneal nerve lies laterally, marked by the forceps in Figure 11-9B.
2. In Figure 11-9C, the anterior tibial tendon is medial, the extensor digitorum communis tendon is lateral to the neurovascular bundle, and the extensor hallucis longus tendon is visible beneath the incompletely removed retinaculum, medial to the neurovascular bundle. In Figure 11-9D, the neurovascular bundle is located after retracting the extensor hallucis longus medially and the extensor digitorum communis laterally.
3. The tendons are retracted along with the neurovascular bundle. Typically this is retracted with the lateral tendons exposing the capsule (**Fig. 11-9E**). A longitudinal incision is made in the capsule. Retractors can be introduced. The surgeon will be able to visualize the anterior ankle from lateral gutter to medial gutter, and, depending on how much distraction and plantarflexion are applied, most if not all of the articular surfaces of the ankle joint (**Fig. 11-9F**).

Posterior Approach to the Distal Tibia/Ankle Joint

Occasionally it is necessary to approach the ankle joint from its direct posterior aspect. Such situations might include tibiotalar or tibiocalcaneal arthrodeses. The patient is positioned prone, and an incision is made directly over the Achilles tendon. The tendon is transected and its ends retracted proximally and distally. The ankle and subtalar joint can be exposed directly by retracting the flexor hallucis medially and the peroneal tendons laterally. Although the posterior aspect of the distal tibia is well exposed via this approach, the posterolateral approach works as well without sacrificing the Achilles tendon.

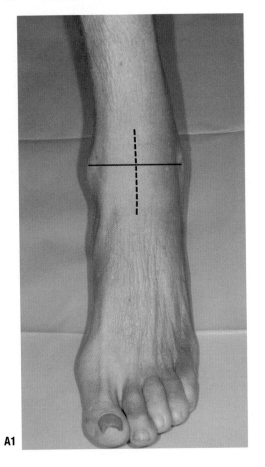

A1

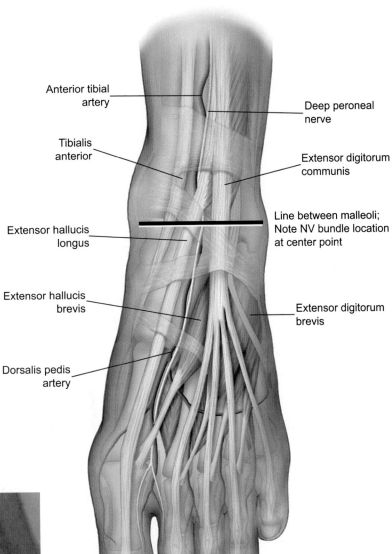

Anterior tibial
artery

Deep peroneal
nerve

Tibialis
anterior

Extensor digitorum
communis

Line between malleoli;
Note NV bundle location
at center point

Extensor hallucis
longus

Extensor hallucis
brevis

Extensor digitorum
brevis

Dorsalis pedis
artery

A2

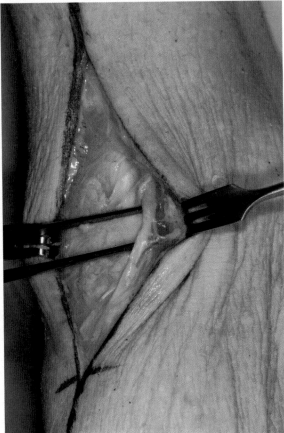

B

FIGURE 11-9

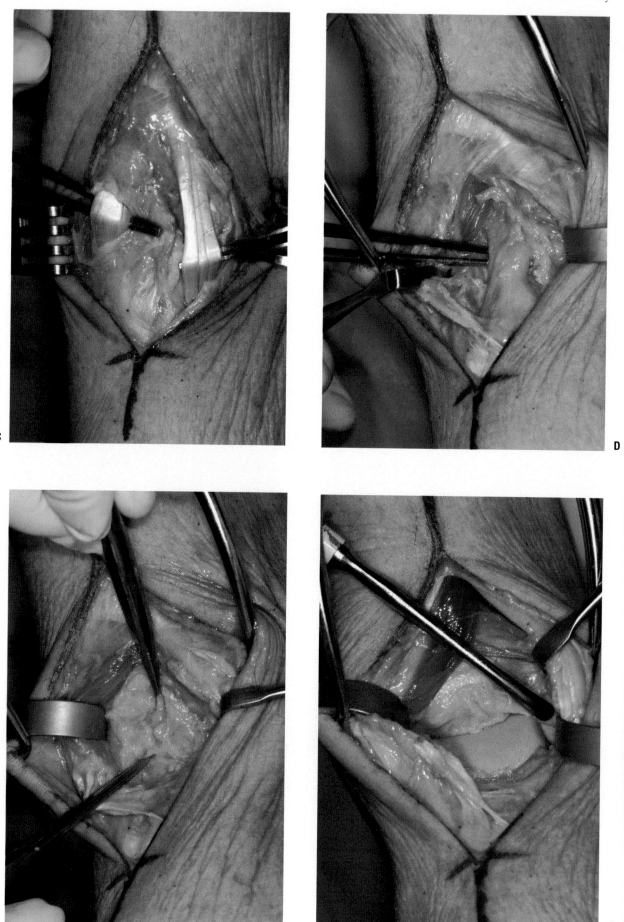

FIGURE 11-9 *(Continued)*

LATERAL APPROACHES TO THE FIBULA/PERONEAL TENDONS

Indications

- Open reduction and internal fixation of fibular fractures.
- Ankle arthrodesis in conjunction with fibular osteotomy.
- Exposure of the posterolateral tibia.
- Exposure of the peroneal tendons.
- Limited exposure of the talus and talocalcaneal joint.

Positioning

The patient is positioned supine, with bony prominences padded. A hip bump placed under the ipsilateral hip may be helpful to facilitate exposure. Alternatively, if this approach is utilized in conjunction with a medial approach for ankle arthrodesis, positioning in the semilateral position with the operative extremity up, may be helpful.

Landmarks

The distal fibula is subcutaneous and is readily palpable.

Technique

1. Incision: for approaches to the distal fibula for open reduction and internal fixation of fractures or for osteotomy for access to the ankle joint, a longitudinal incision of appropriate length is made curving along the posterior margin of the fibula, with the distal limb curving anteriorly (**Fig. 11-10A**). If the pathology to be addressed is in the peroneal tendons, a curved longitudinal incision maybe made paralleling the posterior border of the fibula and curving over the peroneal tubercle.
2. Full thickness flaps are made down to the periosteum, with care to avoid the sural nerve and the short saphenous vein posteriorly. The perforating branches of the peroneal artery lie deep to the distal fibula medially. In addition, the peroneal tendons are at risk, particularly with anterior subluxation.
3. The fibula may be osteotomized to gain access to the joint, as for ankle arthrodesis. The osteotomy should be made obliquely, at a level 4 to 6 cm proximal to the tip of the lateral malleolus. One may lengthen the incision distally to visualize the subtalar joint (3,13,14).

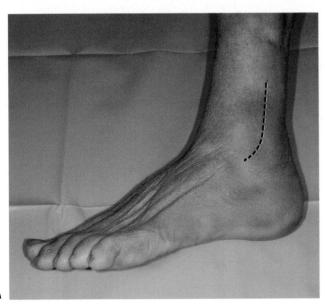

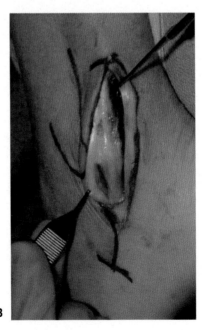

A   B

FIGURE 11-10

4. Alternatively, if the pathology to be addressed lies within the peroneal tendons, the deep fascia overlying the peroneal retinaculum is incised. The retinaculum and the fascial sheath of the peroneal tendons are incised (**Fig. 11-10B**).
   - *Note:* If access to the talus or talocalcaneal joint is needed, the peroneal longus and brevis tendons can be retracted anteriorly to expose the capsule of the talocalcaneal joint, which is then incised. Likewise, the calcaneofibular ligament may be incised to provide further exposure of the talus.

Pearls and Pitfalls

- The sural nerve and the short saphenous vein are at risk in the posterior portion of the field.
- Likewise, the peroneal tendons may be at risk, particularly in cases in which they subluxate anteriorly.

EXPOSURES OF THE TALUS

The talus can be exposed via posteromedial exposure (as discussed previously). Only the posteromedial aspect is satisfactorily seen through this approach. Similarly, a small corner of the posterolateral talus can be seen from the posterolateral approach, although even this amount is compromised by the syndesmotic ligaments just superior to the talus. The talar neck can be exposed dorsally by utilizing the distal part of the anterior ankle exposure, as discussed previously as well.

The utilitarian approaches to the talar neck are primarily the anterolateral and anteromedial approaches. In repair of talar neck fractures the surgeon needs to be cognizant of the potential for varus of valgus malunion of the fracture and so visualization of both the medial and lateral aspects is helpful. For talar body fractures, the aforementioned medial approach to the ankle is useful, with the malleolar osteotomy. In many cases, however, the soft tissues have been avulsed from the medial malleolus as part of the injury mechanism. If that is the case, there is usually enough instability that the talus can be abducted out of the ankle mortise enough to visualize and repair the body fracture. By avoiding the osteotomy, one can avoid further compromise of the vascular supply of the medial malleolus.

Anteromedial Talar Neck Exposure

The incision can be longitudinal along the neck of the talus, or vertically, as an extension of the anteromedial distal tibia exposure. The interval is between the anterior tibial and posterior tibial tendons. The saphenous vein and nerve are at risk. Care should be taken to avoid excessive retraction dorsally or plantarly to avoid further disruption of the talar blood supply. The medial neck is directly visible upon incision the capsule. One can see the anterior articular surface of the calcaneus as well as the sustentaculum via this approach.

Anterolateral Talar Neck Exposure

The incision can be made as a part of the anterolateral distal tibial exposure. The peroneus tertius is retracted dorsally and the neck exposed. One probably will encounter small branches of the superficial peroneal nerve. Through this exposure one can see the anterolateral articular surface of the talus, the lateral process of the talus, the sinus tarsi, and the neck itself. Again, caution should be exercised in stripping soft tissues from the attachment to the talus.

EXPOSURE OF THE HINDFOOT: THE SUBTALAR JOINT

- *Note:* The posterior facet of the subtalar joint can be exposed with a variety of incisions: transverse, longitudinal, or along the skin tension lines. The deeper approach is the same, however. With reflection of the extensor digitorum brevis distally and plantarward, and posterior retraction of the peroneal tendons, the dorsolateral surface of the calcaneus, the lateral talar neck, and the posterior facet can be visualized (15,16).

Technique

1. A horizontal incision is made just distal to the lateral malleoulus and extends anteriorly approximately 5 to 6 cm **(Fig. 11-11A–C)**.
2. The extensor digitorum brevis is retracted distally and anteriorly. The peroneal tendons are retracted posteriorly. The lateral talocalcaneal ligament is identified **(Fig. 11-11D)**.
3. The posterior facet is now exposed with a band retractor holding peroneal tendons posteriorly **(Fig. 11-11E)**.
   - *Note:* With dissection dorsally, one can expose the talar neck. By freeing the EDB from the calcaneus from proximal to distal, one can see all of the lateral anterior process of the calcaneus to the calcaneocuboid joint. By placement of a laminar spreader in the sinus tarsi, or some form of distractor across the talocalcaneal joint, the articular surface of the posterior facet can be visualized.

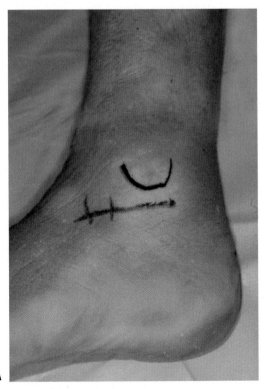

A

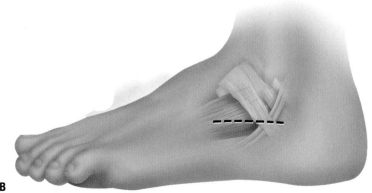

B

FIGURE 11-11

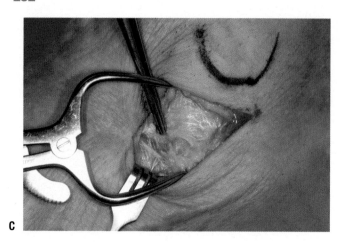

C

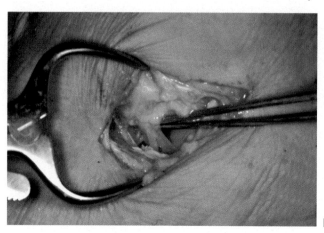

D

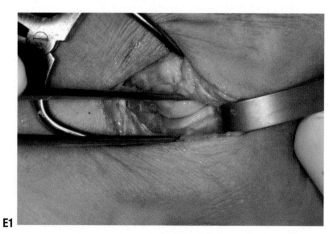

E1

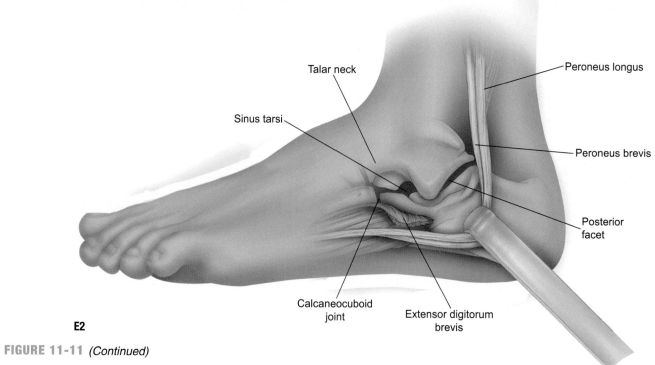

E2

FIGURE 11-11 (Continued)

EXTENSILE TRAUMA APPROACH TO THE LATERAL CALCANEUS

Indications

For operative treatment of fractures of the calcaneus, the standard approach is the loosely L-shaped incision along the posterior and inferior aspect of the lateral calcaneus (17). This is not an incision to be undertaken lightly as the incidence of wound healing and deep infection has been reported to be as high as 30%. Careful soft tissue handling is paramount. Recently, less invasive approaches, which are combinations of lateral sinus tarsi and medial sustentacular approaches have been described.

Position

The patient is positioned laterally, with careful attention to padding of dependent prominences.

Technique

1. The incision proceeds from proximal to distal, beginning lateral to the Achilles tendon. The inferior corner is at the junction of the vertical limb and the glabrous skin of the heel. It is then extended distally along that border, proceeding slightly anteriorly if necessary to access the calcaneo-cuboid joint (**Fig. 11-12A**).
2. The incision is carried directly to bone and the posteroinferior angle and then the soft tissues are stripped directly off of the bone (**Fig. 11-12B**).
3. The surgeon must avoid taking off the tissues in layers. The sural nerve should be dorsal and anterior to the skin incision but plantar branches are routinely encountered. These are severed (**Fig. 11-12C**).
4. The peroneal tendons and sheath, and calcaneofibular ligament are released from the calcaneus. With further dissection, the EDB is elevated from the anterior process (**Fig. 11-12D**). After proper flap mobilization, K-wires can be placed in the talus and fibula as needed for retraction.

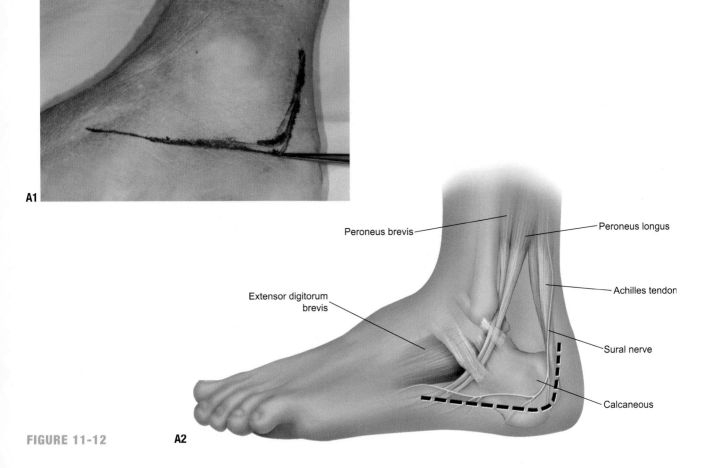

A1

FIGURE 11-12   **A2**

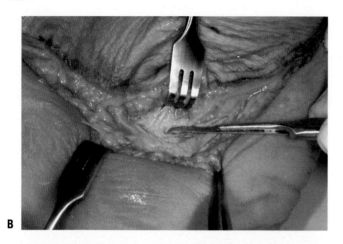

B

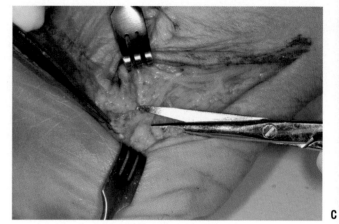

C

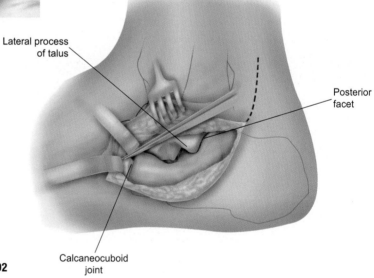

D1

D2

Lateral process
of talus

Posterior
facet

Calcaneocuboid
joint

FIGURE 11-12 *(Continued)*

MIDFOOT EXPOSURES

Dorsal Approach to the Talo-Navicular Joint

The talo-navicular joint can be exposed dorsally as an extension of the anterior ankle joint exposure. It can also be exposed medially as an extension of the talar neck exposure (4,6,16). The dorsal approach is described here.

Technique

1. The interval between the tibialis anterior tendon (AT) and the EHL tendon is identified (**Fig. 11-13A**).
2. The skin is incised and then the retinaculum. Superficial to the retinaculum are found branches of the superficial peroneal nerve (**Fig. 11-13B**).
   - *Note:* These should be handled with care, resected if necessary. Cutaneous neuromas are occasionally a problem after the dorsal approaches to the foot.
3. The retinaculum is incised and the interval between the AT and the EHL developed.
4. The dorsalis pedis and deep peroneal nerve are near, and deep, to the EHL tendon (**Fig. 11-13C**).
5. The capsule is incised and the joint exposed (**Fig. 11-13D**). The naviculo-cuneiform joint can be exposed by extending the approach.

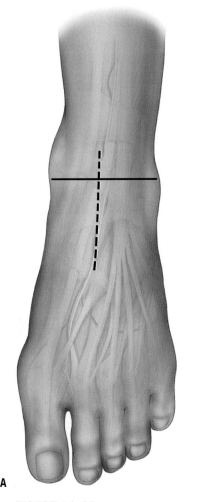

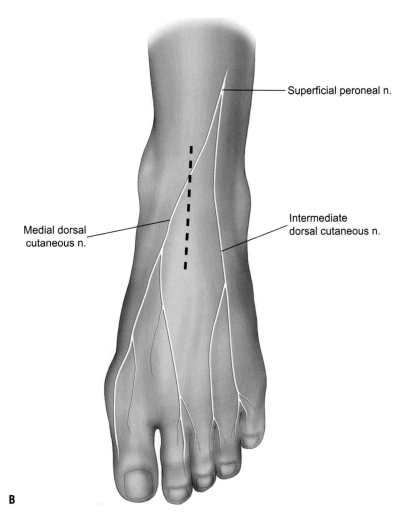

Superficial peroneal n.

Medial dorsal
cutaneous n.

Intermediate
dorsal cutaneous n.

A   B

FIGURE 11-13

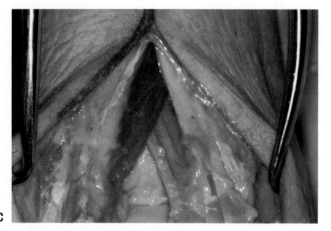 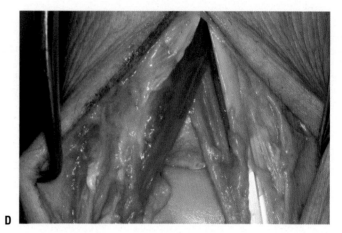

C   D

FIGURE 11-13 *(Continued)*

Lisfranc Joint Exposure

Indications   The five tarsometatarsal joints are exposed via dorsal approaches. One would use these exposures for injuries to the Lisfranc complex, or fusions of these joints. If the procedure is being performed for fracture repair, the image intensifier can be used to center the incisions over the appropriate joints. Typically, one can reach three joints with one longitudinal approach.

- *Note:* Care should be taken in the spacing of these incisions, leaving wide bridges of skin. These longitudinal incisions can be extended distally for dorsal compartment fasciotomies. These approaches are relatively straightforward, the surgeon needs to be aware of the cutaneous nerves and the NV bundle overlying the medial and intermediate cuneiform joint, and then in the first web space.

Technique

1. Skin incision over second tarsometatarsal joint **(Fig. 11-14A)**.
2. The EHL is identified and retracted by scissors; forceps are on the extensor digitorum brevis (EDB) **(Fig. 11-14B)**.
3. The EDB and NV bundles are retracted to the right, EHL to left **(Fig. 11-14C)**.
4. The capsule is exposed and entered. Forceps to bottom in space between first and second metatarsal. Top forceps in medial-intermediate cuneiform joint **(Fig. 11-14D)**.

Exposure of Lateral Lisfranc Joint

Technique

1. Exposure of the 3–5 tarsal metatarsal joints. A longitudinal incision is centered over fourth tarsometatarsal joint **(Fig. 11-15A)**.
   - *Note:* The cutaneous branch of superficial peroneal nerve is in close proximity to this incision **(Fig. 11-15B)**.
2. The EDC is at the left of photo. Joint capsule visible **(Fig. 11-15C)**.
3. The capsule is incised. Tarsometatarsal joints of third (top of photo) through fifth visible **(Fig. 11-15D)**.

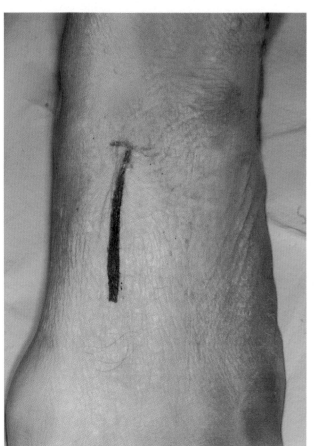

A1

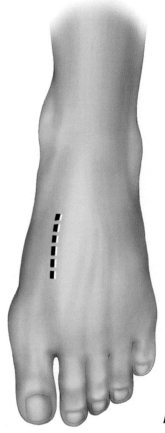

A2

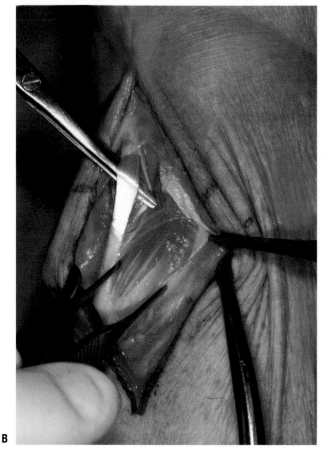

B

FIGURE 11-14

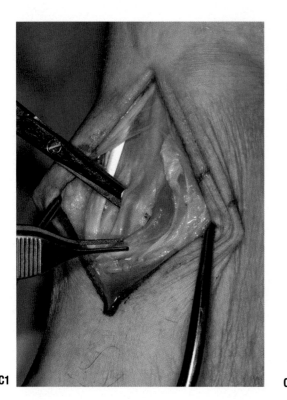

C1

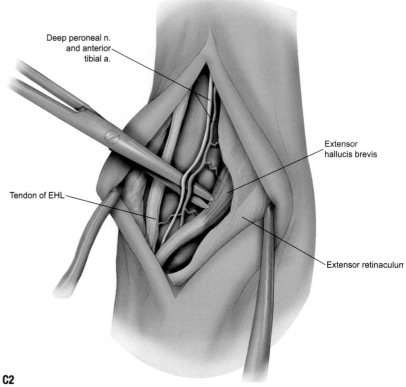

C2

Deep peroneal n. and anterior tibial a.

Extensor hallucis brevis

Tendon of EHL

Extensor retinaculum

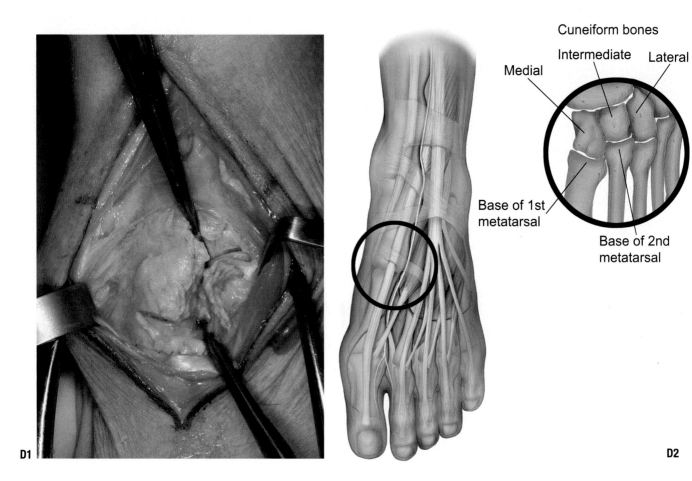

D1

D2

Cuneiform bones

Intermediate

Lateral

Medial

Base of 1st metatarsal

Base of 2nd metatarsal

FIGURE 11-14 *(Continued)*

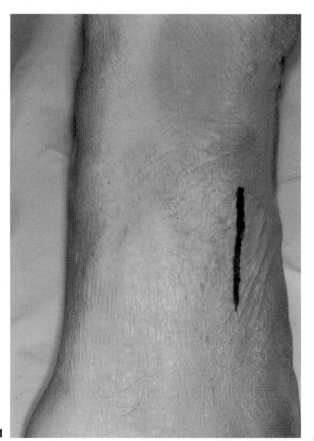

A1

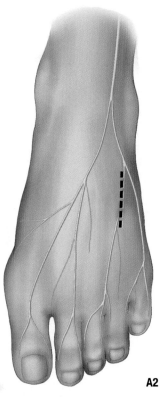

A2

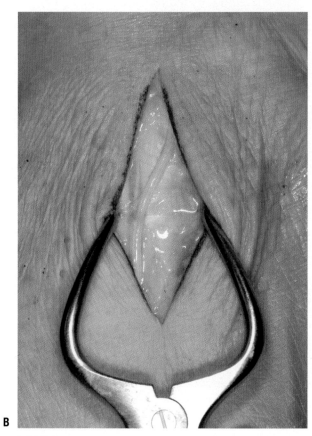

B

FIGURE 11-15

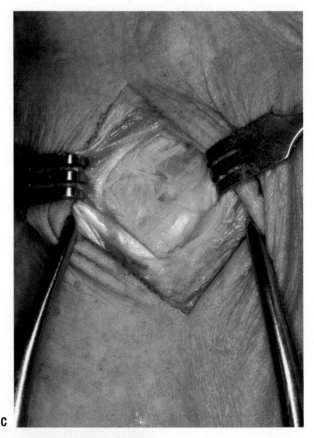

C

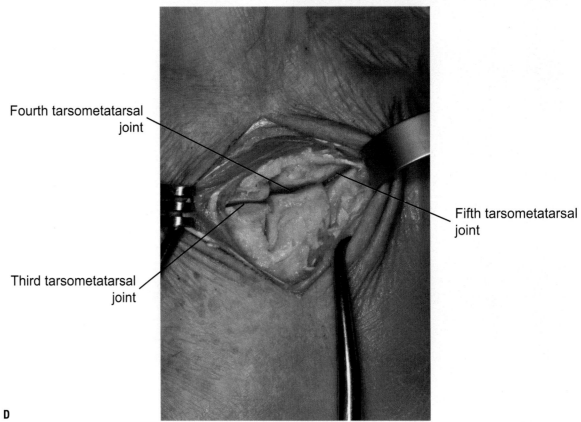

Fourth tarsometatarsal joint

Fifth tarsometatarsal joint

Third tarsometatarsal joint

D

FIGURE 11-15 *(Continued)*

EXPOSURES OF THE GREAT TOE

The exposures of the toes are very straightforward. The most significant is that of the MTP of the great toe.

Great Toe: Medial Exposure of the First Metatarsophalangeal Joint

Indications

- Bunion procedures.
- Removal of exostoses such as for hallux rigidus.

Position   The patient is supine. A sandbag under the ipsilateral hip may be helpful.

Landmarks   The prominence of the metatarsal head, midpoint of the articulation from the medial perspective (**Fig. 11-16A**).

Technique

1. Incision: an Esmarch tourniquet is usually applied just above the ankle. A linear incision is made with a length depending upon the pathology. In most instances this measures approximately 4 to 5 cm. It may be extended somewhat more proximally as needed. It is placed slightly dorsal or less commonly, volar to the mid point of the prominent metatarsal head (**Fig. 11-16B**).

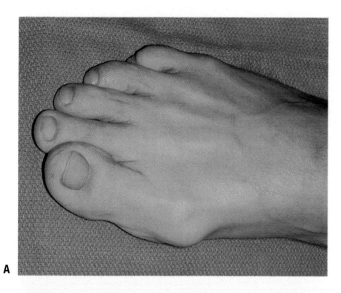

A

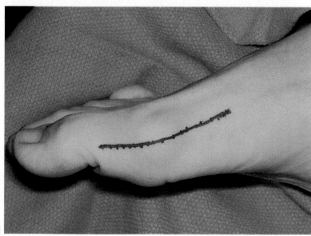

B1

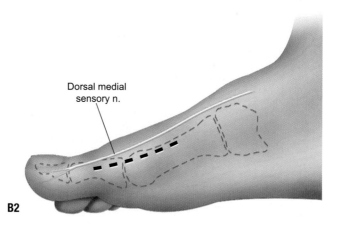

Dorsal medial
sensory n.

B2

FIGURE 11-16

2. The dissection carries to the subcutaneous tissue taking care to avoid the dorsal cutaneous nerve which emerges from the dorsal aspect of the incision **(Fig. 11-16C)**.

3. The bursal tissue and capsule covering the joint is exposed. With incision of the capsule, the metatarsal head or exostosis is exposed. Depending on the procedure, the capsulotomy can be a "U" or "L" shaped distally based flap **(Fig. 11-16D)**. As this flap is elevated the metatarsophalangeal joint is exposed **(Fig. 11-16E)**.

4. Additional reflection of the capsule around the metatarsal head may be required to execute the desired procedure.

5. Closure consists of suturing the lateral capsule to the soft tissue proximally, typically with a 2-0 absorbable suture. Care should be made to avoid prominent knots as this is a site of pressure for shoe wear.

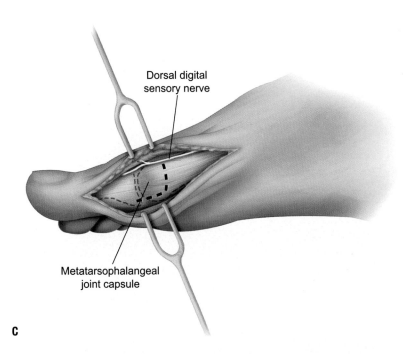

C

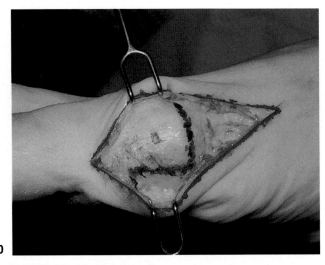

D

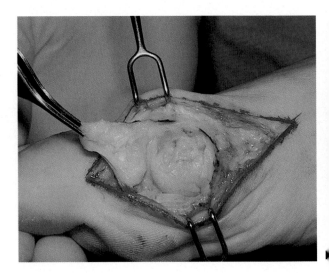

FIGURE 11-16 *(Continued)*

Pearls and Pitfalls

Beware of the cutaneous nerve; a neuroma of this nerve can be quite bothersome in the postoperative period.

Dorsum of the Metatarsophalangeal Joint

Indications   Removal of exostoses.

Position   Supine, an Esmarch tourniquet can be used.

Landmarks   Mid point of the dorsal aspect of the joint.

Technique

1. Incision: a 3 cm incision directed just medial to the midline **(Fig. 11-17A)**.
2. The dissection carries through the skin exposing the long extensor tendon of the great toe **(Fig. 11-17B)**. This is retracted laterally exposing the capsule.
3. The capsule is incised and the exostosis and interarticular pathology may be addressed **(Fig. 11-17C)**.
4. Closure: skin closure is routine. Absorbable sutures without prominent knots are preferable.

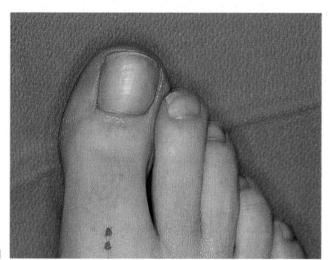

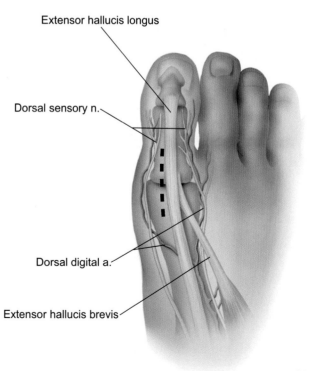

Extensor hallucis longus

Dorsal sensory n.

Dorsal digital a.

Extensor hallucis brevis

A1   A2

FIGURE 11-17

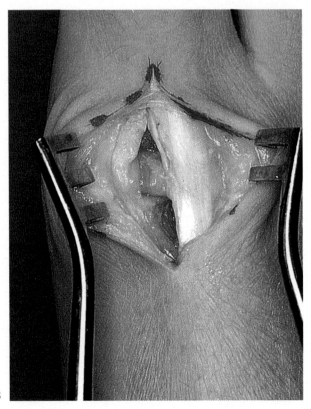

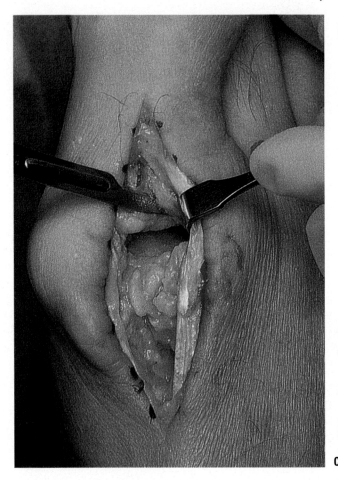

B   C

FIGURE 11-17 *(Continued)*

REFERENCES

1. Acton R. Surgical principles based on anatomy of the foot: Preoperative planning. *Foot Ankle* 1982;2(4):200–204.
2. Anderson T, Montgomery F, Carlsson A. Uncemented STAR total ankle prostheses. *J Bone Joint Surg Am* 2004;86-A Suppl 1(Pt 2):103–111.
3. Weller GG, Graham JL, Kile TA. Anatomy and surgical approaches. In: Morrey BF, ed. *Reconstructive Surgery of the Joints*. Rochester, MN: Mayo Foundation, 1996.
4. Hansen ST. *Functional Reconstruction of the Foot and Ankle*. Philadelphia: Lippincott Williams & Wilkins, 2000.
5. Hoppenfeld S, de Boer P. The foot and ankle. In: *Surgical Exposures in Orthopaedics: The Anatomic Approach*. Philadelphia: JB Lippincott, 1984; 513–576.
6. Kagaya H, Yamada S, Nagasawa T, et al. Split posterior tibial tendon transfer for varus deformity of hindfoot. *Clin Orthop Relat Res* 1996;(323):254–260.
7. Kitaoka HB. Arthrodesis of the ankle: technique, complications, and salvage treatment. *Instr Course Lect* 1999;48:255–261.
8. Michelson J, Amis JA. Talus-calcaneus-cuboid (triple) arthrodesis. In: Kitaoka HB, ed. *Master's Techniques in Orthopaedic Surgery: The Foot and Ankle*. Philadelphia: Lippincott Williams & Wilkins, 2002; 401–424.
9. Penny JN, Davis LA. Fractures and fracture-dislocations of the neck of the talus. *J Trauma* 1980;20(12):1029–1237.
10. Sarrafian SK. Topographic anatomy and surgical approaches to the ankle and foot. In: Jahss M, ed. *Disorders of the Foot and Ankle: Medical and Surgical Management*. Philadelphia: WB Saunders Company, 1991.
11. Konrath GA, Hopkins G, 2nd. Posterolateral approach for tibial pilon fractures: a report of two cases. *J Orthop Trauma* 1999;13(8):586–589.

12. Takakura Y, Tanaka Y, Kumai T, et al. Ankle arthroplasty using three generations of metal and ceramic prostheses. *Clin Orthop Relat Res* 2004;(424):130–136.

13. Rupp RE, Podeszwa D, Ebraheim NA. Danger zones associated with fibular osteotomy. *J Orthop Trauma* 1994;8(1):54–58.

14. Smith RW. Ankle arthrodesis. In: Kikaoka HB, ed. *Master's Techniques in Orthopaedic Surgery: Foot and Ankle*. Philadephia: Lippincott Williams & Wilkins, 2002; 533–549.

15. Kitaoka HB. Talocalcaneal (subtalar) arthrodesis. In *Master's Techniques in Orthopedic Surgery: The Foot and Ankle*. Philadelphia, Lippincott Williams & Wilkins, 2002; 387–399.

16. Younger AS, Hansen ST, Jr. Adult cavovarus foot. *J Am Acad Orthop Surg* 2005;13(5):302–315.

17. Freeman BJC, Duff S, Allen PE, et al. The extended lateral approach to the hindfoot: anatomical basis and surgical implications. *J Bone Joint Surg Br* 1998;80B:139–142.

12 Cervical Spine

Robert K. Eastlack and Bradford L. Currier

The complex and often variable anatomy of the cervical spine mandates careful preoperative planning and an appreciation of the limitations inherent in each surgical approach. Such planning can significantly reduce the technical demands of the surgery, and reduce the likelihood of complications.

With all of the approaches, optimizing patient positioning prior to an incision will lead to a smoother procedure, and may improve the result of the operation. This includes the use of imaging modalities after positioning to ensure adequacy of the image, which can be adjusted much more easily prior to final preparation and draping of the patient.

Indications for a particular approach depend largely on the anatomic levels requiring surgical management, as well as the techniques planned for any reconstruction. **Table 12-1** lists the more common anterior and posterior approaches, and the cervical levels exposed most effectively by each approach. With the advent of fluoroscopically guided techniques (i.e., transarticular C1-2 screws or anterior odontoid screws), one must also consider the trajectories required for placing instrumentation when choosing the surgical approach.

ANTERIOR APPROACHES

Transoral Approach

Indications   This approach is typically used for resection of anterior processes, such as the odontoid with basilar invagination, infection, tumors, irreducible odontoid fractures in chronic dislocations, and congenital disorders of the anterior axis or atlas.

As its name implies, this approach uses the oral cavity as its pathway to the upper cervical spine. Visualization can be difficult due to the constraints of the jaw and oral cavity, but it can allow direct access from the clivus to the upper portion of C3. Although there is little vascularity encountered when approaching the spine through this midline approach, infection and cerebrospinal fluid leakage have been considerable problems in the past. The heightened chance of infection and historically poor outcome of bone grafting with the transoral approach make it a questionable choice for use dur-

TABLE 12-1.   Common Approaches to the Cervical Spine

Approach	Limitis of Exposure
Anterior	
Transoral	C1-2
High retropharyngeal	C1-2 facets to the C2-3 disk space
Odontoid screw placement	Use anterior approach to C5 level
Anterior, transverse incision	C3-T1 (limits affected by body habitus)
	Transverse incision nonextensile; limits exposure to 3 or 4 disc levels
Anterior, longitudinal incision	C2-T1; extensile for exposure of more segments than transverse incision; exposure of T1 or below may require resection of medial clavicle/manubrium
Posterior	
Posterior midline	Extensile from occiput to sacrum, as necessary
Paramedian incisions	Used for percutaneous introduction of transarticular C1-2 screws

ing anterior cervical fusions (1). The limitations in exposure with this approach can be reduced by the use of mandibular osteotomies. Morbidity from these techniques can be substantial; however, the approach does allow unique anterior exposure from the clivus to C6. It is typically useful for lesions within the bodies of C2-3, and when the oral cavity cannot be easily traversed, such as with severe temporomandibular joint arthrosis or an interdental distance less than 25 mm.

Preoperative Planning/Preparation   As with all spine surgery, medical comorbidities should be ascertained, but particular focus must be paid to nutritional status. Total lymphocyte count and albumin are generally useful markers of nutritional status. Dental evaluations should be performed preoperatively to ensure an oral cavity that is free from ongoing infection. Standard preoperative antibiotic recommendations currently include an intravenous cephalosporin and metronidazole.

Position   A padded headrest or Gardner-Wells™ tongs are used to stabilize the head with the patient in the supine position. Awake, nasotracheal intubation may be performed with or without fiberoptic assistance depending on the perceived stability of the cervical spine. Once a neurologic examination is performed, anesthetic can be administered, and then the patient can be placed in a mild reverse-Trendelenberg position to prevent aspiration (2). Various retractors can be used for widening the interdental gap, such as the Codman Crawford or the Spetzler-Sonntag transoral retractors (**Figs. 12-1–12-3**). The soft palate can often be elevated with a malleable self-retainer. Alternatively, two Red Robin catheters can be fed through the nares (one on each side) and brought out through the mouth. Once both catheters have been placed, the two ends on each side are tensioned superolaterally and secured to the drapes. Prepare the oropharyngeal area with betadine solution, and place a throat packing to prevent debris from falling into dependent laryngeal spaces or the trachea. Obtain localizing radiographs once the posterior pharyngeal area is exposed, and then inject epinephrine solution along the site of planned incision. Although surgical loupes with overhead illumination can be used in these cases, an operating microscope provides a clearer image and allows for easier assistant participation.

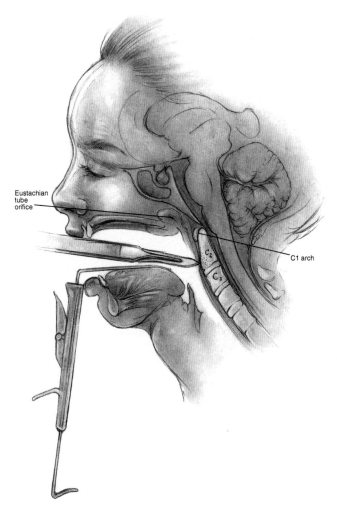

Eustachian
tube
orifice

C2

C3

C1 arch

FIGURE 12-1

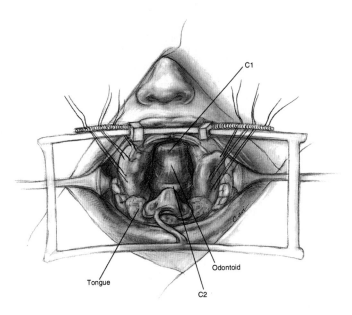

C1

Tongue

Odontoid

C2

FIGURE 12-2

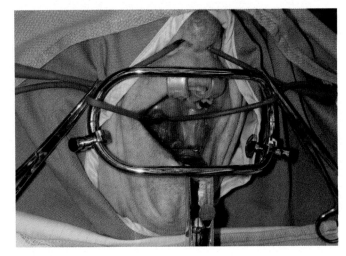

FIGURE 12-3

Landmarks   The tubercle of the atlas can be palpated to discern the midline, and a vertical incision is carried out 1 to 2 cm above and below the tubercle in the midline **(Fig. 12-4)**.

Technique

1. Incision: the incision is made full thickness to bone through the mucosa and pharyngeal musculature. Subperiosteal elevation should be carried out from the midline, which will bring the longus colli muscles and anterior longitudinal ligaments laterally. Lateral elevation on the atlas should be restricted to 1.5 cm from the midline, as the vertebral arteries, internal carotid arteries, and hypoglossal nerves are at risk with more aggressive lateral exposure (3) **(Fig. 12-5).** The internal carotid artery can be quite close to the midline, as suggested by Currier et al, who found it more than 7.5 mm medial to the foramen transversarium in 6% of their subjects (4). The hypoglossal nerve lies approximately 2 to 3 mm lateral to the middle of the anterior aspect of the C1 lateral mass (5) (see Fig. 12-5).

2. If access to the odontoid is desired, the central 1 to 1.5 cm of the atlas may be resected to expose the upper portion of C2. Should the anterior portion of the atlas be removed, attempt to preserve the transverse ligament, if possible. The transverse ligament prevents lateral displacement of the atlas lateral masses, which can lead to craniocervical instability (6). If it cannot be preserved, a posterior occipitocervical arthrodesis may be necessary. Soft tissues, such as pannus, can be resected from the areas surrounding the bony anatomy, but residual amounts adherent to the dura may best be left in place to avoid cerebrospinal fluid (CSF) leakage. The tectorial membrane can be decompressed to allow improvement in CSF flow.

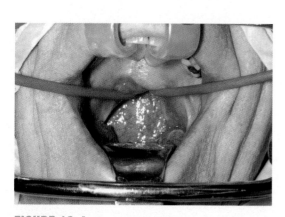

FIGURE 12-4

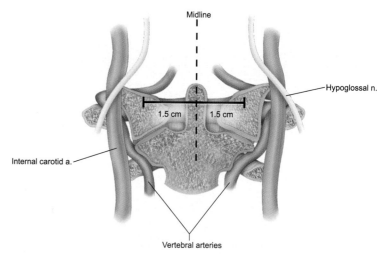

FIGURE 12-5

Postoperative Management   Once the resection portion of the procedure has been completed, CSF containment should be confirmed with a Valsalva maneuver, and then reconstruction or closure can proceed. If possible, the longus colli is reapproximated in the midline, followed by absorbable suture approximation of the pharyngeal layer. Intubation is typically continued for 1 to 2 days due to the risk of swelling postoperatively. Antibiotic regimens vary in the literature, but we typically use cefazolin and metronidazole for 5 to 7 days starting immediately preoperatively. The metronidazole can be administered through a nasogastric feeding tube placed intraoperatively after wound closure. Clear liquids are begun approximately one week after surgery, but a regular diet should be withheld until 3 weeks postoperatively (6).

Complications   Rates of complication with the transoral approach have been quoted between 18% and 26%, including a mortality rate of 6%, according to one source (7). Although early use of the approach led to very high infection rates (above 50%), more recent studies demonstrate infection rates below 3% (8–10). CSF leakage during the procedure should be addressed with attempted closure, grafting, fibrin glue, and a meticulous closure, as the persistence of leakage can result in fistula formation (11). A lumbar drain should be strongly considered in this situation, as the persistence of CSF leakage can be exceptionally troublesome. Other potential complications include bleeding from injury to the vertebral or internal carotid arteries, craniocervical instability, lingual swelling, and postoperative infection.

Anterior Retropharyngeal Approach

Indications   The high retropharyngeal approaches allow access to the anterior upper cervical spine, and may be indicated for debridement of tumors or infection, and stabilization of the atlantoaxial segment. It is possible to expose the C1-2 facet articulations at the upper end of the approach, while the most caudal access afforded by the primary incision is the upper end of C3. An extensile vertical incision can be employed to allow access to the mid and lower cervical regions.

Although this approach can be carried out medial (anterior approach) or lateral (anterolateral approach) to the carotid sheath, we favor the use of the method described by McAfee and colleagues, termed the anterior retropharyngeal approach (12). It is an extension of the Southwick and Robinson approach initially described for use in the lower cervical spine (13). By accessing the retropharyngeal space medial to the carotid sheath, one avoids the risk of injuring the carotid vessels or cranial nerves at the skull base, but there is a higher risk of injury to the superior laryngeal or glossopharyngeal nerves than when approached lateral to the carotid sheath. Additionally, the anterior approach allows access to both vertebral arteries, while exposing lateral to the carotid sheath compromises access to the contralateral vertebral artery. Finally, anterior decompression and reconstructive measures may be more easily performed when visualizing the spine from the anterior approach than the anterolateral approach.

Preoperative Planning/Preparation   Particular attention should be focused on any compromise of swallowing or respiratory function. In the revision setting, it may be necessary to have the patient undergo vocal cord evaluation. A preoperative tracheostomy may be warranted to avoid airway problems, and an otolaryngologist can assist with this determination. When attempting tumor resections, angiography or a CT angiogram should be obtained to define the locations of the vertebral arteries.

Position   The patient is placed in a supine position, and cranial traction should be strongly considered. If postoperative halo-vest immobilization is planned, the use of a halo ring can be substituted for Gardner-Wells tongs. Before traction is applied, baseline evoked potentials from neuromonitoring should be obtained (if used). The patient should be awake for fiberoptic nasotracheal intubation, so neurologic assessment can be performed following the intubation and positioning. Oral placement of tubes or devices should be avoided, as they may inferiorly displace the mandible and compromise maximum exposure of the upper-most aspects of the cervical spine. Finally, place the patient in a slight reverse-Trendelenberg position to aid in visualization and improve venous drainage.

Landmarks   Unlike lower areas of the cervical spine, the side of approach need not be dictated by underlying anatomical variations. A right-sided approach may be easier for those surgeons with right-handed dominance, but if there is a foreseeable need to extend below C5 then one should consider a left-sided approach to avoid injury to the recurrent laryngeal nerve. Tumor location predominantly on one side may also influence the need for approach on a particular side. Mild head rotation can facilitate the exposure. If performing the anterolateral high retropharyngeal approach, the ipsilateral earlobe should be prepped and then sutured to the cheek anteriorly. Otherwise, it will be an obstruction during the exposure.

Technique

1. Incision: the submandibular incision for the anterior approach begins at the tip of the mastoid process and traverses medially to the level of the hyoid bone (modified Schobinger incision) (14). When more caudal exposure is desirable a vertical incision can be made along the sternocleidomastoid to intercept the submandibular incision (**Figs. 12-6 and 12-7**). Once the superficial fascia and platysma are divided, skin flaps can be raised deep to the platysma. Before proceeding more deeply, a nerve stimulator can be used to find the mandibular branch of the facial nerve (**Fig. 12-8**). It generally courses superiorly above the retromandibular vein and should be preserved due to its innervation of the orbicularis oris muscle. The retromandibular vein can be sacrificed by ligation adjacent to its junction with the internal jugular vein.

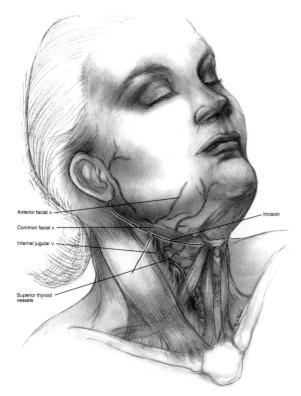

Anterior facial v.
Common facial v.
Internal jugular v.
Incision
Superior thyroid vessels

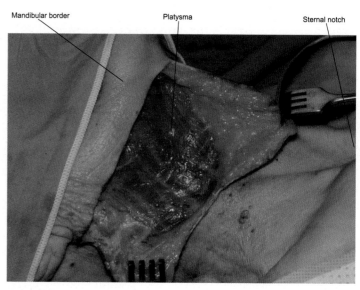

Mandibular border   Platysma   Sternal notch

FIGURE 12-6   **FIGURE 12-7**

12   Cervical Spine   273

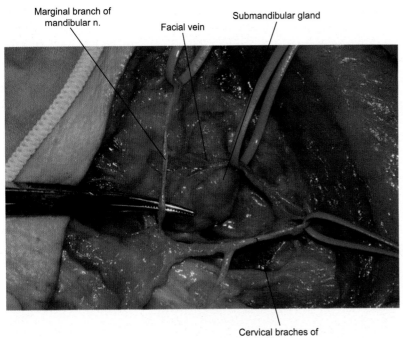

Marginal branch of mandibular n.

Facial vein

Submandibular gland

Cervical braches of facial n.

A

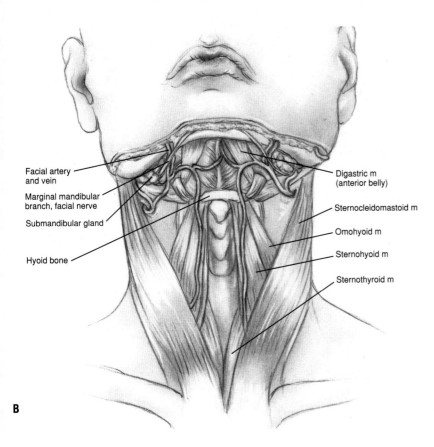

Facial artery and vein

Marginal mandibular branch, facial nerve

Submandibular gland

Hyoid bone

Digastric m (anterior belly)

Sternocleidomastoid m

Omohyoid m

Sternohyoid m

Sternothyroid m

B

FIGURE 12-8

2. The facial vein can be found and ligated just inferior to the submandibular gland (**Fig. 12-9**). It typically courses superficial to the gland and is oriented cephalocaudally. By leaving the ligature on the superior stump of the vein, it can be used to retract the superficial fascia of the submandibular gland and protect the marginal branch of the mandibular nerve as it courses within the fascia. The submandibular gland is then mobilized superiorly, exposing the intersection of digastric and stylohyoid muscles. These muscles are divided at their confluence near the hyoid bone and reflected proximally (**Fig. 12-10**). Occasionally, the submandibular gland must be resected to allow adequate exposure; however, its corresponding salivary duct must then be ligated to prevent fistula formation.

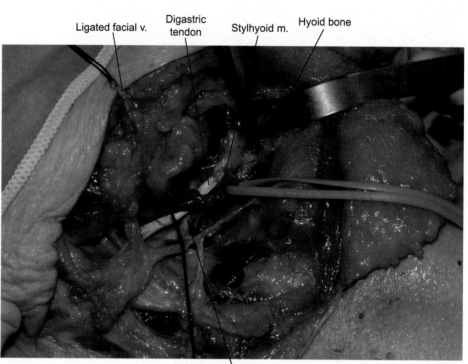

FIGURE 12-9

Transected stylohyoid
and digastric m.   Hypoglossal n.   Facial a.   Superior laryngeal n.

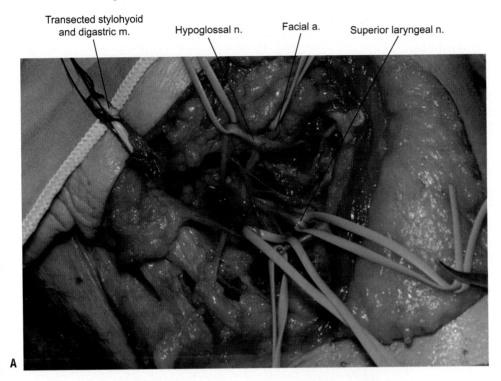

A

Submandibular gland
excised

Hypoglossal n.

Superior
laryngeal n.

Jugular and
carotid vessels

Tendon of digastric

Superior laryngeal
vessels ligated

Sympathetic trunk

Sternocleidomastoid m.   Vagus n.

B

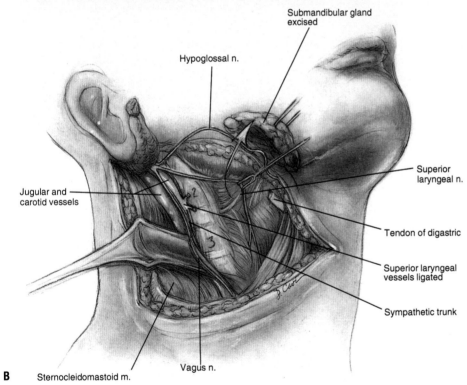

FIGURE 12-10

3. Next, the superior thyroid, lingual, and facial arteries and associated veins are ligated and divided **(Fig. 12-11)**. It is helpful to proceed from inferior to superior during this process, using the hyoid bone as a marker for localizing each artery. The superior thyroid artery is just below the hyoid bone, while the lingual and facial arteries are at and just above it, respectively. The superior laryngeal nerve often travels close to the superior thyroid artery, and injury to it must be avoided.

4. The deep fascia can now be divided along the border of the sternocleidomastoid muscle, and the carotid sheath is localized by palpating the internal carotid pulse. Once the digastric and stylohyoid muscles have been transected, the hyoid bone and accompanying pharyngeal structures can be more easily mobilized medially. Care should be taken not to retract these muscles too vigorously near the mastoid, as the facial nerve courses through this area and may sustain a neuropraxic injury.

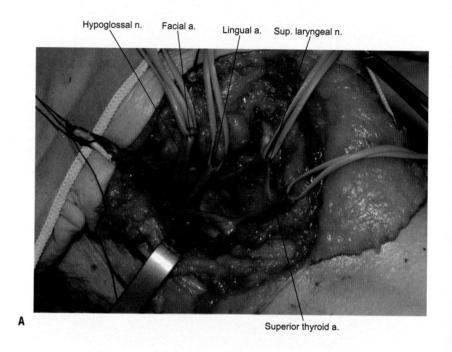

A

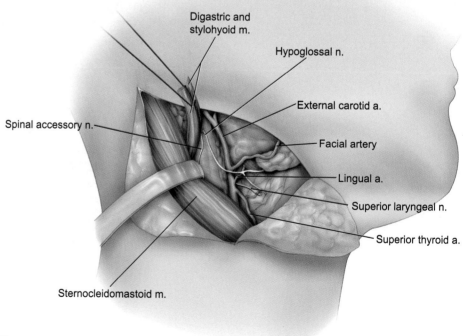

FIGURE 12-11   B

5. The hypoglossal nerve is found more superior than the superior laryngeal nerve; both should be protected by careful dissection and mobilization. Once the hypoglossal nerve is dissected out from its exiting site at the skull base to its insertion near the tongue, it can be retracted superiorly (**Fig. 12-12,** see Fig. 12-10B). The carotid sheath can then be retracted posterolaterally. Although medial retraction of the pharynx is helpful, excessive force can cause iatrogenic injury to the laryngeal and pharyngeal branches of the vagus nerve. Use blunt finger dissection to separate the carotid sheath from the medial pharynx and larynx, and the retropharyngeal space can then be safely entered.

6. A peanut or Kittner dissector can now be used to clear alar and prevertebral fascia away from the longus colli muscle, which is then divided longitudinally in the midline (**Fig. 12-13**). The longus colli muscles insert on the anterior arch of the atlas bilaterally, so they can help define the midline of C1 if adequately exposed. When starting the midline incision, avoid extending beyond the cephalad margin of the atlas, which could violate the anterior occipitoatlantal membrane. The incision is carried down to bone and subperiosteal flaps are elevated laterally. The anterior longitudinal ligament underlying the longus colli should be reflected within these flaps. Limit lateral elevation of these flaps on the atlas to 1.5 cm from midline, as the vertebral arteries can be in significant danger beyond this distance.

7. If decompression is planned, it should generally be performed in a cephalad-to-caudal direction. This reduces difficulty with visualization, as bleeding tends to run in a caudal direction. The posterior longitudinal ligament and uncovertebral joints help identify the posterior and lateral safety margins of the decompression. If reconstruction is to be performed, the head should be carefully repositioned to neutral alignment prior to graft placement and fixation.

8. The transected digastric and stylohyoid muscles should be reapproximated with sutures. Similarly, the origin of the sternocleidomastoid muscle must be repaired at the mastoid process. Before occlusion of the retropharyngeal space, a drain should be placed in this deeper area of the wound. The platysma can be reapproximated with a running absorbable suture, followed by the skin in a routine fashion according to the surgeon's preference.

Postoperative Management   Extubation may be performed immediately after surgery, but longer cases or those with greater likelihood of significant edema should be considered for a day or two of continued intubation. Less commonly, tracheostomy might be required immediately or in a delayed fashion if there is more serious airway compromise or concern. Drains are typically left in for approximately 24 hours, but higher outputs may necessitate longer durations or exploration in cases of persistent heavy bleeding. It is generally advised to keep the head of the bed elevated to encourage more rapid resolution of edema. Dietary advancement should begin with sips of water or clear liquids, and then slow progression may ensue if tolerated on the first postoperative day.

Complications

● Neurapraxias or lacerations of various nerves may occur during the high retropharyngeal exposures. Injury to the mandibular branch of the facial nerve may cause drooping of the ipsilateral mouth corner, but this usually resolves spontaneously over the first few postoperative months in cases of neuropraxia. The hypoglossal nerve typically recovers from neuropraxic injury within several months after surgery (6,15). The superior laryngeal nerve has a role in voice physiology, and injury may result in high-pitch phonation and diminished supraglottic sensation (6). Its recovery from neuropraxia is less predictable. Finally, the spinal accessory nerve can suffer injury during mobilization of structures around the mastoid process, and may result in ipsilateral paralysis of the trapezius and sternocleidomastoid muscles.

- Inadvertent entry into the pharynx or esophagus warrants immediate placement of a nasogastric tube, if not already present. This should be done under direct visualization, and the disruption repaired in two absorbable layers. Postoperatively, the nasogastric (NG) tube should be left in for 7 to 10 days to prevent fistula formation, and an esophagram and/or esophagoscopy should then be performed prior to an oral diet (16). Parenteral or NG tube nutrition will be required during the period of oral dietary restriction. Intravenous antibiotics that cover both aerobic and anaerobic pathogens should be employed for approximately 5 days postoperatively. In the case of delayed discovery or presentation of the perforation, a pedicled sternocleidomastoid muscle flap may be required for reinforcement (16).

- Retraction against the medial pharyngeal structures may induce enough edema to result in airway obstruction. Sustained intubation or short-term tracheostomy may be employed while the edema resolves. Hematoma formation is another possible cause of airway obstruction, so postoperative bulb drainage is generally encouraged.

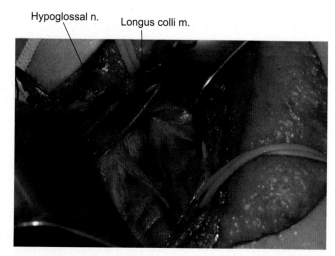

FIGURE 12-12

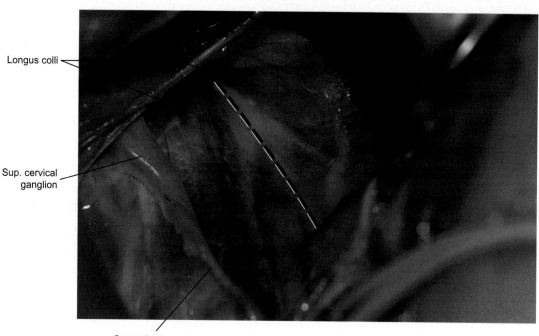

FIGURE 12-13

Mid-Lower Anterior Cervical Approaches

The mid and lower anterior cervical spine can be approached through two skin incisions, depending on the extent of exposure required. A transverse incision can be employed for exposure of three disc levels or two vertebral body resections. When more extensive visualization is required, a longitudinal incision should be used. These anterior approaches typically allow access from C3 to T1, but anatomic variabilities may reduce the extent of this range. By employing the interval between the sternocleidomastoid muscle laterally and pharyngeal structures medially, one is afforded a fairly direct anterior visualization of the cervical spine. This vantage point is ideal for most standard anterior spinal procedures.

Preoperative Planning/Preparation   ENT consultation should be obtained for concerns of swallowing abnormalities, phonation problems, or aberrant anatomy. In the revision setting, preoperative endoscopic assessment of vocal cord function should be strongly considered. If the vocal cord ipsilateral to the original surgical approach is dysfunctional, surgery should proceed through the same side, so inadvertent injury to the remaining functional vocal cord does not occur. If both vocal cords appear to be functioning well, some authors have advocated using an approach from the contralateral side (17). In most cases, a left-sided approach should be employed, as the left recurrent laryngeal nerve takes a less variable course within the tracheoesophageal groove than the nerve on the right side.

While evaluating the patient preoperatively, palpate for the carotid pulses and listen for bruits with a stethoscope. Abnormalities should be evaluated with a carotid ultrasound (Duplex) study, and an appropriate consultation as indicated. Thyromegaly can compromise wound closure, or cause increased external airway pressure following closure. A partial thyroidectomy may be required prior to wound closure in these circumstances.

Plain radiographs and other studies should be scrutinized, so that any unique anatomic features are anticipated and accounted for during the surgical exposure. In the case of odontoid fractures for which anterior screw placement is being considered, pectus carinatum (barrel-chest) may be a contraindication to using the technique. The acute angle required for drilling and placing the screw may be impossible to achieve. However, newer equipment designs such as systems incorporating flexible drill bits have minimized these early problems.

Assess the degree to which the patient can extend the neck without neurologic symptoms.

Position   Place the patient in the supine position on a regular table, and if iliac crest bone is to be taken, place a bump under the ipsilateral hip. Standard preoperative antibiotics are adequate for the majority of anterior cervical procedures. Intubation in patients with spinal cord compression or myelopathic findings should be performed awake and/or with fiberoptic assistance. If neuromonitoring is planned, the set-up should begin prior to patient positioning and intubation. If the spine is stable, position the neck in a safe degree of extension (as determined by preoperative examination). If there are any changes with the electrophysiologic monitoring, reposition the neck to the neutral position and do not proceed unless the changes revert to baseline. A rolled towel, intravenous saline bag (1 L), or other similar-sized bump between the shoulder blades will help maximize cervical extension. Slight cervical rotation away from the chosen side of approach can facilitate visualization during exposure, as the mandible can otherwise partially obstruct an anteroposterior view. The head should be well-padded at its contact point with the table, especially during longer cases.

When anterior decompression is planned, cervical traction with Gardner-Wells tongs can be used in place of operative site distraction (i.e., Caspar distractor). Using external traction rather than local distraction should be more strongly considered in multilevel decompressions, or in cases with poor bone quality. If Gardner-Wells tongs are used for traction, be mindful of the placement of the tongs relative to the axis of occipitocervical rotation in the sagittal plane, as well as the vector of pull. When extension of the cervical spine is desirable, tong position should be slightly anterior within the "safe window" above the ear, and the traction vector from anterior to posterior.

A sheet is folded and placed transversely under the patient's torso. Gel or foam pads are rolled around each arm, ensuring that the patient's skin is well-padded from any prominent intravenous tubing, connections, or neuromonitoring leads. Cotton padding is placed around each wrist underneath straps that can be used for intermittent caudal upper extremity traction during intraoperative radiographs. Avoid traction if the patient has upper extremity deformities or injuries. The pre-positioned sheet can now be folded over the patient's torso and taped in position to secure the arms. The width of the sheet must allow access to both the iliac crest and the upper chest.

Draping of the neck should be expansive and include the area from the clavicles to the mandibular prominences, as well as lateral to the sternocleidomastoid muscles. Ideally, both sides should be draped out and prepped, so that any emergent vascular or respiratory issues can be managed without the need for additional redraping or preparation.

Landmarks   The transverse incision provides more limited access than the longitudinal incision, and must therefore be placed in the neck according to the desired levels of visualization. Palpable landmarks within the neck usually provide adequate guidance for incision placement (**Table 12-2**), however it must be noted that cervical extension may shift the superficial landmarks (hyoid bone, thyroid cartilage, cricoid cartilage) slightly more cephalad relative to their corresponding vertebral levels at a neutral position (**Fig. 12-14**). The hyoid is at the level of C3, the thyroid is at the level of C5 to C6, the cricoid cartilage is at the level of C5 to C6 interspace, and the carotid tubercle is at the level of C6. This requires a mild shift of the incision caudally relative to the palpable landmarks when the neck is extended. Attempt to place the transverse incision within a skin crease, or parallel to Langer lines. It is helpful to mark the planned incision with a marking pen, and then place a sheet of Ioban over the neck region. Attempting to discern skin creases after placement of the Ioban can often be difficult. We also recommend pre-incision subdermal infiltration of epinephrine solution, with or without local anesthetic to diminish bleeding.

TABLE 12-2.	Palpable Landmarks in the Neck
Palpable Landmarks	**Level**
Hyoid bone	C3
Thyroid cartilage	C5-6
Cricoid cartilage	C5-6 interspace
Carotid (Chassaignac's) tubercle	C6 (most reliable; on transverse process of C6)

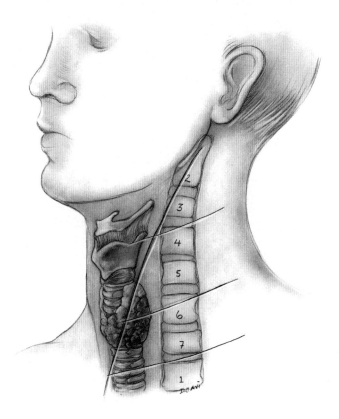

FIGURE 12-14

Technique

1. Incision: the incision should begin around the midline of the neck and extend laterally to the anterior border of the sternocleidomastoid. Although one can extend beyond the midline without significant problems, carrying the incision too far laterally can cause cosmetically displeasing adhesions to the underlying sternocleidomastoid. Typically, a 4 to 5 cm incision is adequate for two-level visualization, but may require extension across the midline of the neck when more exposure is desired (**Fig. 12-15**). A longitudinal incision can be used to provide more extensile access to the anterior cervical spine. This incision is carried out along a line drawn between the sternal notch and the mastoid process, just medial or anterior to the sternocleidomastoid muscle (**Fig. 12-16**). It should be placed over the target vertebrae using the palpable landmarks, and its length will vary according to the extent of exposure required.

2. Because the skin is thin and cosmesis is of greater concern in this area, dermal bleeding is best managed with bipolar electrocautery following the initial skin incision. Skin hooks or rakes are placed for retraction, and the skin edges are lifted away from the neck to facilitate separating the dermis and subcutaneous layer from the platysma with Metzenbaum scissors or electrocautery. If the external jugular vein is encountered, it can be swept aside or ligated as needed. The platysma is identified by noting its longitudinally oriented fibers as seen in **Figure 12-17**, and it (as well as the investing fascia) can be divided parallel to its fibers. Elevate the platysma with two sets of tissue forceps and snip between them through the full thickness of the muscle. While maintaining upward tension with the forceps, the plane deep to the platysma can be developed by spreading with the Metzenbaum scissors, allowing the muscle to be incised without damage to underlying structures. A self-retainer is placed deep to the platysma, exposing the superficial layer of the deep cervical fascia.

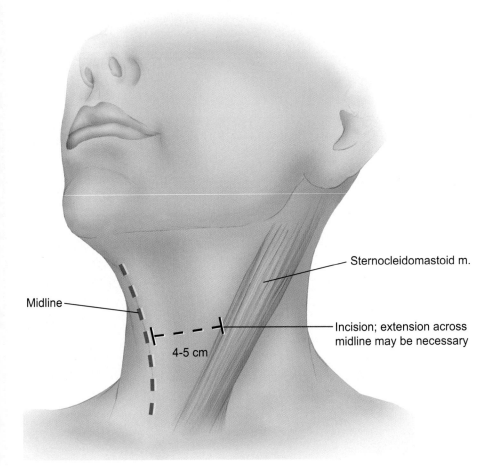

Midline

Sternocleidomastoid m.

Incision; extension across
midline may be necessary

4-5 cm

FIGURE 12-15

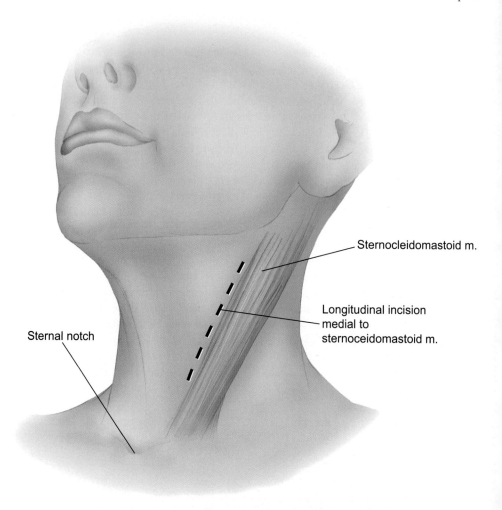

Sternocleidomastoid m.

Longitudinal incision
medial to
sternoceidomastoid m.

Sternal notch

FIGURE 12-16

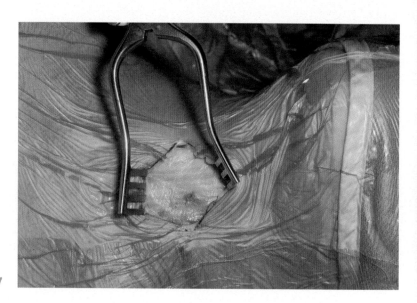

FIGURE 12-17

3. Dissecting scissors can now be used to divide the investing superficial layer of the deep fascia from one end of the incision to the other (**Fig. 12-18**). The superficial jugular branches may be encountered and ligated, if they represent obstruction to further dissection. Enter the next layer of deep fascia along the anterior border of the sternocleidomastoid muscle. This can be accomplished with careful spreading with scissors, as well as blunt finger dissection, until a plane is developed below the muscle. Take care to incise the deep cervical fascia just medial to the medial border of the sternocleidomastoid muscle. Entering the fascia over the substance of the muscle requires dissection through both layers of the investing fascia, as well as the muscle itself (**Fig. 12-19**).

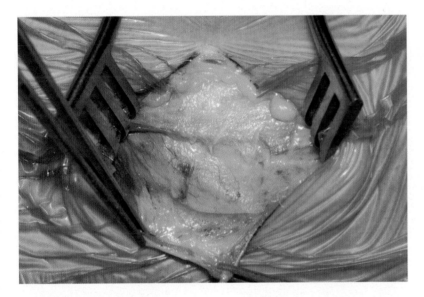

FIGURE 12-18

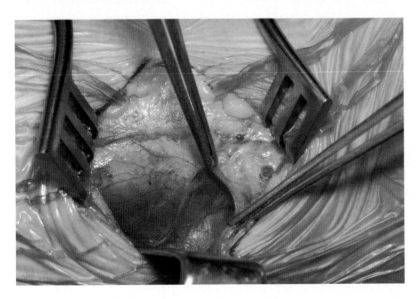

FIGURE 12-19

4. At this point gently palpate for the carotid artery pulse just medial and deep to the sternocleidomastoid. Once the carotid sheath has been identified in this manner, continue with gentle finger dissection medial to the sheath (**Fig. 12-20**). A smooth Meyerding or Richardson retractor
can then be placed medial to the dissecting finger, so that it can be used to retract the trachea
and esophagus (**Fig. 12-21**). In the upper cervical levels, the superior thyroid artery may be identified during this maneuver. The superior laryngeal nerve accompanies the artery and protection
of the artery will help protect the more friable and less visible nerve. Gentle rostral retraction of
both structures will generally afford adequate exposure. In the mid-levels, the middle thyroid
artery and accompanying veins may be identified, and may be transected to allow continued approach to the spine, if necessary. In the lower levels, the recurrent laryngeal nerve can occasionally be seen traversing from caudal to cephalad as it moves medially into the tracheoe-
sophageal groove. The ansa cervicalis may also be appreciated running along the anteromedial
aspect of the carotid sheath.

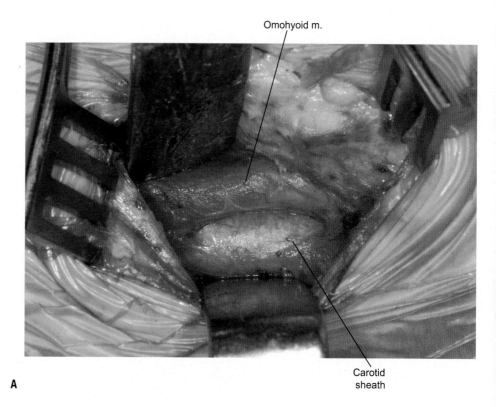

Omohyoid m.

Carotid
sheath

A

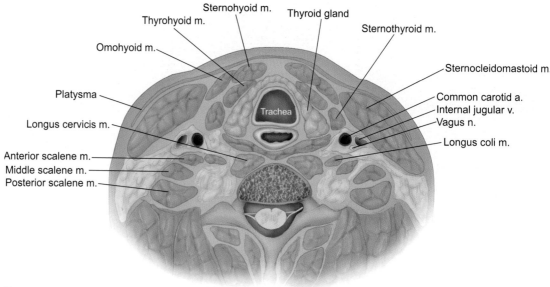

Sternohyoid m.

Thyrohyoid m.

Omohyoid m.

Thyroid gland

Sternothyroid m.

Platysma

Sternocleidomastoid m.

Trachea

Common carotid a.

Longus cervicis m.

Internal jugular v.

Vagus n.

Anterior scalene m.

Longus coli m.

Middle scalene m.

Posterior scalene m.

FIGURE 12-20   **B**

5. The middle layer of the deep cervical fascia should now be visible at the base of the exposure (see Fig. 12-21), and it may invest the omohyoid muscle within the C5 and C7 region. Occasionally, the omohyoid muscle must be transected, but generally it can be retracted rostrally or caudally to provide adequate exposure. Palpate the anterior spine and enter the middle fascial layer over the vertebral bodies with blunt finger dissection while protecting the medial structures with the retractor. The prevertebral fascia (also known as alar fascia) overlying the anterior longitudinal ligament and vertebral bodies should now be in view.

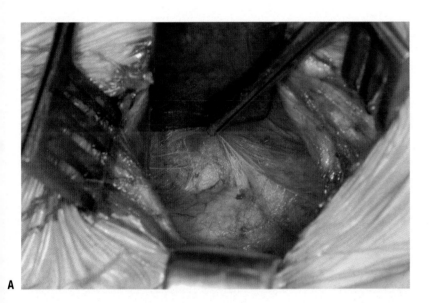

A

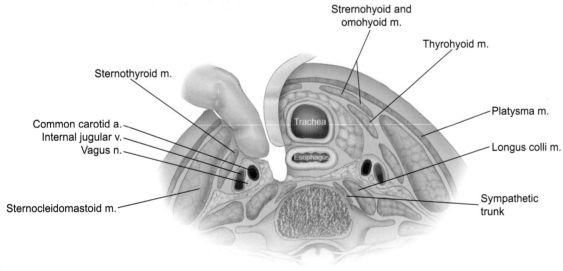

B

FIGURE 12-21

6. Palpate the vertebral bodies through the fascia to determine the approximate location of the midline, and then use a Kittner or peanut dissector to clear the fascia away from the midline of the spine (**Fig. 12-22**). Once a vertebral segment and disk have been exposed by this maneuver, place a radiopaque marker into the disc space. This can be accomplished with a specially designed marking needle or by bending a standard 20-guage needle with two oppositely-directed 90 degree bends, such that the tip of the needle is no more than 1 cm from the first bend (**Fig. 12-23**). A localizing radiograph should then be obtained. Concurrent caudal traction on the patient's arms may be necessary to visualize the lower cervical segments on lateral radiographs. Usually, lateral radiographs or fluoroscopy is adequate; however, lower cervical regions may be obscured by the shoulders and necessitate use of an anteroposterior image. If plain radiography is used and iliac crest bone autografting is planned, the graft harvesting can be performed while waiting for the film to be developed.

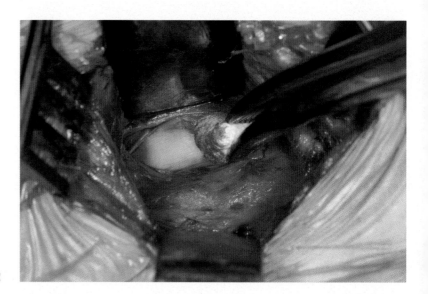

FIGURE 12-22

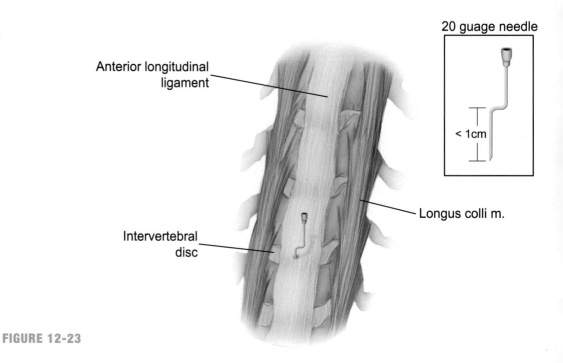

Anterior longitudinal ligament

20 guage needle

< 1cm

Longus colli m.

Intervertebral disc

FIGURE 12-23

7. Once the proper levels are confirmed with imaging, handheld retractors are replaced medially and laterally, and the localizing needle is removed. Additional fascial clearing may be necessary above and below the localized segment using the peanut to uncover the anterior longitudinal ligament. Mark the midline using the longus colli muscles for orientation. Using the bovie electrocautery, elevate the longus colli muscles laterally, superficial to the anterior longitudinal ligament and the annulus. Take care not to use the cautery aggressively over discs that are not planned for removal, and not to damage more superficial structures with the cautery. These flaps must be elevated laterally enough to allow uncovertebral joint visualization, but do not overexpose laterally or the vertebral arteries can be violated, especially at the level of the disc. A small Cobb elevator can be used to elevate the longus colli muscles. Bleeding can be controlled with bipolar cautery or gel foam. Elevation of the longus colli in this manner allows self-retaining retractors to be placed beneath them (**Fig. 12-24**). This maneuver protects the sympathetic chain overlaying the lateral aspect of the longus colli, and also shields the esophagus and trachea from direct retraction forces.

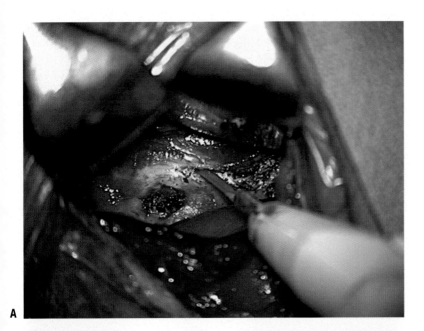

A

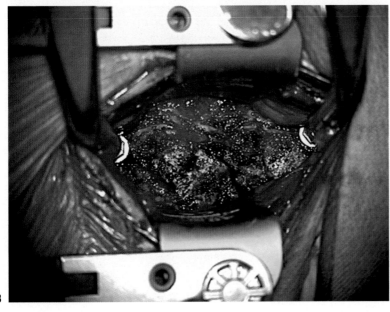

B   FIGURE 12-24

8. Individually place retractor blades medially and a blunt-tooth blade laterally, with blade tips below the longus colli, and then attach the self-retractor apparatus. The anesthesiologist should be asked to deflate the cuff of the endotracheal tube at this point, and then reinflate it to the lowest pressure necessary for maintaining a seal. This may help prevent excessive pressure on the recurrent laryngeal nerve between the retractor and tracheal cuff. Handheld or self-retractors with smooth blades can be used in cephalad and cranial positions to improve exposure. Alternatively, distraction screws may be inserted into the vertebral bodies in the midline. They may be used to apply segmental distraction as needed, and they also facilitate the rostral and caudal exposure.

9. Following the decompressive or reconstructive portion of the procedure, copiously irrigate the wound, and carefully inspect the medial structures for maintenance of integrity. If there is any suspicion of esophageal perforation, methylene blue or indigo Carmen solutions can be injected into the esophagus by the anesthesiologist. Any leakage should be addressed by repair with absorbable suture, copious irrigation, and administration of intravenous antibiotics covering aerobic and anaerobic organisms for 5 to 7 days. If available, consider asking an ENT colleague to inspect the defect intraoperatively and help manage the patient postoperatively.

10. A drain should be placed in the deeper areas of the wound, and may be brought out through the incision or a separate site. The platysma is reapproximated with a running 2.0 absorbable suture through its investing fascia, and the subcutaneous and skin tissue can be approximated according to the surgeon's preference. We typically use 2-0 or 3-0 absorbable suture in the subcutaneous/dermal layer, followed by a subcuticular 4-0 absorbable suture in the skin and steri-strips. A dry, sterile dressing is applied and any external immobilization can then be placed.

Postoperative Management   Extubation may be performed immediately after surgery, but longer cases or those with greater likelihood of significant edema should be considered for a day or two of continued intubation. Less commonly, tracheostomy might be required immediately or in a delayed fashion if there is more serious airway compromise or concern. Although there is no direct evidence to suggest antibiotics are effective at reducing infections beyond the initial preoperative dose, they are typically given for 24 hours postoperatively. Drains are typically left in place for approximately 24 hours, but higher outputs may necessitate longer durations or exploration in cases of persistent bleeding. The head of the bed can be elevated to 30 to 45 degrees, which can encourage resolution of edema and hematoma drainage. Dietary advancement should begin with sips of water or clear liquids, followed by slow progression of the diet on the first postoperative day.

Odontoid Screw Approach   As briefly discussed in the preparation section, anterior odontoid screw placement requires a unique trajectory of insertion. The position of the patient's head may need to be altered during positioning to allow for the appropriate screw trajectory. If the patient has a barrel-chest or large breasts, it may be impossible to achieve the correct trajectory without compromising the alignment of the odontoid fragments. The surgical approach must address this unusually sharp angle of insertion by beginning an anterior approach at the C5 level. The dissection through the anterior neck structures will therefore be no different than as described above, however, once the prevertebral fascia is identified, it will be cleared away from the C2-3 disc level. The caudal portion of the C2 body must be visualized and confirmed with lateral imaging using the marker technique described above.

Complications   Although major complications with the anterior approach are uncommon, many patients complain of temporary hoarseness and swallowing dysfunction. Injury to the recurrent laryngeal nerves (RLN) can cause major problems with phonation or swallowing, and spontaneous recovery from neuropraxia is not a certainty. It had been thought that a left-sided approach may be less likely to result in injury to the RLN; however, a recent series demonstrated similar rates of RLN dysfunction in both right and left-sided approaches (18). A prospective study of RLN function following anterior cervical surgery suggests that clinically symptomatic injury (hoarseness) occurred with an incidence of 8.3%. Laryngoscopy demonstrated that the overall incidence of RLN injury was 24.2%, including those patients with laryngoscopy-evident asymptomatic dysfunction. Fortunately, at 3 months postoperatively only 2.5% of subjects continued to have symptomatic dysfunction (19).

Dysphagia is not uncommon following cervical surgery. In a recent prospective analysis of swallowing after anterior and posterior cervical surgery, nearly one-half of patients undergoing anterior surgery suffered clinically significant dysphagia postoperatively. Most of these patients recovered by 2 to 3 months postoperatively, but 4 of the 38 patients in the anterior approach group required up to 10 months of dysphagia treatment (20).

The sympathetic chain travels longitudinally over the longus colli, and is at risk of injury with aggressive dissection or retraction above the muscle. It is most vulnerable around C6 as it courses around the carotid tubercle, and injury can lead to ipsilateral postoperative Horner's syndrome (ptosis, meiosis, and anhydrosis).

The internal carotid artery (ICA) and jugular vein are in close proximity to the exposure and must be carefully protected at all times. Lacerations should be promptly repaired. Arterial occlusion can be devastating if the contralateral ICA or vertebral arteries have high-grade obstruction or the Circle of Willis is incomplete. Manipulation of these vessels can also cause loosening of arteriosclerotic plaques, and lead to thromboembolic strokes.

Esophageal injuries can lead to retropharyngeal abscesses or mediastinitis if they are not addressed at the time of the index operation. Subsequent surgical debridements and repairs are wrought with difficulty and further complications, so scrutiny for tears during the initial operation is critical.

Injury to the vertebral arteries is very unusual, but excessive dissection lateral to the vertebral bodies may cause this unfortunate event. Pressure at the site of injury can typically control the bleeding, and collateral flow will often be adequate to prevent stroke. If it is known that the opposite vertebral artery is occluded, however, vascular repair or shunting should be considered.

Edema and hematoma formation following surgery may cause significant airway obstruction, and require the replacement of an endotracheal tube. Reintubation is difficult in this setting, especially when the neck cannot be extended. In-line traction, or occasionally, fiberoptic visualization may be necessary. If these are unsuccessful, an emergency tracheostomy may be required. Recognizing and treating the problem early in its course is essential.

Despite this litany of potentially devastating complications, they occur in approximately ≤1% of patients (21).

POSTERIOR APPROACHES

Occipitocervical Approach

Indications   This approach can be utilized for decompression and/or fusion procedures, and may serve as the extensile rostral end of a longer posterior spinal exposure.

Although the midline posterior approach to the occipitocervical region begins with similar principles as utilized in the more caudal areas of the spine, the unique anatomy requires distinct technical considerations. Careful attention must be paid to preoperative positioning so that deeper structures are accessible, and alignment is optimal in cases planned for arthrodesis.

Preoperative Planning   Much of the preoperative evaluation is dictated by the underlying abnormality, as well as the particular plan for correction. Standard plain radiographs of the cervical spine should be obtained, and flexion-extension views can play a critical role in determining which levels below the occipitocervical junction require additional exposure. If the possibility of instrumentation exists, preoperative computed tomography is advised. Using contrast to elucidate the vascular anatomy provides invaluable guidance for safely placing hardware into the bony elements.

Finally, the surgeon must scrutinize the superficial characteristics of the patient's upper neck. Skin conditions that may predispose the patient toward increased infection risk need to be recognized and treated before proceeding with surgery. Rarely, abnormal body habitus can complicate the feasibility of performing an adequate posterior exposure of the occipitocervical junction. This may require consideration of alternative treatment options or anterior surgical approaches.

Position   Neuromonitoring is encouraged for most procedures in this region of the spine. Once baseline monitoring has been established, intubation can proceed. Fiberoptic intubation may be required when strict cervical immobilization must be maintained. Awake intubation can also be employed for situations in which baseline neuromonitoring is not available. The pinion is placed so that it resides a minimum of 1 to 2 cm above the surfaces of the face or nose. Facial edema that occurs during long surgery in the prone position can otherwise cause encroachment onto the pinion, and subsequent skin breakdown may occur. If postoperative halo vest immobilization is anticipated, use a halo ring in place of the pinion. For procedures in the posterior cervical spine, it is helpful to have the arms located at the sides during surgery. A folded sheet can be used to secure the arms to the body once they are wrapped in gel sheets. The patient is then placed in the prone position on an operating table, with dependent areas of the body well-padded. The alignment of the spine must be adjusted and checked with lateral x-rays or the image intensifier before prepping the wound. The relationship of the occiput to the upper cervical spine should be optimized to prevent postoperative swallowing dysfunction, which may result from fusing the occiput cervical area in a nonphysiologic position. Subluxed vertebrae can often be realigned and the orientation of the spine can be manipulated to facilitate exposure and instrumentation. If cables or wires are to be passed under the arch of C1, opening the gap between the occiput and atlas will make the operation easier. If C1-2 transarticular screws are planned, the trajectory of the screws must be checked during positioning to be sure the procedure is feasible. Positioning should be performed with the patient under light sedation to allow a wake-up test following positioning, to assure maintenance of neurologic integrity. Reverse-Trendelenberg position of the operating table facilitates visualization of the occipitocervical junction, and may also reduce venous congestion and bleeding during surgery.

Landmarks   The patient's hair is shaved from the neck to just above the external occipital protuberance (EOP), and then laterally out to the ears. Widely prepare and drape the patient from the mid-thoracic level to just above the EOP by 2 cm, and to the mid-lateral aspects of the neck on either side. Tape placed transversely across the back of the head at the new hairline helps keep longer hair from violating the sterile area during preparation. The incision is marked in the midline from just below the EOP to just below the often palpable and prominent spinous process of C2. We prefer the use of an Ioban sheet for the operative area at this point.

Technique

1. Incision: infiltrate the line of incision dermally using epinephrine solution with or without local anesthetic, and make an incision down to subcutaneous fat. Obtain hemostasis with Bovey electrocautery or self-retractor pressure, and use the cautery to dissect through the subcutaneous fat in the midline. The nuchal fascia should come into view during this maneuver, and finger palpation may be utilized to assure that the incision is in the midline. The C2 spinous process should be readily apparent as the most prominent upper cervical vertebra at this point. It is sometimes helpful to gently clear subcutaneous fat off of the midline nuchal fascia, to aid in identifying the proper planes during closure.

2. Incise the fascia at the midline with electrocautery, taking care to prevent violation of the C2-3 interspinous ligament, unless this segment is planned for inclusion in decompression or fusion. Once division of the fascia has been carried out to the EOP, discern the avascular plane found in the midline. Finger palpation may help if the plane is otherwise unidentifiable. Although access to the deeper structures through this avascular plane is not critical, the reduction in bleeding afforded by this technique facilitates hemostasis and visualization during surgery.

3. Gently palpate the bony anatomy once again and note the depth of the posterior arch of C1 for orientation. Electrocautery can be used to incise down to bone on the occiput, as well as to perform a subperiosteal elevation from the laminae of C2. Muscles released from C2 include the rectus capitis major and the obliquus capitis inferior, but muscles directed caudally from the C2 spinous process (semispinalis cervicis) should be preserved unless access to the caudal aspect of the C2 spinous process is critical (**Fig. 12-25**). Unless the C2-3 segment must be fused, the C2-3 articular capsules should be preserved. This capsular layer is often wispy and difficult to recognize, but it plays an important role in posterior stability. If the semispinalis cervicis must be released, elevate the insertion of the muscle with a thin piece of bone using an osteotome. The muscle attachment can then be repaired anatomically and securely at the end of the case.

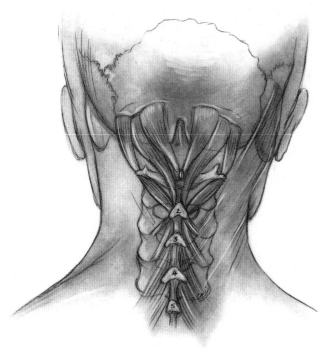

FIGURE 12-25

4. Sharp dissection with a scalpel can now be carried down to the posterior arch of C1 in the midline. This maneuver should only be performed if adequate preoperative computed tomography or intraoperative palpation confirms an intact posterior ring. Rarely, the posterior ring of C1 can be nonconfluent or absent. Use a Cobb elevator to raise subperiosteal flaps off of the occipital bone, and gently from the C1 posterior arch. Extreme caution should be employed when elevating laterally off of the C1 arch, limiting the dissection on the cephalad aspect of C1 to 0.8 cm from the midline, as the vertebral arteries can be easily injured beyond this point.

5. Continue gentle blunt dissection to lift paraspinal musculature away from base of the occiput and off of the atlantoaxial junction superficial to the level of the lamina **(Fig. 12-26)**. If necessary, the atlantoaxial membrane may be carefully elevated from the arch of C1 and lamina of C2 with a curette to expose the dura. The venous plexus surrounding the C2 nerve roots and ganglions become visible as the C1-2 articulation is approached.

6. Under most circumstances we prefer the use of a drain placed in the subfascial lateral recesses of the wound. Closure is performed by approximating the nuchal fascia with absorbable sutures to create a watertight seal. The greater occipital nerve courses through the fascia and can be injured if the exposure strayed from the midline or if fascial sutures are placed too far laterally. Absorbable 2-0 sutures are then applied as a buried dermal layer, followed by a subcuticular stitching with absorbable 3-0 suture. In revision cases, we prefer the use of 3-0 nylon sutures for the skin.

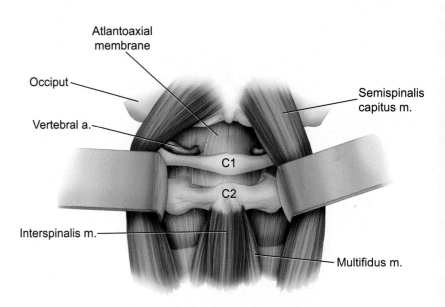

FIGURE 12-26

Postoperative Management   Prone positioning for longer periods of time can lead to significant facial and cervical edema, which may require continued intubation following surgery. Depending on the need for additional postoperative immobilization, the halo ring may be secured to a vest. If a pinion was used, it should be removed after the patient is transferred to the supine position. A collar may be applied before the patient awakens from anesthesia. If necessary, maintaining elevation of the head above the feet during the first 24 to 48 hours after surgery can facilitate edema reduction.

Complications   Infection is the most common complication of the posterior cervical or occipitocervical approach, with rates ranging from 2% to 5% in most series (22–25). However, underlying neural and vascular structures are at slightly greater risk during occipitocervical exposure. The vertebral arteries are in close proximity to the posterior arch of C1, and can be injured during subperiosteal elevation of soft tissues from the posterior surface of the arch. The spinal cord has more limited bony protection between the occiput and C2, and can be more easily injured during exposure. Finally, the exiting C2 nerve root does not have overlying posterior bony protection, and may be at more substantial risk during mobilization of superficial tissue. In general, complications for the occipitocervical approach tend to be related to instrumentation placement, rather than the exposure.

Posterior Approach to the Subaxial Cervical Spine

Indications   This approach through the midline of the posterior neck is simply an extension of a similar approach used both rostrally and caudally in the spine. Indications typically include conditions that require posterior decompression and/or arthrodesis, such as spondylotic myelopathy or radiculopathy, and rarely infectious or neoplastic processes.

Preoperative Planning   Adequate imaging should be obtained before surgery, and may include flexion and extension views to assess for segmental instability prior to decompression or fusion procedures. In general, when instrumentation of the cervical spine is planned, we favor obtaining a CT scan to provide more accurate detail of the bony anatomy.

   The patient's body habitus and posterior neck skin condition must be carefully assessed preoperatively, so adjustments to the planned approach can be made accordingly.

Position   When spinal realignment is planned, or myelopathic changes are present, we prefer to use neuromonitoring during the case. Neuromonitoring ideally begins with baseline potentials prior to intubation or postioning of the patient. The patient can then be intubated, with proper precautions taken in cases of possible spinal cord compression. Pathologic spinal cord compression may occur under various circumstances, such as with destabilizing traumatic injury or spondylotic narrowing of the canal. In these more worrisome situations, fiberoptic and/or awake intubation should be considered. Patients with advanced degenerative change and limited preoperative cervical motion should not be manipulated beyond what they've demonstrated possible in the preoperative clinical setting, unless neuromonitoring is employed during the positioning. Such caution should be heeded during prone positioning, as well. Another option for neurologic assessment during intubation, positioning, or surgery is the wake-up test. In most cases a pinion can be applied after intubation and prior to prone positioning on an operating table. If decompression is planned, the patient's neck should be placed in the position that provides the greatest space for the neural elements. The neck position can be carefully changed to physiologic lordosis after the decompression if a fusion is required. Slight cervical flexion during the initial portion of the procedure also tends to decrease the creasing of the skin at the posterior neck and gives more room for the exposure. All dependent areas of the patient's body in contact with the operating table should be well padded, and for longer cases a urinary catheter is placed. As covered in the occipitocervical section, the arms are usually kept to the sides of the patient with well-padded traction straps extending from the wrists to the foot of the bed. These facilitate intermittent traction on the arms, which provides radiographic access to the lower cervical spine on lateral imaging. Reverse-Trendelenberg position of the operating table reduces venous congestion of neck and epidural venous systems, which may decrease bleeding. Because of the anterior position of the lower cervical spine relative to the upper thoracic spine (as it begins the lordotic curve), the reverse-Trendelenberg position can also provide better visualization of C6-T1 from a posterior vantage point.

Landmarks   Depending on the extent of exposure required in a cephalad direction, the hair should be shaved accordingly. The surgical field should include the posterior iliac crest sites in the event autograft bone is planned, and we prefer the use of iodine-impregnated adhesive sheets over the exposed skin after draping. Palpation of the midline cervical structures can assist in localizing the incision; the spinous processes of C2, C7, and T1 tend to be the most prominent. When small incisions or very limited exposure is desired, fluoroscopy and a needle can be used to localize the area of interest.

Technique

1. Incision: epinephrine solution can be injected in the subdermal layer along the line of the planned midline incision to decrease bleeding from the skin edges. Once the nuchal fascia is identified, sweep the overlying subcutaneous tissue laterally to expose a centimeter-wide stripe of the fascia in the midline.
2. Use electrocautery to divide the nuchal fascia in the midline and elevate the flaps slightly in both lateral directions from the underlying paraspinal musculature. This will expose an avascular plane lateral to the interspinalis cervicis muscles on either side of the spinous process to aid in preserving the interspinous ligaments (**Fig. 12-27**). Once the nuchal fascia has been divided, palpate the spinous processes for orientation. The most prominent spinous process rostrally is C2 and the most distal bifid spinous process is usually C6. An intraoperative radiograph is essential to confirm the level because anatomic variations are common. Lateral imaging may be satisfactory for visualizing the upper cervical spine, but can be problematic below C5 in some individuals. It may be necessary to acquire anteroposterior imaging under these circumstances, using the first thoracic vertebra as a landmark for discerning the vertebral levels.
3. If surgical exposure need only be performed below C2, the muscular origins of the rectus capitis posterior major and obliquus capitis inferior should be left intact on the spinous process of C2. Likewise, the interspinous ligaments between C7 and T1 should also be left intact, as they are important biomechanical restraints to subsequent kyphotic deformity.

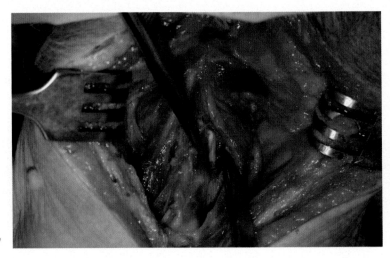

FIGURE 12-27

4. For decompressive procedures alone, including laminoplasty, the subperiosteal elevation should be carried laterally only to the facet capsules. The ligamentous capsular tissue in the cervical region is generally less robust than lower in the spine; however, maintaining capsular integrity may help prevent postoperative kyphotic progression. Otherwise, subperiosteal elevation can be carried out to the lateral margins of the facets/lateral masses. Gentle probing around the lateral mass edge can be used to assess the true lateral margin, rather than continuing subperiosteal electrocautery dissection "around the corner" (**Fig. 12-28**). If one persists with elevation beyond the superficial lateral margin, perforating vessels become more prevalent and bleeding can be problematic. Dissecting anterolateral to the lateral aspect of the facets is rarely necessary and may place the exiting nerve roots at risk of injury.

5. Closure of posterior cervical approaches can be performed with 0-0 or 1-0 absorbable sutures in the nuchal fascia, followed by 2-0 absorbable suture for dermal and subcutaneous approximation. The skin can be closed with subcutaneous absorbable sutures and steristrips, or with nylon sutures. For compromised tissue following infection or radiation, we prefer to use nonabsorbable sutures in all layers. A drain may also be placed prior to closure based on surgeon preference, but avoid placing the drain over any exposed dura or neural elements.

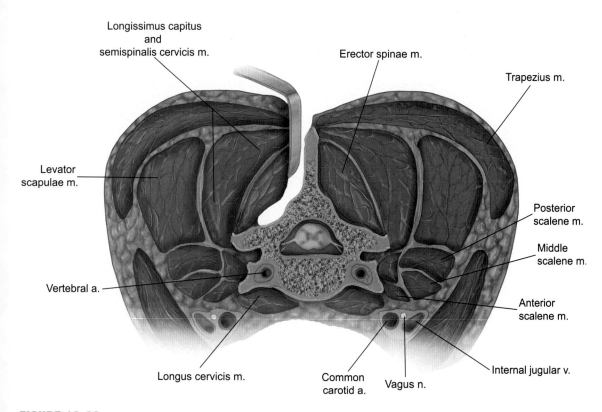

FIGURE 12-28

Postoperative Management   As with other spine surgeries, the duration of the procedure may necessitate continued intubation following surgery. Elevating the head of the patient's bed 30 to 45 degrees can reduce excess facial or cervical edema that occurs during prolonged prone positioning. Postoperative immobilization is individualized.

Pearls and Pitfalls   During exposure of the posterior cervical spine, unintentional damage to the posterior ligamentous complex can lead to debilitating postoperative deformity, which underlines the importance of preserving adjacent ligamentous and muscular restraints to such deformity.

Complications   Most posterior surgical approaches require extensive stripping of the paraspinal musculature from the underlying osseous elements. Such stripping of soft tissue causes more devitalization than one typically must perform during anterior surgery, which may explain the relatively higher wound infection rates seen with posterior approaches. The actual rate of infection with posterior approaches is difficult to ascertain given the variety of surgeries performed with them, and the frequently immunocompromised patients in whom they are often performed. Studies of immunocompetent patients have not demonstrated marked differences between anterior and posterior approaches, however (22,24–28). Several studies of posterior cervical arthrodesis demonstrate infection rates of <5%.

Resection of soft tissue restraints to flexion, such as the occipitocervical musculature and ligamentous structures and the semispinalis cervicis insertion on C2, can lead to development of postoperative flexion deformity (29). As mentioned previously, kyphosis may also occur at the cervicothoracic junction if the interspinous ligament between C7 and T1 is transected, and the segment is not included in the fusion construct (22,29–31).

REFERENCES

1. Bonney G, Williams JP. Trans-oral approach to the upper cervical spine: A report of 16 cases. *J Bone Joint Surg Br* 1985;67(5):691–698.
2. Mendoza N, Crockard H. Anterior transoral procedures. In: An H, Riley LI, eds. *An Atlas of Surgery of the Spine*. London: Martin Dunitz, 1998: 55–69.
3. Clark C, Menezes A. Rheumatoid arthritis: Surgical considerations. In: HN H, SR G, RA B, et al, eds. *The Spine*, 4th ed. Philadelphia: WB Saunders, 1999:1281–1301.
4. Currier B, Yaszemski M. The use of C1 lateral mass fixation in the cervical spine. *Curr Opin Orthop* 2004;15(3):184–191.
5. Ebraheim NA, Misson JR, Xu R, et al. The optimal transarticular C1-2 screw length and the location of the hypoglossal nerve. *Surg Neurol* 2000;53(3):208–210.
6. Biyani A, An HS. Anterior upper cervical spine approaches. In: Herkowitz HN, ed. *The Cervical Spine Surgery Atlas*, 2nd ed. Philadelphia: Lippincott Williams & Wilkins, 2004:69–89.
7. Crockard HA, Sen CN. The transoral approach for the management of intradural lesions at the craniovertebral junction: review of 7 cases. *Neurosurgery* 1991;28(1):88–97.
8. Merwin GE, Post JC, Sypert GW. Transoral approach to the upper cervical spine. *Laryngoscope* 1991;101(7 Pt 1):780–784.
9. Louis R. Anterior surgery of the upper cervical spine. *Chir Organi Mov* 1992;77(1):75–80.
10. Hadley MN, Spetzler RF, Sonntag VK. The transoral approach to the superior cervical spine: A review of 53 cases of extradural cervicomedullary compression. *J Neurosurg* 1989;71(1):16–23.
11. Menezes AH. Transoral approaches to the clivus and upper cervical spine. In: Menezes AH, Sonntag VKH, Benzel EC, et al, eds. *Principles of Spinal Surgery*. New York: McGraw-Hill, 1996:1241–1251.
12. McAfee PC, Bohlman HH, Riley LH, et al. The anterior retropharyngeal approach to the upper part of the cervical spine. *J Bone Joint Surg Am* 1987;69(9):1371–1383.
13. Southwick WO, Robinson RA. Surgical approaches to the vertebral bodies in the cervical and lumbar regions. *J Bone Joint Surg Am* 1957;39-A(3):631–644.
14. Cappucino A, McAfee PC, Gastein CD. Anterior retropharyngeal approach to the upper cervical spine. In: Bridwell KH, DeWald RL, eds. *The Textbook of Spine Surgery*, 2nd ed. Philadelphia: Lippincott-Raven Publishers, 1997:227–236.
15. Sengupta DK, Grevitt MP, Mehdian SM. Hypoglossal nerve injury as a complication of anterior surgery to the upper cervical spine. *Eur Spine J* 1999;8(1):78–80.
16. Orlando ER, Caroli E, Ferrante L. Management of the cervical esophagus and hypofarinx perforations complicating anterior cervical spine surgery. *Spine* 2003;28(15):E290–295.
17. Silber J, Albert T. In: HN H, editor. *The Cervical Spine Surgery Atlas*, 2nd ed. Philadelphia: Lippincott Williams & Wilkins, 2004.

18. Beutler WJ, Sweeney CA, Connolly PJ. Recurrent laryngeal nerve injury with anterior cervical spine surgery risk with laterality of surgical approach. *Spine* 2001;26(12):1337–1342.
19. Jung A, Schramm J, Lehnerdt K, Herberhold C. Recurrent laryngeal nerve palsy during anterior cervical spine surgery: a prospective study. *J Neurosurg Spine* 2005;2(2):123–127.
20. Smith-Hammond CA, New KC, Pietrobon R, et al. Prospective analysis of incidence and risk factors of dysphagia in spine surgery patients: comparison of anterior cervical, posterior cervical, and lumbar procedures. *Spine* 2004;29(13):1441–1446.
21. Bono C, Garfin S. Anterior cervical approaches. In: Bradford D, Zdeblick T, eds. *The Spine*, 2nd ed. Philadelphia: Lippincott Williams & Wilkins, 2004.
22. Wellman BJ, Follett KA, Traynelis VC. Complications of posterior articular mass plate fixation of the subaxial cervical spine in 43 consecutive patients. *Spine* 1998;23(2):193–200.
23. Fehlings MG, Cooper PR, Errico TJ. Posterior plates in the management of cervical instability: Long-term results in 44 patients. *J Neurosurg* 1994;81(3):341–349.
24. Grieve JP, Kitchen ND, Moore AJ, et al. Results of posterior cervical foraminotomy for treatment of cervical spondylitic radiculopathy. *Br J Neurosurg* 2000;14(1):40–43.
25. Shapiro SA, Snyder W. Spinal instrumentation with a low complication rate. *Surg Neurol* 1997;48(6):566–574.
26. Sevki K, Mehmet T, Ufuk T, et al. Results of surgical treatment for degenerative cervical myelopathy: Anterior cervical corpectomy and stabilization. *Spine* 2004;29(22):2493–2500.
27. Bertalanffy H, Eggert HR. Complications of anterior cervical discectomy without fusion in 450 consecutive patients. *Acta Neurochir (Wien)* 1989;99(1–2):41–50.
28. Heller JG, Silcox DH, 3rd, Sutterlin CE, 3rd. Complications of posterior cervical plating. *Spine* 1995;20(22):2442–2448.
29. Yonenobu K, Wada E, Ono K. Laminoplasty. In: Clark CR, ed. *The Cervical Spine*, 4th ed. Philadelphia: Lippincott, Williams & Wilkins, 2005;1057–1071.
30. Albert TJ, Vacarro A. Postlaminectomy kyphosis. *Spine* 1998;23(24):2738–2745.
31. Ratliff JK, Cooper PR. Cervical laminoplasty: A critical review. *J Neurosurg* 2003;98(Suppl):230–238.

13 Thoracic Spine

Matthew Morrey, Mark B. Dekutoski, Steve Cassivi, and Ziya L. Gokaslan

ANTERIOR CERVICAL THORACIC APPROACHES

The four approaches used for the upper thoracic region include first the high thoracotomy at the fourth rib which provides excellent access to the lateral aspect of the anterolateral cervical thoracic junction especially the sympathetic chain. This is, however, a difficult approach for placement of anterior fixation. Second is the modified anterior approach which resects the medial clavicle. This exposure is fraught with significant shoulder morbidity albeit downplayed for patients who are anticipated not to survive their pathology. These exposures have fallen out of favor with the increasing familiarity with the manubrial split accompanied by a lateral traverse sternal split between the third and fourth rib. The full manubrial split cervicothoracic approach allows anterior extension as low as the diaphragmatic attachments. The modified anterior and manubrial split are limited by the aortic arch which traverses approximately T3 vertebra. Fortunately, the aortal caval window approach can be used to reach the anterior aspect of T3-T5, allowing for direct anterior decompression, and by passing the plate under the aortic arch direct anterior plate fixation is possible.

Indications

Anterior approaches of the cervical thoracic junction are often necessary to address tumor pathology, deformity and anterior column support. These approaches are often avoided due to limited familiarity of the surgeon with the approach, which is paramount to successful surgical intervention and avoidance of complications.

Contraindications

Contraindications or limitations to the cervicothoracic approaches are primarily related to the nature of the pathology of spinal structures such as tumor pathology and with vascular involvement post-radiation changes which can substantially increase the risk of intraoperative scarring compromising exposure and esophageal tissue integrity.

Anterior cervical thoracic approaches for tumor involvement may require ligation of vascular and potential for a dysfunctional limb.

Preoperative Planning

Collaboration between the access surgeon and the spinal surgeon is useful. Adequate visualization of the neurologic structures for direct decompression most commonly defines the caudal extent of the exposure. When anterior fixation is only required to T1 or T2 an extensile anterior lateral neck approach may be adequate. However, for decompression of the T1 vertebra, a manubrial split is required to gain adequate anterior access and fixation. The authors' preference is to conduct a right anterior neck approach to avoid the lymphatic duct and the dominant left carotid artery. However, in the final analysis, the specific pathology most commonly determines the approach selection.

High Thoracotomy

Position   Typically the patient is placed prone with an axillary roll and with the arm elevated and flexed anteriorly to allow for full prepping of the arm and axilla.

Technique

1. Incision: with the inferior border of the scapula defined, the incision courses over the mid-body of the scapula (**Fig. 13-1**).
2. The inferior muscular attachments of the scapula are mobilized after transection and/or mobilization of the trapezius dorsally. The latissimus dorsi muscle is retracted laterally through this window (**Fig. 13-2**).

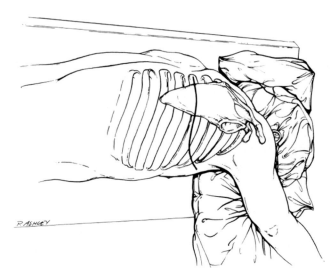

FIGURE 13-1

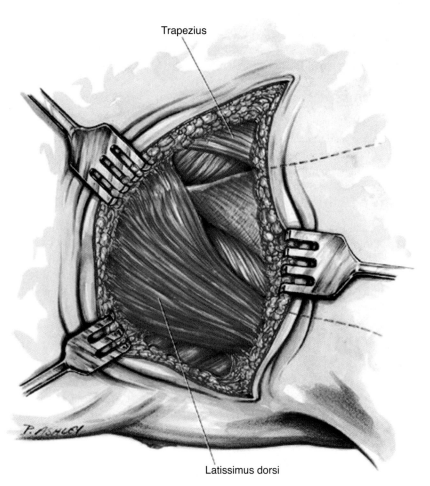

FIGURE 13-2   Latissimus dorsi

3. The rhomboids are released and the fourth rib is identified by palpation.

4. An incision over the fourth rib is conducted while protecting the intercostal neurovascular structures anteriorly and cephalad **(Fig. 13-3)**.

5. A dorsal osteotomy of the rib allows further mobilization and retraction of the scapula. The scapula retractor, along with chest wall retractors, allows for direct visualization from C7 to the diaphragm **(Fig. 13-4)**.

   ● *Note:* The right side of the chest allows for the greatest flexibility of the exposure.

Direct Anterior Cervical Thoracic Approach

This is a modification of the anterior exposure with resection of the medial clavicle. This approach employs the interval between the strap muscles medially the sternocleidomastoid laterally, the esophagus and trachea medially and the carotid sheath laterally. Selection of a right or left approach is based on familiarity of the surgeon and recognition that the recurrent laryngeal nerve is more consistent on the left side than on the right side of the neck. Further, hand dominance, familiarity, and the left sided lymphatic duct all contribute to the decisions of a left or right approach.

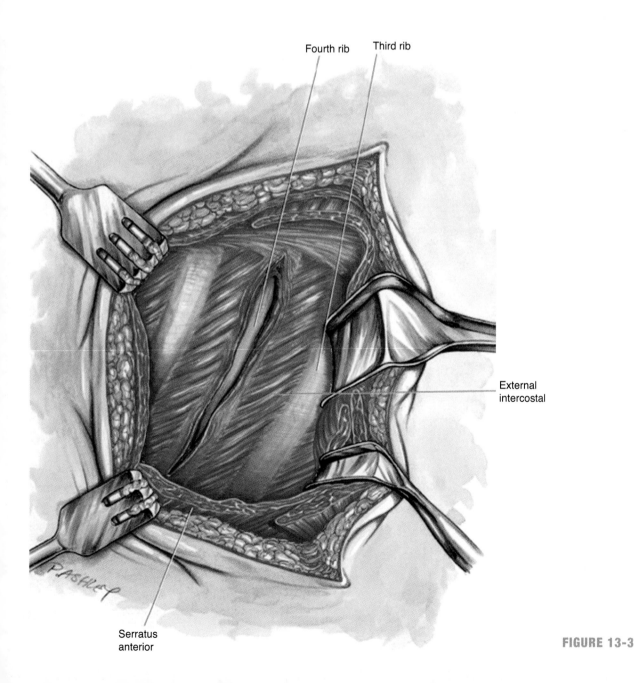

Fourth rib   Third rib

External intercostal

Serratus anterior

FIGURE 13-3

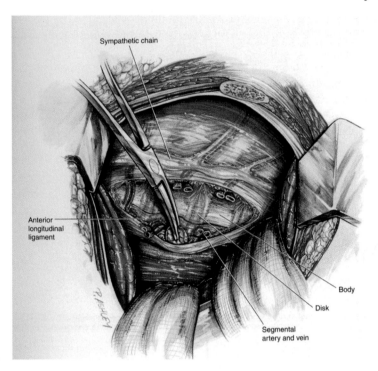

Sympathetic chain

Anterior
longitudinal
ligament

Body

Disk

Segmental
artery and vein

FIGURE 13-4

Technique

1. Incision: the incision may be extensive or more limited as shown in **Figure 13-5**.
2. Once the anterior neck approach is developed and the pharynx is identified and recurrent laryngeal nerve typically deep to it. The inferior extent of this anterior dissection will be the C-7 T-1 disc where upon a more extensile approach is typically needed (**Fig. 13-6**).

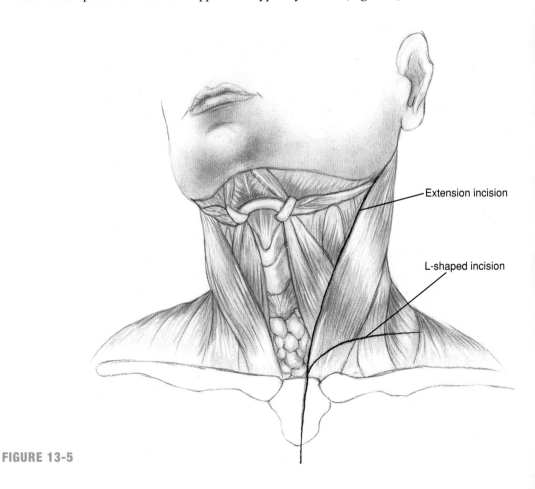

Extension incision

L-shaped incision

FIGURE 13-5

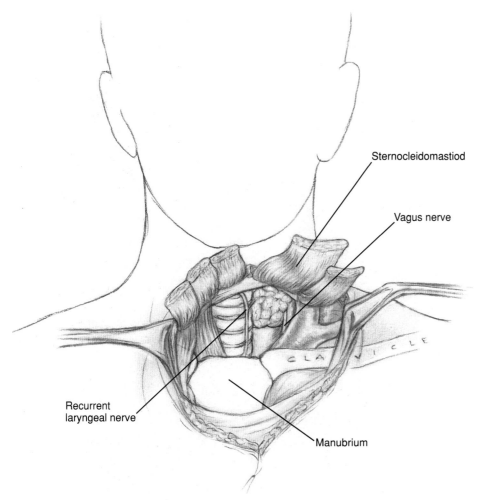

Sternocleidomastiod

Vagus nerve

CLAVICLE

Recurrent
laryngeal nerve

Manubrium

FIGURE 13-6

3. Resection of the medial clavicle is conducted and the dissection is carried down lateral to the anterior strap muscle which allows for continuation down onto the anterior cervicothoracic junction **(Fig. 13-7)**.

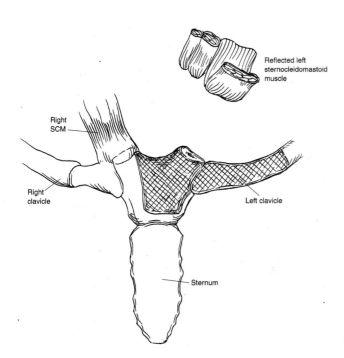

Reflected left
sternocleidomastoid
muscle

Right
SCM

Right
clavicle

Left clavicle

Sternum

FIGURE 13-7

4. Isolation and direct visualization of the recurrent laryngeal nerve as it enters the tracheoe-sophageal group is necessary to avoid transecting this structure **(Fig. 13-8)**.
5. The subclavian vein and phrenic nerve are readily identified and followed directly down to the spine (see Fig. 13-8).

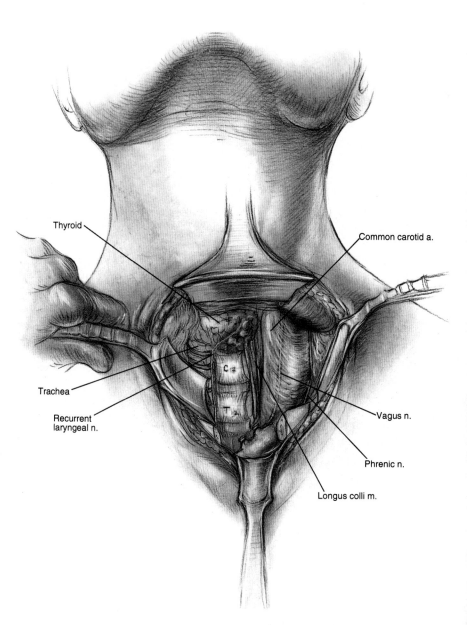

FIGURE 13-8

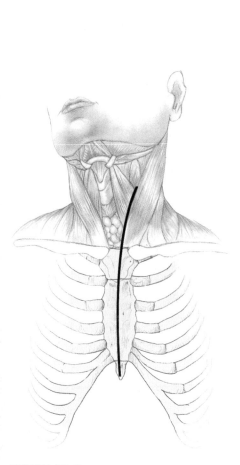

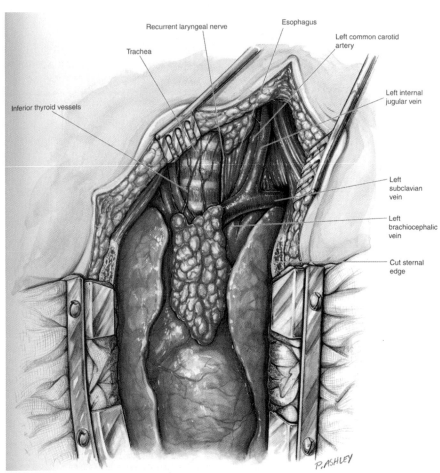

FIGURE 13-9

FIGURE 13-10

Sternal Split

The pathology, morbidity and recovery dictate the selection of the direct anterior access by way of sternotomy. Modification of the sternal split includes splitting the manubrium and emerging laterally between the third and fourth ribs. By emerging between the third and fourth ribs mobilization at this interval allows more direct anterior access to the cephalad aspect of the aortic arch. Should further dissection be necessary, the strap muscles are mobilized taking care to protect the recurrent laryngeal and subclavian nerves. This exposure provides greater consistency to access the anterior anatomy and the most, direct approach for placement of implants and visualization of neurological structures during decompression.

Technique

1. Incision: with the patient supine, incision begins typically over the anterior border of the sternocleidomastoid and extends distally in the midline over the manubrium and the sternum to the level of the zyphoid process **(Fig. 13-9)**.
2. Blunt dissection separates the posterior aspect of the sternum creating a retrosternal space.
3. The sternum is split longitudinally, usually with an oscillating saw.
4. A sternal retractor is used to separate the sternum taking care to avoid tearing the retropleural fascia **(Fig. 13-10)**.

5. The dissection of the retropleural fascia allows exposure of the lower cervical and upper thoracic regions **(Fig. 13-11)**.
6. Closure of the sternotomy is extremely important. Nonunion can be very painful. This is performed in a classical fashion with circumferential wire sutures.

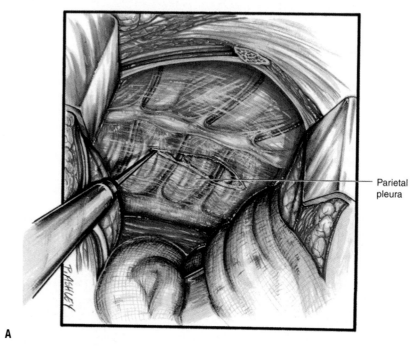

Parietal
pleura

A

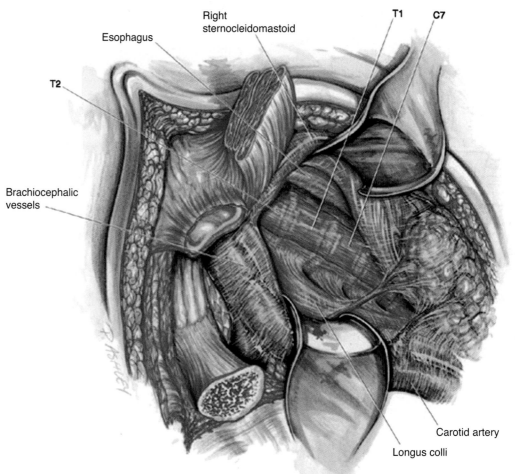

Esophagus

Right
sternocleidomastoid

T1

C7

T2

Brachiocephalic
vessels

Carotid artery

Longus colli

FIGURE 13-11   **B**

Interaortocaval Subinnominate Window

Indications   For proper anterior posterior screw orientation at the level of T3-T5.

Position   The patient is placed supine on the table.

Technique

1. Incision: the incision begins along the anterior border of the sternocleidomastoid muscle and continues distally over the sternum **(Fig. 13-12)**.
2. The medial border of the sternocleidomastoid muscle is identified, the dissection is deepened to expose the trachea thyroid and esophagus which are gently retracted to the right. Note: Care is taken to protect the left recurrent laryngeal nerve and the thoracic duct.
3. Distally, the sternum is divided with an oscillating saw.
4. After splitting the thymus the left innominate (brachiocephalic vein) is isolated to the superior vena cava (Fig. 13-12).

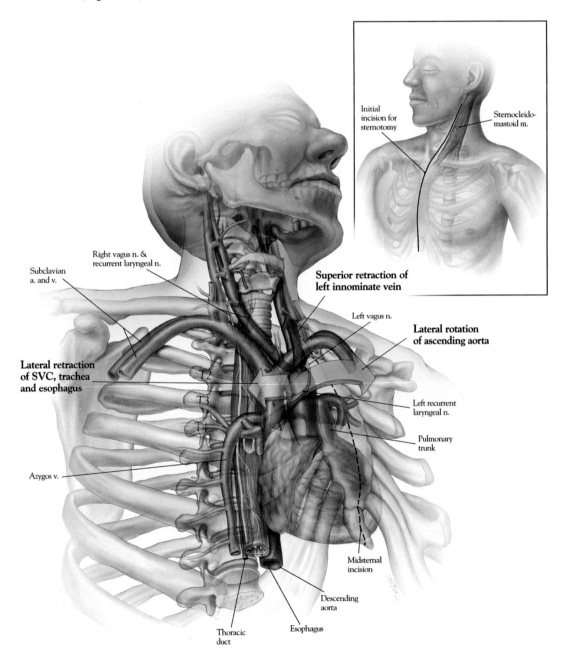

FIGURE 13-12

5. The proximal innominate (bachiocephalic) artery is isolated.
6. The aorta is retracted to the patient's left and the superior vena cava to the patient's right exposing the T1-T3 vertebra. The procedure proceeds according to the nature of the pathology (**Fig. 13-13**).
7. The sternum is repaired with no. 5 titanium wires. The remainder of the closure is routine.

For limited direct anterior decompression within the window the author will use renal vein type rectractor blades. If a drill or screws need to be passed via the aortocaval window a section of 40F chest tube can be used to act as a soft tissue protector. The clear tubing affords visualization and protection from the vascular tissues.

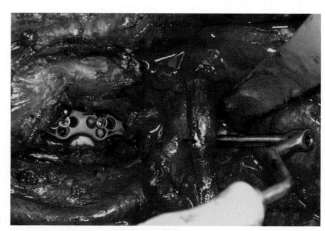

FIGURE 13-13

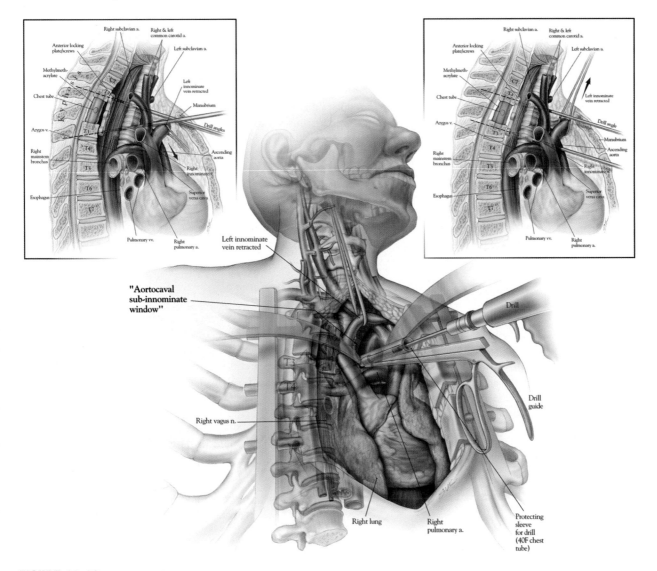

FIGURE 13-13 (Continued)

ANTERIOR THORACOLUMBAR EXTENSILE APPROACH

Indications

- Access to the anterior thoracic spine for an anterior condylar resection tumor
- Anterior thoracic release for deformity and/or reconstruction
  - *Note:* This exposure often requires the collaboration of an access surgeon and spine surgeon. Proficiently in managing some conditions in the prone position, the use of the operating endoscope and inner costal portals is increasing.

Comment

A strong caution is advised against endoscopic procedures for tumor pathology of the thoracic spine. Unfortunately, early local recurrence from iatrogenic spread to the pleural cavity has been documented with this approach. Contamination of the entire pleural cavity will tend to occur from the dependent positioning, bleeding from the tumor site, and by the seeding that results from the piecemeal removal of the tumor.

Position

We typically position the patient with left side up so as to avoid the interference with the liver. Stabilization is achieved with radiolucent bolsters, the right hip is flexed and the left hip extended. Taping of the pelvis and shoulder region reduces intraoperative rolling of the patient. Thoracotomy can also be accomplished in the prone position through a traditional anterolateral approach with the arms in the abducted position most commonly used **(Fig. 13-14)**.

Technique

1. Incision: the curvilinear incision enters through the 9th to 11th ribs depending on the pathology and anticipated length of exposure **(Fig. 13-15)**. The extensile thoracoabdominal approach is typically carried out cephalad to the 9th rib so as to allow for a direct visualization of the dorsal diaphragmatic attachment.

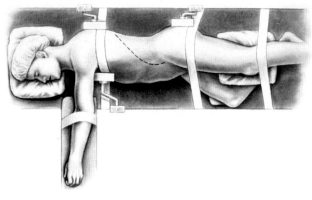

FIGURE 13-14

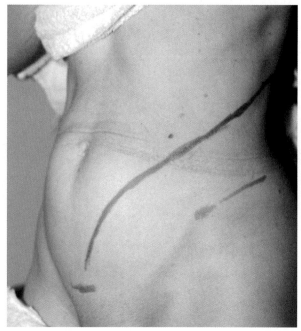

FIGURE 13-15

2. The latissimus dorsi muscle is split and dissection carried down to the intercostal area.
3. The dissection is carried over the rib to protect the neurovascular bundle as in a standard thoracotomy fashion, but with the patient in a prone position.
4. The rib is exposed subperiosteally and as the intercostal nerve and vessels are protected, it is resected **(Fig. 13-16)**.
5. A chest wall retractor is inserted and with clipping and/or tying of intercostal vessels and with gradual spreading, the thoracic contents are retracted away from the spine.
   - *Note:* Direct spinal access typically requires ligation of vessels unilaterally and/or bilaterally. This can be done with safety; however, efforts should be taken to maintain blood pressure above 60 to 70 mm Hg. Further, if the patient has had radiation and/or myelopathic changes, hypotension and vascular ligation can cause relative cord ischemia and/or even paralysis.
6. Distally, the retroperitoneum can be entered over the tip of the 11th rib.
7. The costochondral cartilage is divided.
8. Direct blunt dissection by finger or gauge sponge inferior to the diaphragm is carried out in the retroperitoneum.
9. Carrying the incision more inferiorly into the abdomen requires dividing the internal/external oblique abdominal muscles as well as the transverse abdominal muscle.
10. The reflection continues to the rib and then down the lateral border of the rectus abdominus sheath to the anterior-superior iliac spine.
11. The retroperitoneam is now brought forward, typically with a sponge and a stick.

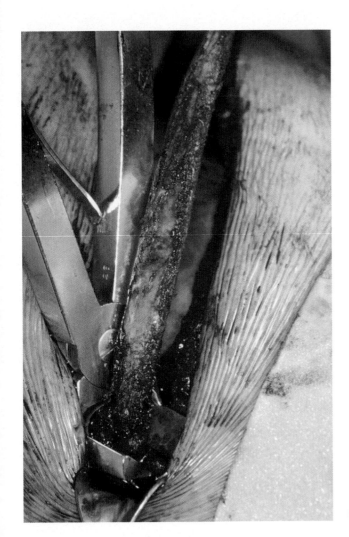

FIGURE 13-16

12. The quadratus lumborum, the femoral nerve, and the iliopsoas muscle are identified coming anterior to the iliac vessels and the bifurcation of the aorta is observed to the left.
    ● *Note:* Segmental vessels can be sectioned at the levels of pathology as necessary.

13. The diaphragm is released at the thoracolumbar junction (**Fig. 13-17**).

14. At this point the nerves to the posterior diaphragm are spared if possible as they have significant contributions to the sympathetic chain. Branches from the T11 and T12 splanchnic innervate the diaphragm but may be taken unilaterally without significant patient morbidity.

15. The iliopsoas typically attaches at L-1 and is reflected from the midline laterally with careful avoidance of dissection in the posterior third of the iliopsoas to avoid entry to the lumbar plexus. The thoracolumbar vertebral bodies are now accessible.

16. Closure: The diaphragm is first repaired with nonabsorbable sutures. The thoracic pleura through the rib bed is closed and the lung inflated.

17. A chest tube is used to maintain the reinflated lung.

18. The viscera is protected while the abdominal musculature is closed in layers. Careful closure will lessen the likelihood of abdominal hernia.

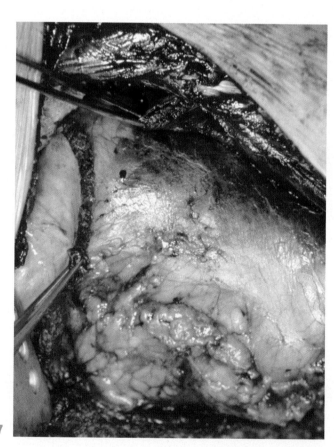

FIGURE 13-17

RECOMMENDED READING

Cohen ZR, Fourney DR, Gokaslan ZL, et al. Anterior stabilization of the upper thoracic spine via an "interaortocaval subinnominate window." Case report and description of operative technique. *J Spinal Disord Tech* 2004;17(6):543–548.

Grossfeld S, Winter RB, Lonstein JE, et al. Complications of anterior spinal surgery in children. *J Pediatr Orthop* 1997;17(1):89–95.

Hollinshead WH, ed. *Anatomy for Surgeons*. New York: Harper and Row, 1966.

Micheli LJ, Hood RW. Anterior exposure of the cervicothoracic spine using a combined cervical and thoracic approach. *J Bone Joint Surg* 1983;65A:992–997.

14 Lumbar Spine

PART 1. Anterior Exposure of the Lumbar Spine

Paul M. Huddleston, Scott Zietlow, and Jason C. Eck

Orthopedic surgeons developed and refined the anterior lumbar exposures early in the 20th century for the treatment of tuberculous spinal conditions and as a method to treat spondylolisthesis (1,2). The anterior lumbar anatomy is complex; as a result, many of these techniques have been developed and performed in close cooperation with General Surgery specialists. This collaboration should continue. During routine exposures, an additional set of seasoned hands will facilitate speeding the case to completion. For more difficult and complex exposures, the same hands may very well mean the difference between a serious but transient intraoperative complication or lasting morbidity and death. Regardless of the difficulty of the case, "the best interest of the patient is the only interest to be considered" (3).

ANTERIOR PARAMEDIAN RETROPERITONEAL LUMBAR EXPOSURE

Indications

- Biopsy
- Arthroplasty
- Arthrodesis

Position

The patient should be placed in the supine position on an operative frame or table that will allow intraoperative x-ray or fluoroscopy in two planes. The use of a bolster under the lower back will accentuate lumbar lordosis and facilitate exposure of the anterior lumbosacral junction. If the patient is obese, the table may be placed in a Trendelenburg position and tape placed upon the upper abdomen and the pannus retracted cranially. The upper extremities are placed on well-padded arm boards in a "90-90" position. The head is secured in a neutral position. All bony prominences are padded. All monitoring lines and catheters are safely secured.

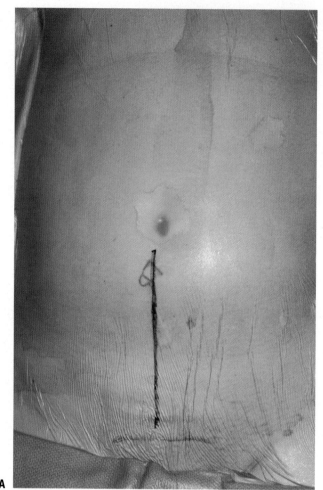

A

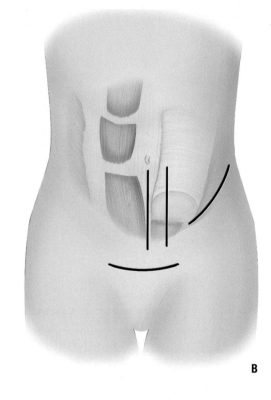

B

FIGURE 14-1

Landmarks

Lines are drawn overlying from below the umbilicus heading inferiorly towards the pubic bones and symphysis **(Fig. 14-1A)**. The symphysis will signify the lower limit of the possible skin and muscle dissection.

Equipment

A minimum of two large bore peripheral IVs should be placed. Additional monitoring with central venous and peripheral arterial lines is used as necessary. The use of headlamp illumination and operative loupes is left to the discretion of the surgeon but is recommended. A bipolar cautery, in addition to a monopolar, should be available for controlling hemostasis near and around the neural elements. If intraoperative neuromonitoring is used, then leads are placed in the lower extremity prior to the prep and drape. Intraoperative x-rays of fluoroscopy will aid in the identification of operative levels and verify the location of any implants placed. Self-retaining abdominal retractors may be used but the authors prefer handheld retractors if available, as these tend to be easier on the tissues.

Technique

1. Incision: to access the lower three levels of the lumbar spine or in patients with a large abdomen, a midline incision is ideal. For visualization of the lowest lumbar level or when cosmesis is an issue, a low transverse incision is preferred. Alternatively, a paramedian longitudinal incision may be placed directly over the rectus abdinus to minimize the development of dead space above the fascia and subsequent possible wound infection **(Fig. 14-1B)**.

2. Dissection progresses through the skin and subcutaneous tissue levels to the fascia. A small skin flap is then elevated over the left abdominal region to provide access to the anterior rectus sheath **(Fig. 14-2)**. The midline is identified and the fascia is divided over the left rectus muscle **(Fig. 14-3)**. The muscle is dissected from its medial fascial border and the various perforating vessels are ligated, divided, and cauterized as needed **(Fig. 14-4).**

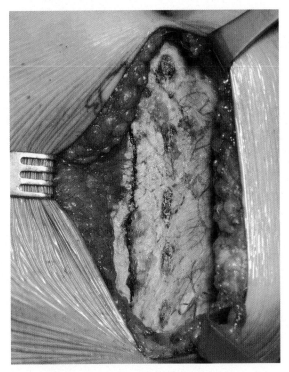

FIGURE 14-2

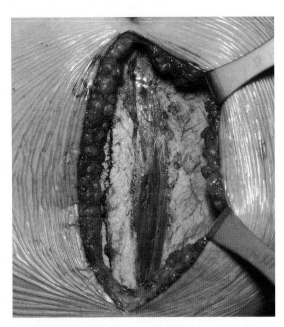

FIGURE 14-3

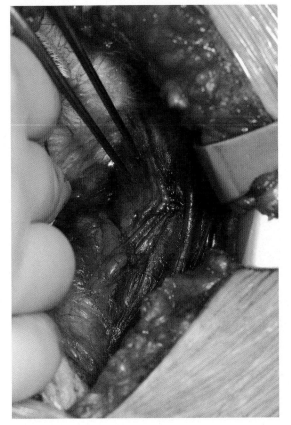

FIGURE 14-4

3. The posterior rectus fascia is visualized and the arcuate line identified **(Fig. 14-5)**. Using surgical forceps to elevate the posterior rectus fascia, a small incision is made through this using an electrocautery or knife **(Fig. 14-6)**. Care is taken not to incise the peritoneum and abdominal viscera. Development of this potential space allows access anterior to the peritoneum through to the retroperitoneal space **(Fig. 14-7)**. This is a critical portion of the surgical approach and the surgeon must be confident they are in the correct tissue plane to avoid injury to the abdominal contents and/or damage to the lateral abdominal lumbar neurovascular structures.

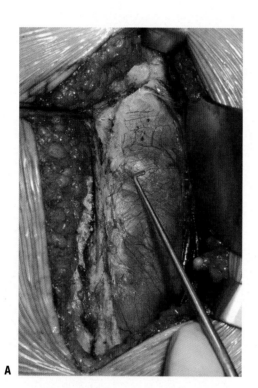

A

FIGURE 14-5

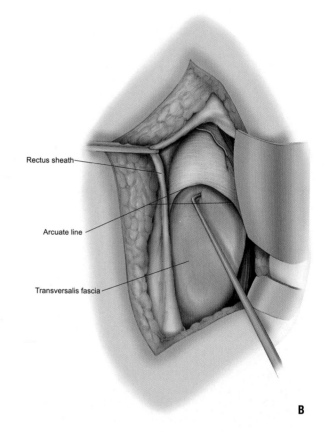

Rectus sheath

Arcuate line

Transversalis fascia

B

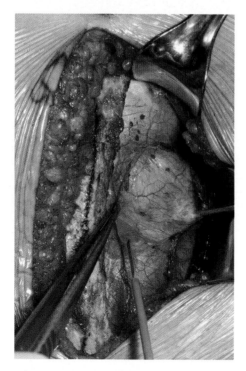

FIGURE 14-6

FIGURE 14-7

4. The dissection is developed laterally towards the retroperitoneal space. This can be performed by manual blunt dissection, using a "sponge-on-a-stick" if necessary. Peritoneal tears, if encountered, should be repaired with an absorbable suture on a tapered needle as they are recognized. The abdominal structures are then mobilized from patient's left to right direction within the abdominal cavity.

5. As the retroperitoneal dissection progresses laterally, retroperitoneal fat may be encountered as well as the round ligament or vas deferens. If necessary, the round ligament may be divided to assist in mobilization (**Fig. 14-8**). The blunt dissection should continue cranial to these structures. If the patient has a larger body habitus and/or the exposure is difficult, the posterior rectus sheath can be divided cranially in a "north to northeast" fashion. This need not be repaired upon subsequent closure and facilitates more generous mobilization of the abdominal contents and/or visualization of the mid to upper lumbar spine if necessary.

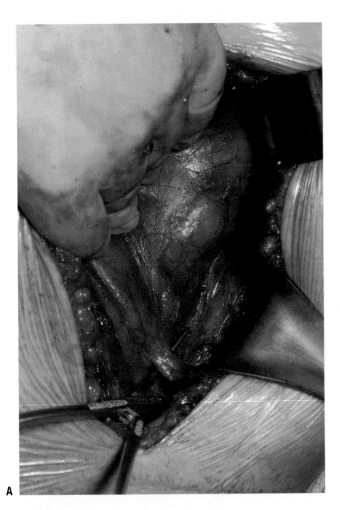 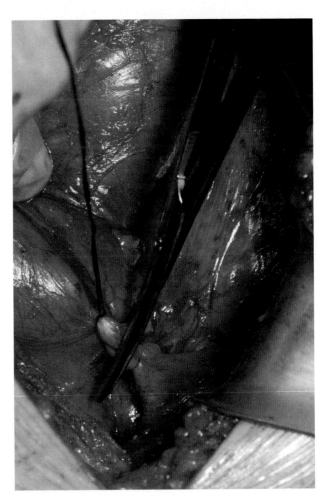

A   B

FIGURE 14-8

6. Care is taken to identify the ureter **(Fig. 14-9)**. This will be seen as a small, white structure within the retroperitoneum. This can be identified by very carefully observing its peristalsis or gently inducing or testing for the peristalsis by compression with a small forceps.

7. The iliopsoas becomes visible within the field and the anterior neural structures upon it can be appreciated **(Fig. 14-10)**. Care again should be taken not to damage these with electrocautery, or pressure from surgical retractors.

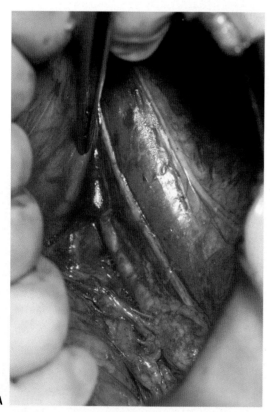

FIGURE 14-9

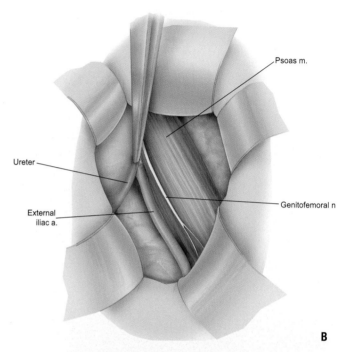

Psoas m.

Ureter

External
iliac a.

Genitofemoral n

B

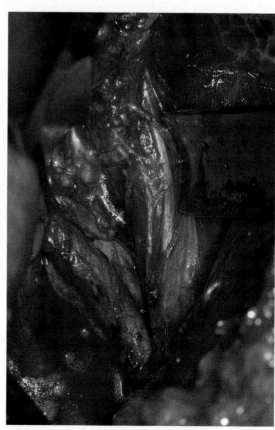

FIGURE 14-10

8. If exposure to the upper lumbar spine is necessary, exploration and mobilization of the external iliac vein and artery will be necessary to identify and ligate the ascending or recurrent iliolumbar vein (**Fig. 14-11**). These vessels appear as short, medium, or multiple lateral insertions into the common iliac vein from a cranial direction. These branches are deep within the abdomen near the pelvic brim where visibility is poor. They should be doubly ligated prior to be being divided (**Fig. 14-12**). The obturator nerve and lumbosacral trunk are especially at risk in the area below the recurrent iliolumbar vessels over the lateral aspect of the sacrum (**Fig. 14-13**).

9. The sympathetic chain is most easily moved laterally, away from the midline. This is most easily accomplished by blunt dissection with a small sponge. Large branches of the sympathetic chain may be ligated and divided with any attendant vessels if necessary.

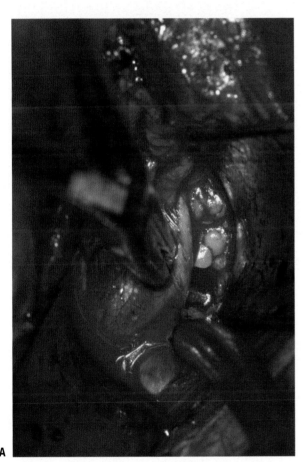

A

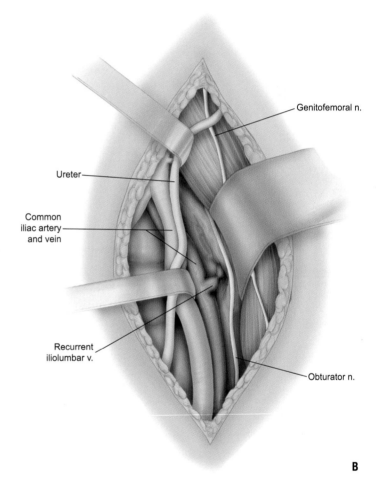

B

FIGURE 14-11

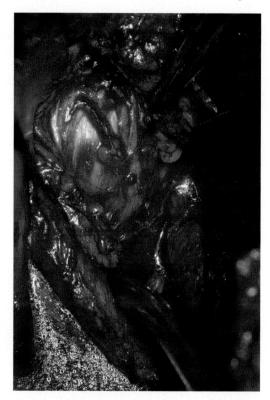

FIGURE 14-12

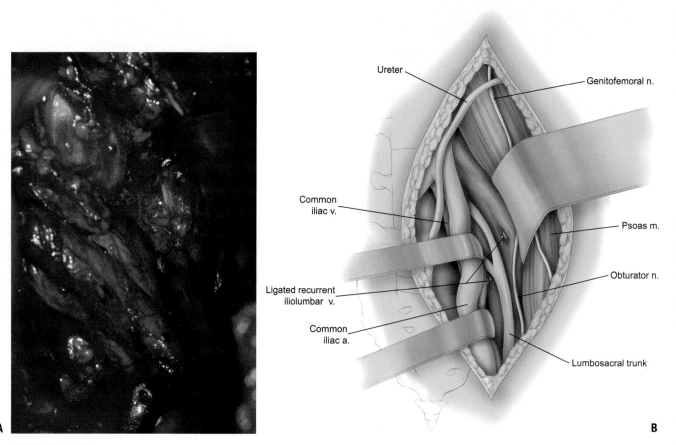

Ureter

Genitofemoral n.

Common
iliac v.

Psoas m.

Ligated recurrent
iliolumbar v.

Obturator n.

Common
iliac a.

Lumbosacral trunk

A

B

FIGURE 14-13

10. To access the lumbosacral junction, below the confluence of the common iliac veins, the middle sacral artery and veins should be identified and ligated (**Fig. 14-14**). Divide the hypogastric plexus in a vertical fashion with a sharp blade and use a small sponge to blunt dissect the filmy, plexus laterally towards the iliac vessels. Careful placement of self-retaining or handheld retractors will protect the great vessels and allow clear visualization of the disc space (**Fig. 14-15**).

11. Following the operative procedure, a final sponge and needle count is performed. The fascial layer is closed in a watertight fashion using a running suture. The subcutaneous layer is repaired and the skin approximated. In the presence of a large dead space, the use of a suprafascial drain is optional.

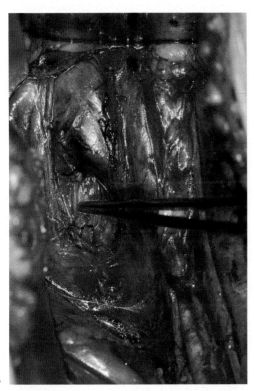

A

B

Aorta

Sympathetic chain

Superior vena cava

Hypogastric plexus

Ligated middle sacral artery and vein

Ureter

Psoas m.

Genitofemoral n.

External iliac a.

FIGURE 14-14

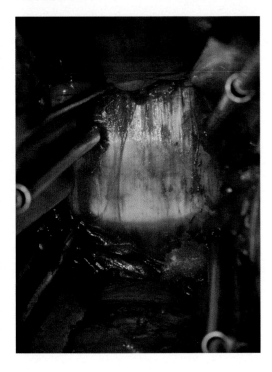

FIGURE 14-15

Pearls and Pitfalls

- If cosmesis is an issue, the low transverse incision can be utilized to expose the lumbosacral junction in a thin patient. The lateral paramedian vertical incision uses a smaller skin flap with less chance of subcutaneous hematoma and concomitant healing issues. For exposure of more cranial levels or in patients with complicating anatomy, a lateral abdominal incision will be the most extensile.

- Extremely large peritoneal tears offer the surgeon the option to repair or not repair as it is unlikely that significant compression and compromise of the abdominal viscera will occur. With smaller defects, identify and repair them as they are encountered.

- If there is a question about identification or injury of the ureter, indigo carmine can be given to the patient intravenously in the operating room. This will manifest itself as a very dark, red color in a few minutes that is easily visible within the ureter, the bladder, or abdominal cavity if a ureter injury is present. In revision cases and approaches or areas where significant scarring and adhesion are present such as infection or tumor or radiation field, then preoperative ureter stents can be placed to assist in identification and protection of this vital structure.

- Injury to the sympathetic chain may cause sympathetic dysfunction in the lower extremity. Side effects include increased warmth to the leg, increased hair growth and sweating with subsequent maceration of the foot and/or the development of allodynia. Injuries can be lessened by using blunt dissection around the chain and avoiding the use of electrocautery.

- The genitofemoral and lateral femoral cutaneous nerves can be damaged as they course over and through the iliopsoas muscle. Care must be taken in the placement of retractors within this area. The lumbosacral trunk and obturator nerve are at great risk near the recurrent iliolumbar vessel in the lateral aspect of the sacrum. Because of this, "blind" cauterization must never be used to attempt to control bleeding in this area.

- While exposing and dissecting over and around the anterior lumbar spine, avoid the use of electrocautery if possible and utilize blunt dissection to minimize the neural trauma to the hypogastric plexus. Abdominal ileus and trouble with micturition can be expected following an extensive anterior vessel dissection. In males, additional risks include sexual dysfunction and sterility secondary to retrograde ejaculation.

LATERAL LUMBAR APPROACH

Indications

- Biopsy
- Arthrodesis
- Arthroplasty
- Trauma

Position

The patient should be placed in the sloppy lateral position with the operative side up on an operative frame or table that will allow intraoperative x-ray or fluoroscopy in two planes. The use of a bean bag under the down side will allow manipulation of the patient's torso as necessary to gain better visualization from both anterior and lateral perspectives, if necessary. If the patient is significantly over their ideal BMI, the table may be placed in a Trendelenburg position and tape placed upon the upper abdomen and the pannus retracted cranially. The upper extremities are placed in an "over-under" position. The head is secured in a neutral position. All bony prominences are padded. All monitoring lines and catheters are safely secured.

Landmarks

The surgical landmarks include the 12th rib, umbilicus, pubic bones and upside iliac crest.

Equipment

A minimum of two large bore peripheral IVs should be placed. Additional monitoring with central venous and peripheral arterial lines is used as necessary. The use of headlamp illumination and operative loupes is left to the discretion of the surgeon but is recommended. A bipolar cautery in addition to a monopolar should be available for controlling hemostasis near and around the underlying neural elements. If intraoperative neuromonitoring is to be used, then leads are placed in the lower extremity. Intraoperative x-rays of fluoroscopy will aid in the identification of operative levels and verify the placement of any implants placed. Self-retaining chest wall and abdominal retractors are used with additional handheld retractors added as needed.

Technique

1. Incision: lines are drawn overlying from over or just below the 12th rib to just below the umbilicus.
2. The dissection continues down through the skin and subcutaneous tissue to the level of the fascia. The fascia is divided in line with the skin incision in a muscle splitting fashion and the approach continues as described with the anterior approach.

Pearls and Pitfalls

- Advantages include a different angle of approach to the anterior lumbar spine in situations where a direct anterior transperitoneal or retroperitoneal approach has been previously performed. Specialty and technique-specific instruments can allow the possibility of anterior spinal discectomies and placement of interbody devices even in situations where the scarring of the great vessels might otherwise seem too onerous.
- This approach is very extensile. It is possible to visualize the lumbar spine from the lumbosacral to thoracolumbar junction through a single incision.
- Denervation of the abdominal wall with pseudohernia is an infrequent but disappointing complication of the approach. It is tolerated poorly by patients and often recalcitrant to surgical treatment.
- Closing this approach will be much more time consuming than the anterior approaches. Due to the muscle-dividing nature of the lateral approach, the subsequent patient recovery tends to be more painful.
- Confusion may occur with variations in segmentation of the lower lumbar sacral spine. It is strongly recommended that operative levels be confirmed with nontraumatic radiographic markers placed for identification with intraoperative x-ray.

PART 2. Posterior Exposures of the Lumbar Spine

Paul M. Huddleston and Jason C. Eck

The surgeon has many options for approaching the posterior lumbar spine. For biopsy, decompression, arthrodesis, and/or instrumentation, many of these exposures may seem to be simple variations of a common theme. Only when the surgeon has considered the balance between visualization and morbidity will the differences be clearer. From "new," minimally invasive techniques to more established "old school" maximally invasive revision work, each technique has evolved along the spectrum of this balance. We should constantly remind others and ourselves that these approaches are but another tool for the surgeon and that the key to success will always be "the decision, not just the incision."

POSTERIOR EXPOSURE FOR UNILATERAL LUMBAR DECOMPRESSION

Indications

- Discectomy
- Hemilaminotomy

Position

The patient should be placed in the prone position. The use of either longitudinal bolsters at the patient's sides or any operative frame that allows the abdomen to hang free can reduce intra-abdominal pressure. This decreases epidural venous pressure and blood loss during the case **(Fig. 14-16)**. The upper extremities are placed on well-padded arm boards in a "90-90" position. The head is secured in a neutral position. All bony prominences of the extremities are padded.

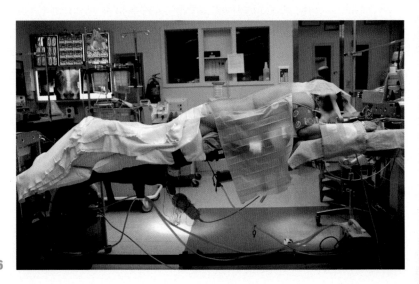

FIGURE 14-16

Landmarks

A line is drawn connecting the superior most point of the iliac crests. This roughly identifies the L4-5 disc space **(Fig. 14-17)**. The spinous processes are typically easily palpable. A spinal injection needle may be used to mark the site for potential surgical incision and a lateral intraoperative x-ray taken to assist in minimizing the skin incision.

Equipment

The use of headlamp illumination with operative loupes or an operative microscope is left to the discretion of the surgeon but is recommended. A bipolar cautery in addition to a monopolar should be available for controlling hemostasis near and around the underlying neural elements.

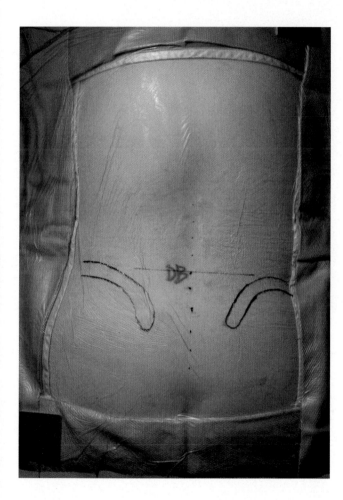

FIGURE 14-17

Technique

1. Incision: a midline longitudinal incision is made over the spinous process above the operative level.
2. The incision is taken down to the fascial layer. The spinous process should be easily palpable. The paraspinous muscles of the affected side are then subperiosteally elevated off the spinous process and lamina using a periosteal elevator **(Fig. 14-18)**. Dissection should be carried lateral to the facet joint. Care should be taken not to violate the capsule of the facet joint. A hand-held or self-retaining retractor can be used to maintain the exposure **(Fig. 14-19)**.

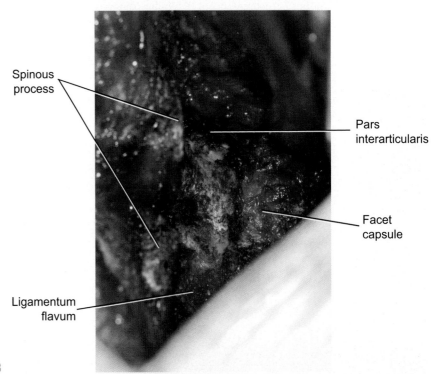

Spinous process

Pars interarticularis

Facet capsule

Ligamentum flavum

FIGURE 14-18

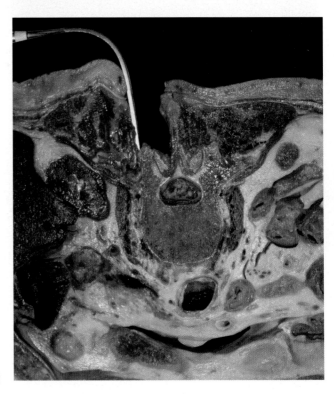

FIGURE 14-19

3. Intraoperative fluoroscopy or radiographs should be taken to verify the appropriate level by placing a radiographic marker. These may be orthogonal but a lateral projection is usually satisfactory. To accomplish this, the ligamentum flavum is then dissected off the superior edge of the inferior lamina using either a curette or elevator. A small periosteal elevator is then placed just medial to the lumbar pedicle in question. This will identify the operative level even in the most degenerative or distorted of cases. The intraoperative radiograph may then be obtained **(Fig. 14-20)**.

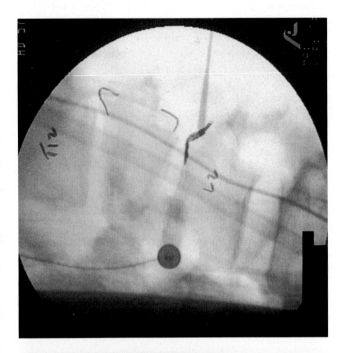

FIGURE 14-20

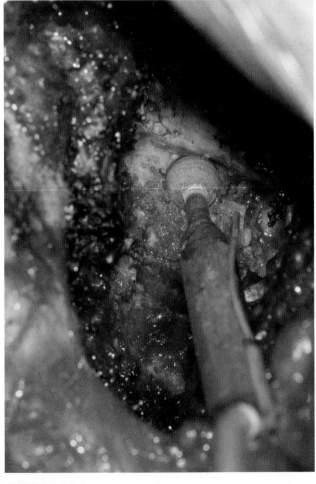

FIGURE 14-21   **FIGURE 14-22**

4. A rongeur or high-speed burr is then used to remove the inferior portion of the superior lamina and superior portion of the inferior lamina **(Fig. 14-21)**. This will allow release of the insertion of the ligamentum flavum from the superior lamina of the caudal vertebra **(Fig. 14-22)**. Immediately underneath this ligament is the epidural fat, thecal sac, and exiting nerve roots **(Fig. 14-23)**. In some cases the medial portion of the facet joint must be removed to provide sufficient visualization. An adequate amount of facet joint should be preserved to maintain adequate post-operative motion segment stability. Lateral decompression should be carried flush to the medial wall of the pedicle to ensure adequate decompression of the lateral recess and traversing nerve root.

5. After sufficient bone and ligamentum flavum have been removed the exiting nerve root should be visualized **(Fig. 14-23)**. If the exposure is being performed for discectomy then the nerve root can be carefully retracted toward the midline to expose the disc space. A bipolar cautery may be used to coagulate obstructing epidural veins.

6. The approach to the disc space is completed with an annulotomy. A scalpel on a long handle or a small freer can puncture the annulus. Small rongeurs or punches can be used to remove any free or extruded disc material. The remaining disc space is irrigated with sterile saline solution injected with any small catheter and syringe.

7. A ball-tip probe or flat elevator is used to prove the foramen to assure an adequate decompression has been performed. If necessary, additional bone can be removed at this time. A final irrigation is performed. The dura is visualized to verify it remains intact.

8. The fascial layer is meticulously closed in a watertight fashion using interrupted and running suture. The subcutaneous layer is repaired and the skin approximated. The use of a drain is optional.

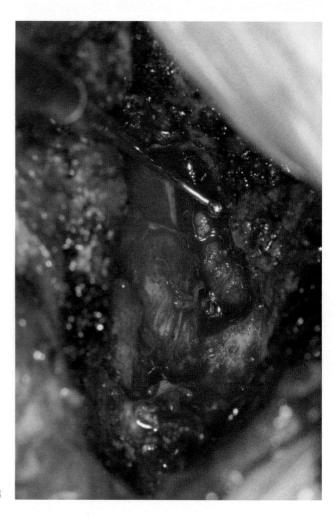

FIGURE 14-23

Pearls and Pitfalls

- Dissecting only on the affected side eliminates contralateral soft tissue destruction and leads to faster recovery.
- Assisted illumination by either head lamp or operating microscope will greatly improve visualization, especially if smaller incisions are utilized.
- An extension-type operating room table may be used for lumbar spinal decompressions but the approximation of the lamina and spinous processes that occur with these devices may make visualization more difficult. Subsequently, the surgeon will be working through an extended lumbar spine, which may make accessing the spinal canal and disc space a challenge.
- The increased visualization achieved by using an operative microscope will improve the visualization and participation of an assistant or student, if present.
- Any suspicion of the presence of an incidental durotomy created during the surgical approach should be put to rest prior to wound closure. Bad news never gets better with age!

POSTERIOR BILATERAL EXPOSURE OF THE LUMBAR SPINE

Indications

- Laminectomy
  - Central stenosis
  - Bilateral stenosis
- Posterolateral arthrodesis
- Posterior instrumented arthrodesis

Position

The patient should be placed in the prone position. The use of either an Andrew's table with the patient in the knee-chest position or a Wilson frame can allow the abdomen to hang free and reduce intra-abdominal pressure. This decreases epidural venous pressure and blood loss during the case. The upper extremities are placed on well-padded arm boards in a "90-90" position. The head is secured in a neutral position with padding over the eyes. All bony prominences of the extremities are padded.

Landmarks

A line is drawn connecting the superior most point of the iliac crests. This roughly identifies the L4-5 disc space. The spinous processes are typically easily palpable. A spinal injection needle may be used to mark the site for potential surgical incision and a lateral intraoperative x-ray taken to assist in minimizing the skin incision.

Equipment

The use of an operative microscope or loupes as well as intraoperative monitoring is left to the discretion of the surgeon. A bipolar cautery in addition to a monopolar should be available for controlling hemostasis near and around the underlying neural elements.

Technique

1. Incision: a midline longitudinal incision is made over the spinous process above and below the planned operative level **(Fig. 14-24)**.
2. The incision is taken down to the fascial layer. The spinous process should be easily palpable. The paraspinous muscles of both sides are then subperiosteally elevated off the spinous process and lamina using a periosteal elevator **(Fig. 14-25)**. Dissection should be carried out to the facet joint. Care should be taken not to violate the capsule of the facet joint unless fusion is planned at that level. In cases of laminectomy alone there is typically no need to violate the facet capsules.

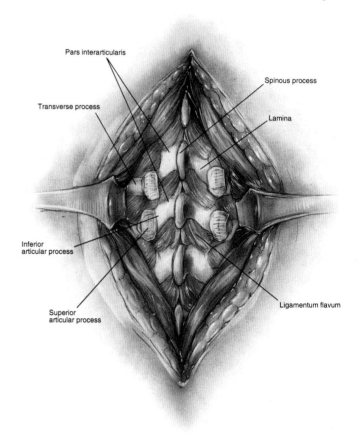

FIGURE 14-24

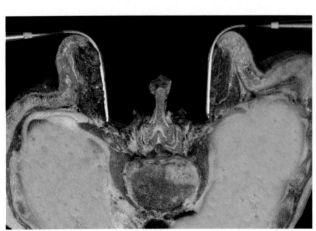

A

FIGURE 14-25

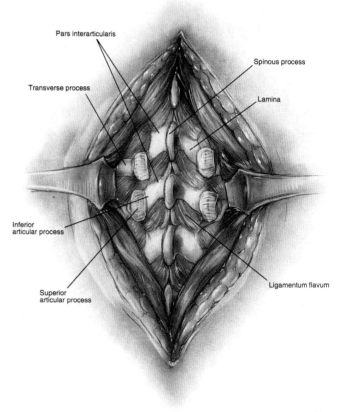

B

3. Care should be taken to maintain the facet capsule until proper levels have been radiographically confirmed. A clamp can then be placed on the spinous process and an intraoperative lateral radiograph taken to confirm the appropriate level.

4. The rongeur may be used to remove the spinous processes if indicated and attached soft tissues. Otherwise, care should be taken to preserve as many of the anatomic structures (spinous processes, facet capsules) until it is necessary to sacrifice them.

5. To completely visualize the thecal sac, the decompression should effectively undermine the origin of the ligamentum flavum on the under-half of the inferior aspect of the superior vertebrae and the lateral recess allowing complete visualization of the neural elements. A high-speed burr or Kerrison rongeurs is used to remove the lamina and medial portions of facet joints. No more than 50% of either facet joint should be removed at a given level to maintain stability (see Fig. 14-21).

6. The decompression should extend from the pedicle above to the pedicle below, including any encroaching facet complex on either side.

7. If posterolateral fusion is planned then the dissection progresses over the facet joint to the tips of the transverse processes. Decortication of the transverse processes may be performed using curettes, periosteal elevators or a high speed burr. If present, the lateral aspect of the pars and facet joint should be decorticated to provide additional surfaces for arthrodesis.

8. The ideal visualization of the posterolateral transverse processes will be obtained from the opposite side of the operating table. Working on the contralateral lateral gutter will minimize surgeon fatigue and minimize the overall length of the wound and soft tissue dissection.

9. If entry into the lumbar vertebral pedicle is planned, either in anticipation of biopsy or instrumentation, it is critical for the entry point to be adequately visualized. The entry site into the pedicle and the trajectory of any implants can be confirmed by the anatomy and by using intraoperative radiographs or fluoroscopy. Direct visualization of the medial aspect of the pedicle through a lamino-foraminotomy can assist with orientation if necessary. Care should be taken to avoid breach of the medial and inferior pedicular walls, as these are most likely to lead to nerve root irritation or injury.

10. At this point any necrotic or devitalized tissue is removed. Irrigation of the operative field and a careful sponge and needle count is performed.

11. The dura is inspected to verify that it is intact. A ball-tip probe or flat elevator is used to verify adequate decompression of each foramen.

12. The fascial layer is meticulously closed in a watertight fashion using interrupted and running suture. The subcutaneous layer is repaired and the skin approximated with either skin closure performed in a style consistent with the preference of the surgeon. The use of a drain is optional.

Pearls and Pitfalls

- The use of an extension table can assist in achieving sagittal plane balance when more than one motion segment is being considered for instrumentation.
- It is highly recommended that for more lengthy cases that direct pressure over the face and eyes be avoided by use of a cranial pinion. Preoperative positioning of the patient's head at an elevation higher than the heart may decrease facial and neck edema.

EXPOSURE OF THE LUMBAR SPINE FOR TRANSFORAMINAL LUMBAR INTERBODY FUSION

Technique

1. A traditional midline longitudinal approach is made to the lumbar spine. Care is taken to keep the supraspinous and interspinous ligaments intact. The paraspinous muscles are subperiosteally elevated from the dorsal surface of the lamina out to the tip of the transverse process, allowing the dorsal aspect of the vertebral bodies to be exposed (see Fig. 14-26).

2. The decision is made to approach the canal and disc space unilaterally. Usually the side with a symptomatic radiculopathy is chosen. If there is a degenerative or developmental curve present then the side of the concavity is chosen. Pedicle screws are placed as described above. An inferior hemilaminectomy and total facetectomy are performed. This allows complete exposure of the lateral spinal canal, thecal sac, foramen, and exiting nerve root.

3. The superior and inferior pedicles, thecal sac with traversing nerve root, and the exiting root compose a "vascular triangle." The lower nerve root is protected by sliding a nerve root retractor along the upper surface of the pedicle of the inferior vertebra. The upper nerve root lies along the inferomedial surface of the pedicle and can be directly visualized (**Fig. 14-26**).

4. A knife or elevator is used to enter the outer annulus and complete discectomy is performed. Endplate preparation is completed with specialized instruments.

5. Distraction across the disc space can then be performed. An implant is then impacted into place to the middle of the disc space. Graft position can be confirmed using fluoroscopy. The posterior two-thirds of the disc space are then packed with bone graft. The distraction across the interspace is then relaxed and the rods are the attached to the pedicle screws and the interspace can be compressed.

6. Posterolateral intertransverse process fusion can then be performed as described.

7. Copious irrigation is then performed. A layered close is performed as described above.

8. For a more minimalist approach, a unilateral subperiosteal dissection is performed on the side where the facetectomy is to be performed. A muscle splitting Wiltse type approach may be performed on the contralateral side (**Fig. 14-27**).

9. Blunt dissection down to the level of the facet complex minimizes soft tissue trauma and provides a relatively bloodless exposure (**Fig. 14-28**).

10. The transverse processes and the intertransverse ligament are then identified (**Fig. 14-29**). Pedicle fixation is then placed after adequately identifying and preparing the entry point into the pedicle.

Pearls and Pitfalls

- The surgical approach for a transforaminal lumbar interbody fusion (TLIF) is useful for all levels of the lumbar spine.
- Correct exposure of the interbody space through the vascular triangle should allow interbody arthrodesis with minimal or no retraction on the thecal sac or the exiting nerve root. This is especially critical at the L1-2 and L2-3 lumbar levels as the spinal cord will terminate in this region in most adults.

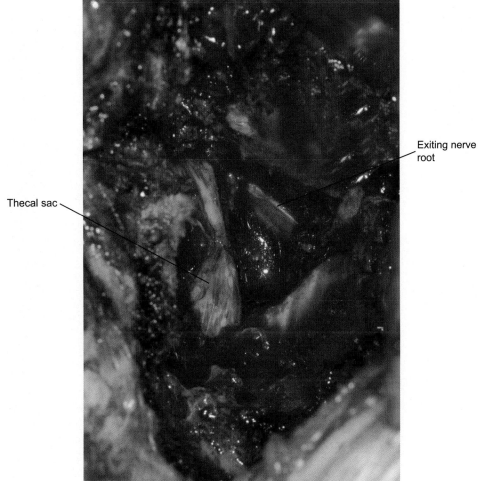

Exiting nerve root

Thecal sac

FIGURE 14-26

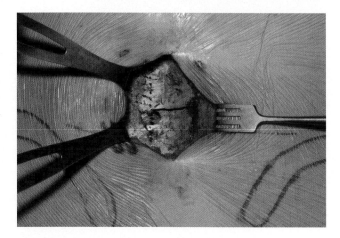

FIGURE 14-27

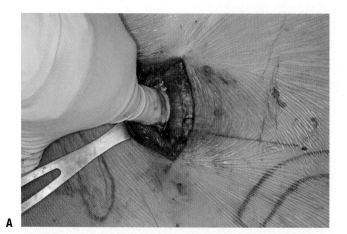

A

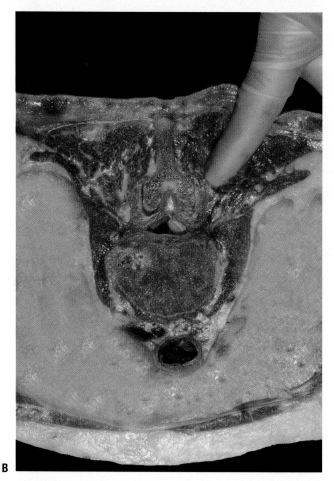

B

FIGURE 14-28

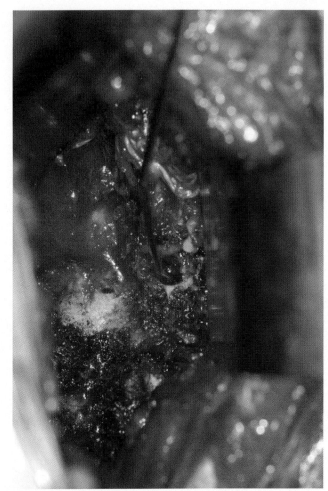

FIGURE 14-29

Acknowledgment

The editors acknowledge with appreciation the time and expertise contributed by Drs. Harold Gregory Bach and Mark Mikhael in the preparation of the material used in this chapter.

PART 1 REFERENCES

1. Ito H, Tsuchiya J, Asami G. A new radical operation for Pott's diseases. *J Bone Joint Surg* 1934;16:499–515.
2. Capener, N. An operation for spondylolisthesis. *Lancet* 1932; I:1233.
3. Mayo WJ. Commencement address. Rush Medical College, Chicago, 1910.

Index

339